mar's **COMPREHENSIVE**

MEDICAL ASSISTING

Administrative and Clinical Competencies

2nd Edition

nstructor's Manual

Wilburta (Billie) Q. Lindh, CMA
Marilyn S. Pooler, RN, CMA-C, MEd
arol D. Tamparo, CMA-A, PhD
oanne U. Cerrato, BS, MT (ASCP), MA

dited by
thel Morikis, BSN, RN-C, CMA
atricia Schrull, RN, MBA, MEd, CMA

DELMAR

THOMSON LEARNING

Australia Canada Mexico Singapore Spain United Kingdom United States

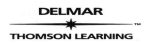

DELMAR

THOMSON LEARNING™

Instructor's Manual to Accompany
Delmar's Comprehensive Medical Assisting: Administrative and Clinical Competencies, 2nd Edition
by Wilburta (Billie) Q. Lindh, Marilyn S. Pooler, Carol D. Tamparo, and Joanne U. Cerrato
Edited by Ethel Morikis and Patricia Schrull

Business Unit Director:
William Brottmiller

Executive Editor:
Cathy L. Esperti

Acquisitions Editor:
Maureen Muncaster

Senior Developmental Editor:
Elisabeth F. Williams

Editorial Assistants:
Jennifer Frisbee
Jill Korznat

Executive Marketing Manager:
Dawn F. Gerrain

Production Coordinator:
John Mickelbank

Art/Design Coordinator:
Mary Colleen Liburdi

Project Editor:
David Buddle

Cover Design:
The Drawing Board

NOTICE TO THE READER

Publisher does not warrant or guarantee any of the products described herein or perform any independent analysis in connection with any of the product information contained herein. Publisher does not assume, and expressly disclaims, any obligation to obtain and include information other than that provided to it by the manufacturer.

The reader is expressly warned to consider and adopt all safety precautions that might be indicated by the activities described herein and to avoid all potential hazards. By following the instructions contained herein, the reader willingly assumes all risks in connection with such instructions.

The publisher makes no representation or warranties of any kind, including but not limited to, the warranties of fitness for particular purpose or merchantability, nor are any such representations implied with respect to the material set forth herein, and the publisher takes no responsibility with respect to such material. The publisher shall not be liable for any special, consequential, or exemplary damages resulting, in whole or part, from the readers' use of, or reliance upon, this material.

Contents

SECTION III: CLINICAL PROCEDURES

Unit 6: Integrated Clinical Procedures

Unit 7: Assisting with Specialty Examinations and Procedures

Unit 8: Advanced Techniques and Procedures

Unit 9: Laboratory Procedures

SECTION IV: PROFESSIONAL PROCEDURES

Unit 10: Office and Human Resource Management

Unit 11: Entry Into the Profession

To the Instructor

One of our major roles as educators of medical assistants is to prepare students to be proficient in their profession upon graduation. To attain that goal, we can facilitate student learning to perform the skills of medical assistant as accurately and efficiently as possible.

To help prepare your students for work in today's dynamic health care setting, we have developed a complete learning system through various learning media. Student supplements for *Delmar's Comprehensive Medical Assisting: Administrative and Clinical Competencies,* 2nd edition, include two skills CD-ROMs packaged with the textbook, a comprehensive *Student Workbook*, a video series—Delmar's Medical Assisting Video Series, 2nd Edition—and Delmar's Medical Assisting CD-ROM. These supplements have been carefully developed to complement and enhance the student's learning process through a variety of media and learning opportunities. The videos and Medical Assisting CD-ROM illustrate procedures and portray issues and concepts in a situational context for the student. Both the videos and Medical Assisting CD-ROM are accompanied by their own *Instructor's Manuals* to help you incorporate multimedia technology in your curriculum. The *Workbook* allows for interpretive exercises in which the student must apply chapter knowledge, using critical thinking skills. The supplements work together to build upon and reinforce the material to be learned, avoiding duplications and redundancies. Each supplement creates a new and exciting learning experience for the student, maximizing the potential of each medium—written, interactive, and video—to engage the student and stimulate the learning process. Each workbook chapter references appropriate video topics.

OUTCOME- OR COMPETENCY-BASED EDUCATION

The American Association of Medical Assistants (AAMA) *Role Delineation Study: Occupational Analysis of the Medical Assisting Profession* and the *Registered Medical Assistant Competency Inventory* from the American Medical Technologists (AMT) specify that students must achieve entry-level competency by the time they graduate.

Outcome-based education, or competency-based education, has become an integrated part of medical assistant programs and is used to describe (1) the knowledge a student must have and (2) the performance and skill levels a student must possess to be considered competent and at career-entry level for employment. When students have the opportunity to participate in a program of study that is outcome- or competency-based, they know exactly what is expected of them and the transition from the classroom to the world of work is made easier.

With this type of education, performance is the primary source of evidence of the competency achievement. The students' education is directed toward preparing them to perform prescribed tasks of medical assisting (tasks actually performed by employees in the medical assisting profession) under the conditions of the real world and at a level of competency (accuracy and time requirements) necessary of entry-level medical assistants. Our goal as instructors is to facilitate student learning and achieving competency in the skills and tasks of their profession before leaving their educational program.

Four major components of competency-based education include (1) behavior statements, (2) subject matter content, (3) opportunities for learning, and (4) evaluation.

1. Behavior statements describe what the student must be able to do and the conditions and standards of acceptable performance (criteria for success). These behavior statements can be in the form of performance objectives. Performance objectives simulate the work environment and incorporate a specific behavior required on the job, conditions present on the job, and the same standards of a worker on the job.
2. Subject matter content consists of concepts needed to attain the objectives specified.
3. Opportunities for learning must enable students to gain the required knowledge and attitudes to be able to practice the desired behaviors while being supervised.
4. Evaluation takes place when students are measured against the standards in the objectives, not against other students. This type of education is called criterion-referenced or criterion-based.

Outcome-based or competency-based education is concrete and measurable and includes specific outcomes, goals, and criteria needed to be successful. Students must know what is expected of them and how well they will be expected to perform. They know in advance what the competencies are that they must attain, and they include not only psychomotor skills, but cognitive and affective skills as well. The steps are sequentially arranged and students advance to new learning when previous tasks have been conquered. Students must have a copy of the performance objectives, a performance checklist of steps to follow, and the conditions and standards to accomplish the task. These tools must be clear to students in order for them to know how they can obtain competency and whether or not they have met the objectives. The Skills Competency Assessment Checklists are the tools that will help you and your students measure the required competency outcomes.

SKILLS COMPETENCY ASSESSMENT CHECKLISTS

The Skills Competency Assessment Checklists are designed to set criteria or standards that should be observed while a specific procedure is being performed. They follow the same steps of the procedure as the textbook procedures. As each procedure is performed, the Evaluation Section of this sheet can be used to judge the student's performance. You or another evaluator can use this sheet to grade student competency for each skill. A Skill Tracking Sheet is also provided in the *Student Workbook* to use as an overview for all competency assessment checklists included in the *Workbook*. This tracking sheet can work as a table of contents of all checklists as well as a grid for students and you to easily see where each student stands with all assessments. The tracking sheet together with the student's completed checklist sheets can be combined in a three-ring binder and taken by the student to the externship site.

The format of the Skills Competency Assessment Checklist is designed to provide specific conditions, standards, skill steps, evaluation sections, and documentation sections for essential skills necessary for an entry-level medical assistant. A description of the parts of each Competency Assessment Checklist follows:

Conditions

Conditions give clues to students about *how* and *when* to perform a task. Conditions should be stated in actual terms used in current medical practice. For example, when performing venipuncture, the tourniquet must be removed *before* removing the needle from the patient's vein.

Standards

Standards of time and accuracy are usually measures of efficiency. Where appropriate, the time standard pertains to how much time the student will be allowed to complete a set of tasks. Accuracy deals with how many times the task must be performed and the degree of correctness with which the task must be performed based on the conditions given for each skill, or may indicate a specific score deemed acceptable by the instructor. For some laboratory procedures, the exact time required for the student to complete the procedure competently will vary according to the student's preparation and skill, the instructor's plans for laboratory testing to be done in the classroom on any given day, and the equipment and supplies available in the laboratory.

Skill Step Checklist

There are two columns provided for each task step of the procedure, one to indicate if a student has successfully completed a step, the second with a suggested point value. If the student performs a step of the procedure correctly, the evaluator or you, the instructor, will place a check in the box and count the points. If the student does not perform a step of the procedure or performs a step incorrectly, the evaluator will not place a check in box. Rationales are included if a step of the procedure requires certain knowledge. At the completion of a skill, the evaluator tallies the student's points and compares this number to the possible points attainable for that skill set. For grading purposes, instructors may have their own methods however it may be decided that a satisfactory score (minimum passing grade) for the procedure checklist is 85% or 87% with some procedures requiring 100% (example: injection of medication).

Evaluation Summary

The evaluation will include the actual time needed by the student to complete the specific procedure and will be graded by the evaluator based on student's performance of procedure steps and whether standards were met based on conditions. There is also an area in this section where you may provide and document suggestions for improving the student's performance.

Documentation

Charting is an extremely valuable part of performing clinical or laboratory procedures. This section will help provide students with hands-on charting experience based on actual procedures performed. Because the process of charting is a part of the Skill Competency Assessment, it will help students associate performing a procedure with the immediate charting of it—which comes close to the experience in the workplace.

A GUIDE FOR GRADING SKILLS COMPETENCY ASSESSMENT CHECKLISTS

Instructors can modify the rating system for use with the *Student Workbook* to reflect the needs of their individual medical assisting program. By preparing a master manual of skills competency assessment checklists and assigning a point value to procedural steps, the checklist can be compiled in a binder and left in the skills laboratory for students to use. They can transfer the information from the master binder to their own checklist in the *Workbook*.

If a student does not at first achieve competency, he or she must be re-evaluated until competency is achieved. On subsequent evaluations, however, a standard number of penalty points should be deducted to reflect the student having to repeat the assessment and not achieving competency previously. If a student must repeat several procedures throughout the course, the final grade may indicate which students must retake the course.

Student competency must be achieved prior to the students being placed in an externship program where they will be required to perform in the workplace.

Because regulations vary from state to state regarding which procedures can be performed by a medical assistant, it will be important to check specific regulations in each state. A medical assistant should never perform any procedure without checking legal responsibilities, without correct instruction, and without proper authorization.

EXAMINATION AND ACCREDITATION INFORMATION

For information on medical assisting examinations or accreditation, contact:

American Association of Medical Assistants (AAMA)
(administers the CMA Examination)
20 N. Wacker Drive
Chicago, IL 60606-2963
Tel 800-228-2262
Fax 312-899-1259
Web site http://www.aama-ntl.org

American Medical Technologists (AMT)
(administers the RMA Examination)
710 Higgins Road
Park Ridge, IL 60068-5765
Tel 847-823-5169
Fax 847-823-0458

FREE MEDICAL ASSISTING CURRICULUM FROM DELMAR

Download the latest Medical Assisting Curriculum for the second edition of Lindh free of charge from Delmar. Please visit

http://www.delmaralliedhealth.com/resources/macur.html

Use the user name user and the password teachlindh to reach the download page.

If you cannot download the curriculum, contact your local sales representative and request a print copy of ISBN 0–7668–3297–X or call 1-800-477-3692.

Transition Guide

This transition guide is designed to help you convert your class and lecture notes from the first to the second edition of *Delmar's Comprehensive Medical Assisting.*

NEW TOPICS FOUND IN SECOND EDITION (continued)

xii • Transition Guide

NEW TOPICS FOUND IN SECOND EDITION (continued)

Examination Format and Content	Ch. 47, pp. 1037–1038
Application Process	Ch. 47, p. 1038
Application Completion and Test Administration Scheduling	Ch. 47, p. 1038
Certified Medical Assistant (CMA)	Ch. 47, p. 1038
Examination Format and Content	Ch. 47, pp. 1038–1039
Application Process	Ch. 47, p. 1039
Eligibility Categories and Requirements	Ch. 47, p. 1039
Grounds for Denial of Eligibility	Ch. 47, pp. 1039–1040

Chapter 1

Medical Assisting as a Profession

OVERVIEW

Students learn how the role of the medical assistant has expanded in recent years to include an ever-increasing number of administrative and clinical duties. Students begin to recognize the formal requirements of the medical assisting profession and to think of themselves as professionals. With this as a goal, the concept of professionalism is explored as the students discover the range of opportunities open to them in the field of medical assisting.

KNOWLEDGE EVALUATION OUTCOME ASSESSMENT

The student's attitude toward class attendance and study skills can be applied to his or her personal orientation toward professionalism and a willingness to meet the requirements necessary to enter the profession of medical assisting. Students are encouraged to evaluate themselves and compare this evaluation with the one supplied by the instructor. Specific areas to target for improvement are identified for students. Categories of assessment included in the workbook "Evaluation of Chapter Knowledge" include attendance/ punctuality, personal appearance, effort, self-motivation, courteousness, positive attitude, and completing assignments on time.

SUPPLEMENTARY RESOURCES

Medical Assisting Videos: Appropriate content is available on Delmar's Medical Assisting Videos, 2nd ed., Tape 1, for the following topics:

> Your Career as a Medical Assistant
> Display Professionalism
> Work as a Team Member
> Career-Seeking Skills
> Examinations and Certification through AAMA
> RMA/AMT
> Communication Skills

ANSWERS TO TEXT REVIEW QUESTIONS

1. c. 1978
2. b. 1956
3. d. The AAMA's series of home study courses
4. d. American Medical Technologies (AMT)
5. c. Managed Care's emphasis on ambulatory care

ANSWERS TO TEXT CRITICAL THINKING QUESTIONS

1. Students will look for persons whom they know: family, friends, church community members, and others who possess the attributes of a professional, as described in Chapter 1.

2. Patients today are better informed about health care, and they seek the highest quality health care possible. Formal education for medical assistants ensures that standard can be met. Physician-employers want to employ certified medical assistants because they recognize that there is a lesser likelihood of patients being prone to engage in lawsuits. This is so because certified medical assistants have been educated and are competent to perform administrative and clinical procedures and have passed the national certification examination.

3. Certification is of primary importance. The CMA credential is a testimony to the attainment of knowledge and skills to a competency level. Many employers hire only certified medical assistants. Recertification is testimony to medical assistants' desires to continuously pursue excellence through education.

4. Certification is voluntary and conferred upon an individual by a nongovernmental agency or professional association. Individuals must be qualified to take the examination and must pass the examination to be certified. This form of practice requirement is used by most professional associations. Licensure is mandated and legislated by each state. It is the most restrictive form of regulation. Individuals must be qualified to take the state examination and pass it as well. Registration is voluntary and is conferred upon individuals by their professional association. Their names are listed on an official roster. Passing the examination is not always a requirement. It is the least restrictive form of regulation.

5. Externship is the transition stage between the classroom and actual employment. It provides an opportunity to apply theory learned in the classroom setting to a health care setting through practice, hands-on experience.

   The medical assistant student benefits from the externship experience because of the following opportunities to
   • Apply classroom knowledge in a practical way in a medical setting.
   • Realize improvement in efficiency and proficiency.
   • Observe that there may be more than one acceptable method of performance.
   • Begin to establish a network of colleagues for support.
   The externship site benefits include
   • Currently employed staff will be more alert because of their training responsibilities.
   • Facility/staff workload may be eased by the "work" of the student; however, the student cannot be used as unsupervised staff, nor can the student be paid while at the site.
   • Facility/staff will have the opportunity to observe students who will soon be seeking employment.
   • Facility/staff have the opportunity to learn about the medical assisting profession.

ANSWERS TO WORKBOOK EXERCISES AND ACTIVITIES

Vocabulary Builder

    multiskilled/versatile
    outpatient facilities/ambulatory care settings
    lawsuit-prone/litigious
    recognizes qualifying standards for/accredits
    practical applications of theory/practicums
    proficiency/competency
    guarantee/certify
    official credit/credential
    agreement/compliance
    4-year undergraduate/baccalaureate
    combine/integrate
    characteristics/attributes
    temperament/disposition
    allows for easy/facilitates
    an insight into another's feelings or emotions/empathy
    performing without previous preparation/improvising
    legally authorized to practice/licensed
    granting of licenses to practice/licensure

Learning Review

1. The nine personal attributes of an MA are empathy, attitude, dependability, initiative, flexibility, desire to learn, physical attributes, ability to communicate, and ethical behavior.

2. The four reasons why the medical assisting profession has grown to require more formal, skilled education and credentialing for medical assistants are
   (1) Nurses could not perform the variety of duties required in medical offices and ambulatory care centers.
   (2) Informed patients require educated and credentialed MAs.
   (3) In today's litigious atmosphere, employers recognize the need to employ MAs who are professionally prepared through formal education.
   (4) Dependable MAs allow physicians to focus their time on the medical decisions, treatments, and techniques for which they are educated and licensed.
3. Three anticipated benefits are
   (1) Safeguard the quality of care to the consumer.
   (2) Ensure the CMA's role in the rapidly evolving health care delivery system.
   (3) Continue to promote the identity and stature of the profession.
4. A. Accumulate approved continuing education hours.
   D. Retake the certification examination.
5. The eight settings are offices, clinics, hospitals, medical laboratories, insurance companies, government agencies, pharmaceutical companies, and educational institutions.
6. B. Employee preparedness.
   D. High-quality medical assisting education.
7. A. Maintaining medical records
   A. Coding/insurance claims
   C. Basic laboratory procedures
   G. Patient education
   C. Assisting with minor surgery

   G. Medical law and ethics
   A. Scheduling appointments
   G. Anatomy and physiology
   C. Cardiopulmonary resuscitation
   C. Pharmacology

Multiple Choice Questions

1. b. ethics
2. d. empathy
3. d. five years

4. c. medical terminology
5. a. licensure

Investigation Activity

1. American Association of Medical Assistants
   20 North Wacker Drive, Suite 1575
   Chicago, IL 60606-2963
   800-228-2262 or 312-899-1500

   American Medical Technologists Association
   710 Higgins Road
   Park Ridge, IL 60068
   800-275-1268 or 847-823-5169

2. As a classroom activity, designate several students who will be responsible for gathering information. When materials arrive, have the students break into groups to read and discuss them. Students should exchange their interests and ambitions with one another and tell why they are interested in medical assisting as a profession.

   To follow up, ask the class to decide on the three medical assisting employment settings that are the most interesting or challenging to them. Invite CMAs from each setting to join the class for a special panel discussion, with questions and answers from students.

ANSWERS TO WORKBOOK CASE STUDY QUESTIONS

Instructors may use both Case Studies from Chapter 1 as the basis for classroom discussions. See the role-playing suggestions listed with each case.

Case 1

The purpose of Case 1 is to help students explore why they are interested in pursuing a career as a medical assistant, how the aspiring medical assistant fits into a professional environment, and how various health care settings require different skills and personal qualities from medical assistants. Instructors can use this case history as a springboard for students' own creative investigations of their personal interests and aptitudes, allowing them to consider the range of settings available in which to work instead of maintaining a narrow view of the choices open to them, and to determine what kind of setting best suits their individual personalities, goals, and skills.

1. The medical assisting student must match their personal strengths, goals, and ambitions to the working requirements of a professional setting.
2. The student identifies with the formal structure of working in a professional health care setting and recognizes the need for exhibiting professional behaviors in interactions with both health care professionals and patients.
3. The student identifies work skills, such as a willingness to ask questions, neatness, and accuracy.

4. The student begins to consider the scope of practice of the medical assistant as well as legal and ethical issues involved with clinical procedures medical assistants commonly perform, and the importance of obtaining patient consent.
5. Students explore the different personal qualities and ambitions relevant to specific medical settings.

Role-playing: Students divide into pairs. One student takes the role of the CMA and the other the role of the volunteer. Both students take turns portraying professional and unprofessional attitudes.

Case 2

The purpose of Case 2 is to encourage students to study professional health care settings. Students use their experiences as patients to come to a new understanding of professionalism. They discover how the role of the medical assistant contributes to a successful relationship between patients and the health care professionals who administer care. Students also remember that the goal of the health care professional is to provide the best care to patients in a safe and professional setting.

1. By examining the physician's office and staff from the patient's viewpoint, the medical assisting student reinforces an understanding of the need for professional behaviors.
2. Medical assisting students must sharpen and apply their powers of observation.
3. Medical assisting students apply their powers of observation to a CMA at work in a professional setting.

Role-playing: Students divide into pairs. One student takes the role of the CMA and the other the role of the patient. The student playing the CMA presents to the patient the advantages, services, and office policies offered by a professional health care setting. The patient asks questions about the advantages, services, and office policies and describes what, from the patient's perspective, makes up a professional health care setting.

Case 3

1. Michelle's shy, quiet nature may not be a natural fit at Inner City Health Care. Her difficulty in meeting new people may make it hard for her to interact with a diverse patient population and a large staff of health care professionals. However, Michelle is a bright student with a definite goal in mind. The challenge of the working environment she is seeking could be just what she needs to continue her personal and professional growth. An externship at Inner City Health Care could help Michelle discover whether this setting is the right one for her professional career as a medical assistant, or whether she would be happier elsewhere.
2. Students' responses will vary. However, students should acknowledge the importance of setting new goals outside of their current level of knowledge and experience and of working hard to achieve them.

Chapter 2

Health Care Settings and the Health Care Team

OVERVIEW

Students learn to place themselves in the context of the health care team, recognizing the major medical management models and the wide range of health care professionals medical assistants may come into contact with during their careers. Students understand the difference between medical and surgical specialties of physicians, the allied health professions, integrative medicine, and other health care professions. Students gain a respect for the important role of the medical assistant as a vital link in the health care team with an emphasis on professionalism, proper training, and appropriate behavior in patient communications.

KNOWLEDGE EVALUATION OUTCOME ASSESSMENT

Students are evaluated by the instructor for their understanding of performance objectives, including their understanding of managed care, ability to distinguish medical management models, empathy with patient experience of medical settings, ability to identify members of the health care team, respect for professionalism, and understanding of the medical assistant's role. Use of the "Investigation Activity" and "Case Study" sections of the workbook as classroom activities can serve as a forum for instructor evaluation.

SUPPLEMENTARY RESOURCES

Medical Assisting Videos: Appropriate content is available on Delmar's Medical Assisting Videos, 2nd ed., Tape 1, for the following topics:

> Your Career as a Medical Assistant
> Display Professionalism
> Work as a Team Member
> Career-Seeking Skills
> Communication Skills

ANSWERS TO TEXT REVIEW QUESTIONS

1. c. ambulatory care settings
2. a. managed care operation
3. b. all health care settings
4. d. is made up of physicians, nurses, allied and other health care professionals, patients, and sometimes a practitioner of nontraditional medicine
5. a. are increasingly accepted as complementary to traditional health care
6. c. phlebotomist
7. d. both b and c
8. d. group or partnership
9. c. establishes a primary care physician as gate-keeper
10. d. naturopathy

ANSWERS TO TEXT CRITICAL THINKING QUESTIONS

1. Most medical assistants are likely to work in an ambulatory care setting, which can include a small medical office (either a solo physician or group practice), an urgent care center, or one of the managed care operations, such as an HMO. Students should identify their own personal characteristics in discussing the pros and cons of working in each setting; a solo physician office may call on medical assistants to use their full range of skills, whereas a larger practice in either an HMO or urgent care center may allow medical assistants to develop specialized skills.

2. Just as medical assistants may choose one health care setting over another because of their personality preferences, patients too may find their choice of health care dictated by personal preferences. The benefits of a setting may be determined by what the patient wants and requires from a physician. In a smaller practice, the patient may be appreciative of the long-term, one-to-one relationship that can develop between patient and physician; larger ambulatory care centers may be able to offer more specialized care and more on-site services.

3. The three most common forms of medical management models include sole proprietorships; partnerships of two or more physicians; and professional service corporations with physician shareholders and HMOs and other medical centers where physicians have employee status.

   While a sole proprietorship may be appealing because it gives physicians independence in decision making, it is more and more difficult for one individual to assume the costs and liabilities of starting and maintaining a solo practice. In partnerships, physicians can share expenses; in group practices, physicians can also take turns being "on call." Corporations confer income and tax advantages; they also remove some of the risk from the individual and place it on the corporation. When physicians work for some HMOs, they often work as employees, a situation that provides them with the advantages of a salary and benefits and removes some of the accountability of being an owner of a practice.

   Medical assistants need to look at each facility on its own merit. As a general statement, it may be true that corporations and larger medical centers can offer more fringe benefits such as life and health insurance, educational allowances, and profit sharing or pension plans. On the other hand, small practices may be just as generous with long-term employees and give the medical assistant a sense of loyalty and security.

4. Managed care is a system designed to contain the costs of health care while still providing access. Under managed care, some say that health care access is more restricted for patients because preapprovals are often necessary and some services are denied. Critics also allege that managed care places another burden on providers for they must provide quality care at reduced reimbursement and that paperwork such as for treatment plans is cumbersome. Yet others contend that managed care is the only way to revive our medical delivery system by keeping costs in line and emphasizing preventive as well as sick-person care.

5. Refer to Tables 2-1, 2-2, and 2-3 of the main text.

6. In ambulatory care settings, the medical assistant is the most important allied professional on the health care team and is the link between the physician and the patient.

   Medical assistants will perform administrative tasks, clinical tasks, or both, depending on the setting. Administrative responsibilities may include serving as a receptionist, secretary, transcriptionist, bookkeeper, insurance coder, and patient educator. As clinical assistants, medical assistants may administer injections, perform venipuncture, prepare patients for examinations, assist the physician, and perform electrocardiography and laboratory tests.

   It is important that medical assistants project a positive attitude, be excellent communicators, and display a professional image and pride in their work.

7. In the medical field, the term *doctor* is used to address persons qualified by education, training, and licensure to practice medicine. A doctor of medicine, or MD, is what we typically think of as conferring the title *doctor*. However, other medical degrees grant the title of doctor, including doctor of osteopathy (OD), doctor of chiropractic (DC), and doctor of naturopathy (ND). In nonmedical disciplines, persons who have earned a doctor of philosophy (Ph.D.) or doctor of education (Ed.D.) also are entitled to the term *doctor*.

8. The Commission on Accreditation of Allied Health Education Programs (CAAHEP) recognizes a number of allied health professions.

9. Students should recall some of the allied professionals from Table 2-3 of the textbook and create a scenario based on one of the ambulatory care settings. The "team" could include a physician, patient, clinical and/or administrative medical assistant, and one or more of the other allied professionals who may work in the same setting or in another facility.

10. Integrative medicine or alternative forms of health care are increasingly perceived as complements to traditional health care. The students should recall some forms of alternative therapies from Table 2-4 of the textbook and describe their potential uses. Some of the more well-known therapies include acupuncture, biofeedback, and hypnotherapy.

ANSWERS TO WORKBOOK EXERCISES, ACTIVITIES, AND CASE STUDIES

Vocabulary Builder

1. E.
2. K.
3. D.
4. L.
5. G.

6. F.
7. C.
8. N.
9. A.
10. M.

11. J.
12. B.
13. H.
14. O.
15. I.

Learning Review

1. Managed care is creating an emphasis on ambulatory care settings, as more services are performed on an outpatient basis. Solo medical practices are giving way to group practices and networks where equipment, skills, and resources are shared to provide more services to patients on a cost-effective basis, while maintaining high-quality care. As the clinical and administrative demands on group practices increase and patient management becomes more complex, the medical assistant's role as a link between health care providers and a reassuring contact for patients becomes vital to providing seamless care.

2. **Sole Proprietorships:**
   A. Medical Settings: Primary care physician's or specialist's office.
   B. Patient Experience: Direct, one-on-one contact between physician, staff, and patient, establishing a long-term bond of care.

   Partnerships:
   A. Medical Settings: Group practice, primary, or specialized care centers.
   B. Patient Experience: Staff with flexibility to allow urgent appointments and 24-hour access to care. Offer of specialized care; for example, oncology or women's care. Access to more than one physician, allied health care or other professional, or specialist. Rapport with members of group practice, including the medical assistant.

   Corporations:
   A. Medical Settings: HMOs, PPOs, IPAs, urgent care centers.
   B. Patient Experience: Less personal contact with one specific health care provider. Services may need preapproval from the primary care physician, and second opinions are often required for care.

3. Three creative methods of keeping costs down are
   (1) Using technology more effectively.
   (2) Collaborating on new, cost-effective delivery methods.
   (3) Emphasizing prevention and lifestyle changes for patients.

4. A. The six administrative duties are receptionist, secretary, transcriptionist, bookkeeper, insurance coder and biller, and patient educator.
   B. The five clinical duties are administer injections and perform venipuncture, prepare patients for examinations, assist the physician with examinations and special procedures, perform electrocardiography and various laboratory tests, and triage and assess patient needs when scheduling appointments and tests.

5. A. MD: Doctor of medicine; requires a doctorate in medicine and/or a license to practice that allows a person to diagnose and treat medical conditions.
   DPM: Doctor of podiatric medicine; diagnoses and treats diseases and disorders of the feet.
   DC: Doctor of chiropractic; practices manipulative treatment of disorders originating from misalignment of the vertebrae.
   ND: Doctor of naturopathy; believes healing is accomplished through attention to the natural processes of the body.
   DO: Doctor of osteopathy; accomplishes therapeutic restoration through manipulation of the skeleton and muscles using physical, medicinal, and surgical methods.
   OD: Doctor of optometry; measures the accuracy of vision to determine if corrective lenses are needed and prescribes and fits those lenses.
   DDS: Doctor of dentistry; diagnoses and treats diseases and disorders of the teeth and gums.

   B. (1) Radiation oncologist: A physician with special training in the treatment of cancers using radiation techniques.
   (2) Obstetrician/gynecologist: A physician with special training in the care of pregnant women, including childbirth; a physician with special training in the health care of women, including sexual and reproductive function.
   (3) Neurologist: A physician with special training in conditions and disorders of the nervous system.
   (4) Gerontologist: A physician with special training in the care of older people.
   (5) Ophthalmologist: A physician with special training in the care of diseases and disorders of the eye.
   (6) Pediatrician: A physician with special training in the development and care of children, including diseases and conditions particular to children, and the prevention thereof.

6. Answers to the crossword puzzle:

ACROSS
1. Respiratory therapist
6. Histologic technician
7. Nurse practicioner
12. Medical illustrator
13. Medical laboratory technologist
15. PTA
18. Health unit coordinator
20. OAT
22. CRTT
23. Nurse
24. EMTP
26. Ophthalmic medical technician
30. Anesthesiologist assistant
31. Phlebotomist
32. Perfusionist
34. Diagnostic medical sonographer
35. Occupational therapist
37. Nuclear medicine technologist

DOWN
2. Electroneurodiagnostic technologist
3. Licensed practical nurse
4. Cardiovascular technologist
5. Radiation therapist
8. Pathologist's assistant
9. Registered nurse
10. Clinical laboratory scientist
11. Health information technician
14. Athletic trainer
15. Physical therapist
16. Health information administrator
17. Orthotist/prosthetist
19. Registered dietitian
21. Clinical laboratory technician
25. Medical assistant
27. Cytotechnologist
28. Pharmacist
29. Radiographer
33. SBB
36. PA

7. The seven alternative forms of health care are acupuncture, biofeedback, holism, homeopathy, hypnotherapy, naturopathy, and therapeutic touch.

Multiple Choice Questions

1. c. corporation
2. b. 9 years
3. a. anesthesiology
4. b. medical laboratory
5. d. naturopathy

Investigation Activity

A. Students identify community medical settings and relate each to its proper model of medical practice management, reinforcing the definition of each model: sole proprietorship, partnership, and corporation.
B. As a class, compile a questionnaire to gather data about medical settings. Areas to cover include the nature and description of services or specialties provided, the number of physicians and other health care professionals employed by the practice, the number of patients currently seen by the practice, medical equipment located at the facility, and the hours and location of the facility.

Additional Activity: As a class, choose one community example from each model of medical practice management. Elect three student volunteers and assign one community model to each student. Each volunteer will contact and request a visit to their assigned community model of medical practice management to obtain information about the practices, completing the questionnaire the class devised in Exercise B, above. The three students present their findings to the class, with discussion following to compare the different medical practice management models.

ANSWERS TO WORKBOOK CASE STUDY QUESTIONS

Instructors may use case scenarios as the basis for classroom discussion. Students are encouraged to role-play the scenarios, with one student taking the part of the medical assistant and one the patient.

Abigail Johnson:
1. The patient can give specific information about her diet, so the health care team can target trouble spots and make suggestions for improvement.
2. Listen, provide encouragement, gather as much information as possible about diet, personal habits, and symptoms of diabetes to assist the physician in treatment.

Herb Fowler:
1. The patient can be made aware of the physical risks of continued smoking and weight gain and can be encouraged to develop new behaviors to address them.
2. Patient education and empathy for patient's condition.

Juanita Hansen:
1. The mother can be encouraged to continue bringing the child to the clinic as problems arise.
2. Listen, gather as much information as possible about the nature of the eating problem and the circumstances of the previous accidents, with an eye toward potential child abuse.

Lenore McDonell:
1. The patient should be helped to understand the importance of maintaining regular office visits to preserve her health.
2. Offer comfort, empathy, and gentle reinforcement of the need to maintain medical care.

Chapter 3

History of Medicine

OVERVIEW

Medical assisting students learn to place themselves within the context of the history of medicine, recognizing the individual contributions of physicians and other health care professionals from various cultures and disciplines around the world and throughout history. The student gains a respect for differing philosophies of health care and treatment that may be held by patients, and understands the need for mutually respectful communication between health care professionals and patients. Reviewing this chapter, the student appreciates the many significant discoveries made throughout history to advance the practice of medicine and improve health care. The student begins to see the medical assistant's role in the present and future as a part of continued advances in meeting the health challenges of today and tomorrow.

KNOWLEDGE EVALUATION OUTCOME ASSESSMENT

Students are evaluated for their understanding of performance objectives. Not only should students demonstrate a functional, working knowledge of the history of medicine, they should also demonstrate an ability to apply this knowledge. Students should reach an empathetic sensitivity to the cultural, ethnic, and religious views of patients, which shape patients' expectations regarding the health care received.

SUPPLEMENTARY RESOURCES

Medical Assisting Videos: Appropriate content is available on Delmar's Medical Assisting Videos, 2nd ed., Tape 1, for the following topics:

> Your Career as a Medical Assistant
> Display Professionalism
> Work as a Team Member
> Career-Seeking Skills
> Communication Skills

ANSWERS TO TEXT REVIEW QUESTIONS

1. a. a book describing drugs and their preparation
2. b. care only for women and to assist in childbirth
3. a. Leonardo da Vinci
4. c. the father of medicine
5. d. Elizabeth Blackwell

ANSWERS TO TEXT CRITICAL THINKING QUESTIONS

1. Students might discuss how culture may determine the family members' involvement in health care, whether a female may be examined by a male physician, whether medications are preferred to a more "natural" approach, how often a physician is called for care, circumcision of both males and females (the latter in only a few societies), and how medical expenses are paid.
2. The medical specialist today is an individual who is highly prepared and educated in a specific field of study or technique. The neurosurgeon, for instance, will practice only neurosurgery and has long left the practice of general surgery or general medicine. Specialists in the past were more generalists in that they often treated more than one aspect of a person's illness or disease.
3. To solve the dilemma of not being allowed to treat a female patient (as a male physician), call on the closest female physician in the hospital. If there are none available, calmly explain the situation to the husband, the seriousness of the hemorrhaging, and that a female will be present at all times (such as a surgical nurse). If that does not work, you might invite the husband to attend the surgery. This, however, is risky. It is difficult for loved ones to watch the surgery of someone so close to them.
4. As a medical assistant, I would explain to my physician what I heard. If allowed to do so, I might also explain to the patient the hazards of not following my physician's directions. It would be helpful if I could also explain that my physician would be happy to work in conjunction with the family's acupuncturist. Not all physicians would agree to do so, however.
5. There are far more women in medicine today than in previous years. The female physician, however, still must endure persecution in medical school. Female physicians by their actions, however, have encouraged their peers to spend more time treating and caring for the "total person." Female health care practitioners of 100 years ago were far less fortunate; most were not allowed to practice at all, and if they were, it was only to serve as midwives.
6. Answers will depend on who the students select for their report. Make certain that they carefully document their resources in the reports.

ANSWERS TO WORKBOOK EXERCISES AND ACTIVITIES

Vocabulary Builder

1. Pluralistic
2. Moxibustion
3. Acupuncture
4. Septicemia
5. Bubonic plague, yellow fever, typhus, malaria
6. Allopathic
7. Pharmacopoeias
8. Asepsis

Learning Review

1. A. *Religion* encouraged the calling of a god(s) for a cure through ceremonies, prayers, and sacrifices.
   Magic formed an important part of many early societies and was seen as an essential ingredient to chase away evil spirits.
   Science encouraged experimentation in the use of plant, animal, and mineral substances for medicinal purposes.
   B. 1. R   3. S   5. M
      2. M   4. S   6. R
2. (1) *Cure the spirit:* Recent medical studies into the connection between body and mind show that patients with a more hopeful attitude or sense of spirituality respond better to treatment.
   (2) *Nourish the body:* The medical community is increasingly aware of the impact of diet on the prevention of disease.
   (3) *Give medications:* Allopathic medicine relies on medical and surgical interventions to cure or relieve illness.
   (4) *Treat the whole body:* A holistic approach to treatment and patient care takes into account the full situation of patients, recognizing them as whole people instead of isolating a particular illness or condition without regard to the total person.
   (5) *Use acupuncture and moxibustion:* Acupuncture is known to be effective in the control of pain or treatment of drug dependency; the ancient Chinese practice of moxibustion is not used by allopathic physicians today.
3. **Primitive Societies:** Women were accepted as healers and often performed functions that also served the welfare of the entire community or village. Later cultures reduced women's status to that of caring only for other women and/or assisting in childbirth.
   Chinese: The first reference to a female Chinese physician is mentioned by name in documents from the Han Dynasty (206 B.C. – A.D. 220).
   Muslim: The reluctance of Arabic physicians to violate social taboo and touch the genitals of female strangers encouraged relegating the practice of obstetrics and gynecology to midwives.
   Italian: Italy granted women the status of physician earlier than other countries in Western culture.

American: The first woman to be awarded a medical degree, in 1849, was Elizabeth Blackwell. She was snubbed by the public, but earned the respect of her colleagues. Women have grown in stature in the medical professions throughout the twentieth century.

4. **Prehistoric:** Cultures relied on magic, and the average lifespan for humans was 20 to 40 years. Skeletal remains of humans show advanced arthritis, toothless jaws, and trephination of the skull.

   Ancient Times: In Mesopotamia, Babylon, and China, physicians began to use science to develop pharmacopoeias. Greeks and Romans relied on classical learning. The Chinese studied the pulse and developed the practices of acupuncture and moxibustion. The Egyptians used emetics to cleanse body channels. Plastic surgery was practiced in ancient India.

   Seventh Century: Early Christian monks, such as St. Benedict, held great control over medicine during the rise of Christianity, placing emphasis on the soul rather than the body. In Islam, however, religious leaders moved to preserve the classical teachings of medicine begun by the Greeks and Romans, and medical study was encouraged.

   Ninth Century: Medical education in established universities began—Salerno in southern Italy, the University of Montpelier in southern France, and the University of Paris.

   Renaissance: Physicians were now licensed and received great societal status and income. Art and science were closely linked: Michelangelo studied the human anatomy through dissection and Leonardo da Vinci produced accurate drawings of body systems.

   Nineteenth Century: Women began to achieve a higher status in Western medicine. Anesthesia and asepsis were discovered. Science was heavily relied on as new discoveries revolutionized the practice of medicine and led to the institution of new public health and sanitation measures.

   Twentieth Century: Antibiotics are discovered. Vaccinations for smallpox, poliomyelitis, and other infectious diseases are developed. Insulin is used for the treatment of diabetics. Life expectancy increases. AIDS, for which there is no cure, challenges researchers. Infectious diseases, such as cholera, remains endemic to developing nations with poor sanitation. New drug-resistant strains of malaria, tuberculosis, and other diseases are not responding to traditional medications.

   Twenty-first Century: Gene manipulation may have the potential benefit of reversing the progression of many debilitating diseases.

5. A. In Native American cultures, suicide among the infirm and elderly was considered heroic in times of famine. The Eskimos abandoned the elderly. Greeks and Romans did not treat the hopelessly ill or deformed and left unwanted infants to die. Today, Western society debates the morality, ethics, and legality of physician-assisted suicide and the right to choose life or death.

   B. In the past, ill people were often shunned because sickness was thought to denote a moral failing or disfavor with the gods. The forced isolation may have been beneficial to the community by unwittingly increasing public health standards. Today, AIDS confuses and frightens many people, and those with the disease are often poorly treated by society. In Cuba, those who test positive for HIV are quarantined.

   C. The importance of religion led many early cultures to link illness with spiritual failing, leading to the refusal to treat such individuals and to isolate them from mainstream society. With the rise of Christianity, emphasis was placed on purity of the soul over soundness of body. Today, the roots of illness are known to have scientific, genetic, or environmental causes.

   D. Some Native Americans believe survivors of serious illness hold extraordinary powers. Today, as more people survive serious illnesses, such as cancer, survivors experience increased self-esteem and confidence, though they are not thought to have supernatural instincts or abilities.

   E. Ancient Greeks and Romans did not treat the deformed or disabled. Today, with the institution of the Americans with Disabilities Act (1990), individuals with disabilities are mainstreamed into society and given the same opportunities as others.

6. Students' choices could consist of any of the following diseases or conditions referenced in the textbook chapter: bubonic plague, cholera, diabetes, diphtheria, dysentery, leprosy, malaria, poliomyelitis, septicemia, smallpox, tuberculosis, typhus, venereal diseases, yellow fever.

7. (1) To instruct other qualified students in the practice of medicine.
   (2) To give proper treatment for the benefit of the sick, according to the physician's training and judgment, and to keep the sick from harm.
   (3) To refuse abortive remedies to women or to assist in the death of any person.
   (4) Only trained and licensed surgeons should perform surgical procedures.
   (5) Physicians will not act in an irresponsible, unethical, or illegal manner with patients and will not have sexual relations with patients.

8.
   1. J. 16th century
   2. D. 20th century
   3. N. 19th century
   4. F. 13th century B.C.
   5. C. 18th century
   6. L. 19th century
   11. R. 19th century
   12. M. 19th century
   13. O. 17th century
   14. P. 19th century
   15. Q. 18th century
   16. T. 19th century

7.	E.	19th century	17.	I.	15th century
8.	H.	19th century	18.	K.	19th century
9.	B.	5th century B.C.	19.	A.	20th century
10.	G.	18th century	20.	S.	20th century

Multiple Choice Questions

1. c. Mesopotamian
2. a. Shaman
3. d. 9th

4. b. Cuba
5. d. Banting and Best

INVESTIGATION ACTIVITY

As a class, discuss the various cultural, ethnic, and religious beliefs held by students and their families. Consider how these beliefs may make an impact in fulfilling the role of the medical assistant as well as determining care from the patient's point of view. Share the folk or home remedies held as tradition by students and their families. Collect them to form a class pharmacopoeia.

Collect the one-page reports on significant persons contributing to the history of medicine assigned in the "Text Critical Thinking Questions" to create a class biographical encyclopedia of medicine.

Role-playing: To link student knowledge of medical history with the practical experience of communicating with patients, use this role-playing exercise. One student takes the role of a significant figure in the history of medicine, chosen from the class encyclopedia, and another student takes the role of a patient with a specific problem. The class analyzes the role-playing session to determine historical and cultural attitudes toward illness and treatments and consider how medical advances have changed the lives of people throughout history.

Have the class choose a medical specialty and invite a specialist from that field to speak to the class about the history of that area of medicine as well as its past, present, and future challenges.

ANSWERS TO WORKBOOK CASE STUDY QUESTIONS

The purpose of the case study is to give an example of a contemporary medical situation that evokes the challenges medicine faces today in devising new treatments and possible cures, framed within the context of strongly held cultural and religious beliefs. The role of women in society and in medicine is also explored. Medical assistants begin to see themselves as a part of medical history as it unfolds, recognizing the potential impact of changing current medical practices on the lives of patients and the need for respectful communication between patients and health care professionals when deeply rooted cultural beliefs are held.

1. Margaret Thomas chooses to see a female physician, feeling more comfortable confiding in another woman about her health concerns. The prospect of fetal tissue research for Parkinson's evokes not only Margaret's religious convictions, but also her status as a mother and grandmother. The role of women in society as mothers, sacred protectors of life, factors into Margaret's fears about the experimental treatment. Her daughter, from a younger generation, may have less resistance to the idea of fetal tissue treatments. As health care professionals, medical assistants must recognize that medical advances may challenge traditional roles, such as motherhood, and must come to terms with their own inner convictions and personal ethics while considering the challenge of medical ethics for the twenty-first century.

2. As a medical assistant, it is beyond Audrey's scope of practice to comment speculatively on treatment options for Mrs. Thomas. Audrey should restate Dr. King's explanation about effective drug therapies and the need to see a neurologist for further testing. She should display a compassionate and reassuring tone and demeanor to calm Mrs. Thomas's feelings of distress. Then, Audrey should ask Dr. King to return to answer any questions Mrs. Thomas's daughter may have about experimental treatments.

3. Mrs. Thomas's strong religious beliefs may help her confront the possibility that she may have Parkinson's disease and sustain her through traditional treatment with drug therapies. However, participation in any fetal tissue research program for Parkinson's would go against Mrs. Thomas's religious convictions and present a severe strain on her personal belief system, possibly also causing personal conflict within her daughter or other family members.

4. When potential medical breakthroughs involve controversial or radical ideas that challenge long-held cultural viewpoints or beliefs, society must confront the new issues raised and arrive at a system of medical and personal ethics that deal with the situation effectively. Many times government intervention is necessary to devise new regulations or laws, such as in the case of the issue of fetal tissue research, discussed in this case study. Health care professionals and their patients need to examine their personal ethics and beliefs, weighing the potential benefits of a medical advance against long-held cultural values.

Chapter 4

Therapeutic Communication Skills

OVERVIEW

Medical assisting students learn the importance of effective therapeutic communication for establishing and maintaining successful relationships with other health care professionals and with patients. Students analyze the communication cycle, studying both verbal and nonverbal components, in order to gain confidence and to cultivate objective observation skills that will allow them to assess patients' needs and facilitate care with empathy and impartiality. The need to adapt messages to the receiver's ability to understand is explained and stressed. The unique requirements of both face-to-face and telephone communications are outlined and discussed.

KNOWLEDGE EVALUATION OUTCOME ASSESSMENT

Students are evaluated for their understanding of performance objectives. Students should be able to assess their own communication skills and styles, identifying both personal strengths and areas for improvement. Students hone a keen sense of observation, while recognizing the importance of verbal and nonverbal cues in sending and receiving messages. Whether communicating face-to-face or on the telephone, medical assisting students recognize that successful therapeutic communication is essential to providing good and professional care to patients.

SUPPLEMENTARY RESOURCES

Medical Assisting Videos: Appropriate content is available on Delmar's Medical Assisting Videos, 2nd ed., Tape 1, for the following topics:

> Your Career as a Medical Assistant
> Display Professionalism
> Work as a Team Member
> Career-Seeking Skills
> Communication Skills

ANSWERS TO TEXT REVIEW QUESTIONS

1. d. b and c only
2. b. creating the message to be sent
3. a. is used to express feelings and emotions
4. d. 4 to 12 feet
5. c. a roadblock to communication
6. a. sublimation
7. c. a response that permits the patient to elaborate
8. c. are expendable words used in answering a telephone call

ANSWERS TO TEXT CRITICAL THINKING QUESTIONS

1. "We'll ask the doctor if there is anything that can help you with your complexion concerns. Going out for sports is a good way to keep your weight down."
2. "I'm sorry to hear that, Bill. I'll change the address and phone number. Is there anything I can do for you? You might find one of the pamphlets in the rack over there to be beneficial."
3. "I'm sorry, Edith. We have to get these just right for a good picture for the doctor. Tell me what is the easiest way for you to move into position."
4. "It is always possible that we made a mistake. Let me check your social security number against our laboratory slip to make certain."
5. "You are correct; you move around very smoothly. I did not mean to offend you, only to offer assistance if needed."
6. "Changing to a period of time when you will be less busy is a little frightening, isn't it? I was just talking to a friend who works at the hospital this weekend; they are desperate for volunteers. Is that something that might interest you?"
7. "Martin, this has to be very difficult for you. It is, however, what the doctor recommends. Do you want to discuss it further with the doctor?"
8. "This conversation is going to be very difficult for you, doctor. As painful as it is, it must be comforting to the family to have a doctor who knows them so well and is so sensitive to their needs.

ANSWERS TO WORKBOOK EXERCISES AND ACTIVITIES

Vocabulary Builder

A.
1. Therapeutic communication
2. Buffer words
3. Interview techniques
4. Posture
5. Hierarchy of needs
6. Closed questions
7. Roadblocks to communication
8. Position
9. Kinesics
10. Indirect statements
11. Communication cycle
12. Active listening
13. Biases
14. Prejudices
15. Message
16. Body language
17. Territoriality
18. Open-ended questions
19. Receiver
20. Gestures/mannerisms
21. Touch
22. Masking
23. Sender
24. Cluster
25. Congruency
26. Decode
27. Encode
28. Feedback
29. Modes of communication
30. Perception
31. Facial expressions

B.
1. Denial
2. Rationalization
3. Regression
4. Displacement
5. Repression
6. Sublimation
7. Projection

Learning Review

1. *Ethnic heritage* may indicate a slant toward the Eastern influence in medicine as opposed to the traditional Western style more commonly taught and practiced in the United States today.

   Geographic location and background may reveal that a person is more comfortable with a family physician in a very small clinic than in a large metropolitan multispecialty practice.

   Genetics can predispose individuals to certain conditions and illnesses that run in families. An awareness of a family history of a condition or illness can affect patients' comfort levels and influence physicians' treatment plans.

   Economics may influence the comfort level if office staff and patients have different perceptions about how billing is managed and when and how payments are expected.

   Educational experiences will determine, in part, how patients react to their care.

   Life experiences allow patients to have more empathy in certain situations. For example, patients with family members being treated for a chronic illness will have more knowledge and understanding of that illness in their own lives.

   Personal value systems bring personal preferences, biases, and even prejudices into many physician-patient relationships.

2. (1) A.
   (2) C.
   (3) D.
   (4) F.
   (5) B.
   (6) E.

3. *Sender:* Martin Gordon, patient
   Receiver: Ellen Armstrong, medical assistant
   Message: The patient wants to schedule a follow-up appointment and is anxious and depressed when he learns that the physician will not be available quickly.
   Feedback: The medical assistant recognizes the patient's concerns and schedules the first available appointment on the physician's return. She uses a reassuring tone and comforting words to acknowledge the patient's feelings and needs.

4. (1) Speaking   (3) Gestures or body language
   (2) Listening   (4) Writing

5. A. "You are concerned because your father takes several medications and is no longer able to keep them straight. He's stopped taking any medication at all. I know you are frustrated and concerned about your father's health; I'll make sure the physician knows what is happening so that you can discuss the situation and find a solution."

   B. "You don't have your insurance card and you don't remember the name of the insurance company, but you've used your insurance at this office before. Let me look in our records to see who the insurance carrier is so that we can call to find out more information about this situation."

   C. "You are nervous because the physician referred you to a facility where a patient received the wrong care. I understand that this kind of situation could be upsetting; I'll have the physician speak to you again about your procedure and what you can expect at the hospital when you go for treatment."

   D. "I know you are apprehensive about having blood taken; the physician has ordered the blood tests to find out more about your condition. Would you like to lie down during the procedure in case you get dizzy?"

6. (1) D. Pain.   (3) B. Sad.
   (2) C. Confused.   (4) A. Happy.

7. The five Cs of communication are complete, clear, concise, courteous, and cohesive.

8. *Survival or physiological needs:* shelter and clothing, food and water, air.
   Safety needs: structure, law and order, boundaries.
   Belongingness and love needs: family, friends, community.
   Prestige and esteem needs: mutual respect, integrity, honesty.

9. (1) Reasurring clichés   (5) Defending/contradicting
   (2) Moralizing/lecturing   (6) Shifting subjects
   (3) Requiring explanations   (7) Criticizing
   (4) Ridiculing/shaming   (8) Threatening

10. *Closed question:* "Mrs. Leonard, did the ophthalmologist remove your cataract?"
    Open-ended question: "How well are you seeing now out of the right eye?"
    Indirect statement: "Tell me how you are getting along at home now that your vision has improved."

11. The four tools of communication essential to conducting successful telephone conversations are
    (1) Use a warm greeting and sustain a caring tone throughout the conversation.
    (2) Use words that will be easily understood and ask questions to verify that the patient has understood the message being conveyed.
    (3) Hold the mouthpiece of the telephone 1 to 2 inches away from the mouth. Project the voice at the mouthpiece and then project another foot farther.
    (4) Use buffer words.

Multiple Choice Questions

1. b. perception
2. d. Maslow
3. a. rationalization

4. c. telephone
5. c. clustering

Investigation Activity

Perform Exercises A and B as group class activities, or encourage students to practice nonverbal communication skills at home in front of a mirror or with a partner.

Members of the deaf community are experts at expressing and interpreting nonverbal messages. Invite a deaf person and a sign language interpreter to class to hold a workshop with students to discuss nonverbal communication, fine-tune students' observation skills, and increase students' comfort levels in communicating through the use of natural gestures, body language, and facial expressions.

Role-playing. Have students role-play the Case Studies from the textbook and workbook to discover how nonverbal messages can be conveyed in each situation. Notice how nonverbal cues can influence or alter the verbal message. Practice sending congruent and incongruent messages.

ANSWERS TO WORKBOOK CASE STUDY QUESTIONS

1. Wayne's (the patient) slight retardation requires patience and special attention to the message communicated by the health care professionals and understood by the patient. Care on the part of the health professionals must be taken to put the patient at ease in an environment that might be frightening or intimidating. A comforting tone and non-threatening, welcoming body language should be used by the physician and medical assistant. However, the physician's role as an authority figure can be used to convince the patient of the importance of following the treatment plan.

2. When addressing the physician, Wanda (the medical assistant) will use proper medical terminology, maintain eye contact, and exhibit a professional demeanor. When addressing the patient, the medical assistant will use words consistent with the patient's ability to understand. She will exhibit a comforting and courteous professional demeanor. Eye contact with the patient should be encouraged. However, the medical assistant should not stare at the patient, which may be perceived by the patient as too threatening or aggressive.

3. Wanda uses active listening to ensure that Wayne has understood the physician's instructions regarding the treatment with antibiotics. Wanda's open-ended questions and indirect statements prompt the patient to explain how the antibiotics should be taken and why. Wanda's use of these interview techniques allows her to be sure that the patient understands the message communicated to him. The patient's wandering attention and inability or unwillingness to maintain eye contact are nonverbal cues that signal the medical assistant's need for precision and understanding in facilitating therapeutic communication. Wanda should recognize the patient's nonverbal cues and exhibit patient and encouraging facial expressions and body language to put Wayne at ease and help him concentrate.

4. The health care team meets Wayne's survival or physiological needs by properly administering treatment with antibiotics. The health care team meets Wayne's safety needs by ensuring that the patient understands the importance of following the physician's instructions. Wayne's belongingness or love needs are met as the health care team encourages him to feel comfortable and welcome in the health care setting. The patient's prestige and esteem needs are met as Wayne gains confidence when he realizes he is capable of understanding and following the physician's instructions. Wayne is self-actualized in this situation when he reaches his potential to understand and follow through with the physician's treatment plan.

5. Medical assistant Wanda acted appropriately by exhibiting professional, patient, and compassionate behavior in administering care to the patient. She did not condescend or ignore the patient's special needs due to his slight retardation. She used verbal and nonverbal communication skills to facilitate successful therapeutic communication that was respectful of the patient's situation and that met his health care needs.

Chapter 5

Coping Skills for the Medical Assistant

OVERVIEW

Medical assisting students define stress and the physiological effects of stress on the body. Stressors common in the ambulatory care setting are identified, and coping mechanisms for dealing with each are discussed. The importance of setting realistic short- and long-range goals is emphasized as a primary method of reducing stress. Students are encouraged to examine their own personal goals and aspirations. Inner- and outer-directed personality traits and the positive or negative influence of each on making effective life decisions are explored. The concept of burnout is introduced; students discover personality traits that promote burnout and identify ways to reduce the risk of burning out in the workplace environment. Burnout does not occur suddenly as does stress.

KNOWLEDGE EVALUATION OUTCOME ASSESSMENT

Students are evaluated for their understanding of performance objectives. Students should be able to assess realistically the potential stresses and stressors common in the ambulatory care setting and describe the physiological effects of stress. By analyzing their personal responses to stress, students begin to see how they may respond to stress in a workplace setting and to consider what kind of setting—group practice, urgent care center, HMO—best fits their individual personalities. Encouraging students to set short- and long-range goals builds self-esteem and confidence as they prepare to enter the challenging and demanding profession of medicine and health care.

SUPPLEMENTARY RESOURCES

Medical Assisting Videos: Appropriate content is available on Delmar's Medical Assisting Videos, 2nd ed., for the following topics:

     Tape 1: Your Career as a Medical Assistant
              Display Professionalism
              Work as a Team Member
              Career-Seeking Skills
              Communication Skills
     Tape 3: Perform Administrative Duties
              Triage Skills

ANSWERS TO TEXT REVIEW QUESTIONS

1. a. it does not occur suddenly
2. c. 4 stages
3. c. burnout.
4. c. an individual has certain personality traits

5. c. feelings of accomplishment and pride in work
6. b. prioritizing your tasks and employing time-management techniques
7. b. Abraham Maslow
8. b. they are divided into a series of short-range goals

ANSWERS TO TEXT CRITICAL THINKING QUESTIONS

1. *Plan ahead* by reviewing the next day's schedule before leaving the office. Maintain an accurate inventory of supplies and order before the last items are used. Participate in continuing education activities and read current medical journals. *Arrive early* and check to be sure that each examination room is equipped and ready for the day. Get plenty of *rest*, *exercise* regularly, and *eat balanced meals*. Learn to *laugh* at life's little problems. Establish an appropriate level of humor with other staff members. Use *color* and *light* to create a calm atmosphere. Play soft background *music* for relaxation. Build morning and afternoon *breaks* into the schedule. Close the office during the lunch hour and, if possible, leave the facility. Complete one task before moving on to another. Learn to *prioritize* tasks and do not procrastinate.
2. Participate in self-analysis activities as described within the text.
3. Goals will vary, depending on each individual.
4. Developing negative work attitudes, such as being hard to get along with or having a lack of motivation and having poor personal appearance and hygiene. Having a high need to achieve and not reaching established goals. More motivation to dominate and lead than peers; less motivation to defer to authority. Manifestations include chronic fatigue, anger, self-criticism, hair-trigger display of emotions, a sense of constantly being under attack, and an inability to keep even daily frustrations in perspective.
5. **Role Conflict:** When employees have conflicting responsibilities they feel pulled in many directions. The perfectionist tries to do everything well without setting priorities. Fatigue and exhaustion associated with burnout begin to set in after a period of time.
    Role Ambiguity: The employee does not know what is expected and how to accomplish it because there may not be a role model to follow or ask or established guidelines to follow.
    Role Overload: If the employee cannot say no and continues to accept more responsibility than they can handle, burnout is sure to set in.

ANSWERS TO WORKBOOK EXERCISES AND ACTIVITIES

Vocabulary Builder

1. D.
2. A.
3. I.
4. H.
5. G.

6. C.
7. F.
8. E.
9. B.

Learning Review

1. The five ways the body uses to restore homeostasis are blood pressure, heart rate, respirations, peristalsis, and the amounts of nutrients in the circulating blood supply.
2. The four stages of the GAS theory and the physiological manifestations of each are
    (1) *Alarm:* In this stage, the body perceives the awareness of stress. A slight rise in blood pressure may be evidenced. A person may be experiencing stress caused by physical pain.
    (2) *Fight-or-flight:* The sympathetic nervous system prepares the body for fight or flight. The eyes dilate, the mouth becomes dry. Heart rate, respirations, and pulse increase. Blood vessels in the skin constrict and blood vessels in the heart and brain dilate. Motility in the gastrointestinal and genitourinary tracts decreases.
    (3) *Exhaustion:* Blood vessels weaken after repeated episodes of dilation and relaxation. Blood vessels may burst if dilated to an extreme or are significantly weakened in areas.
    (4) *Return to normal:* Parasympathetic nervous system is activated, and the body returns to normal. Eyes constrict, salivary glands function. Heart rate, pulse, and respirations decrease. Blood vessels dilate in the skin and constrict in the heart and brain. Gastrointestinal and genitourinary tracts begin to function again.
3. 1. E.
    2. C.
    3. D.
    4. A.

    5. B.
    6. F.
    7. G.

4. A. The five considerations important in determining a goal are: it should be (1) specific, (2) challenging, (3) realistic, (4) attainable, and (5) measurable. Specific goals are focused and have very precise boundaries. Challenging goals create enthusiasm and an interest in achievement. Realistic goals are practical or beneficial for the present and for future self-actualization. An attainable goal is a goal that is possible to fulfill. Measurable goals achieve some form of progress or success.

    B. Students' responses regarding individual goals will vary.

5. | 1. | R. | 6. | P. | 11. | R. |
    |----|----|----|----|-----|----|
    | 2. | R. | 7. | P. | 12. | P. |
    | 3. | P. | 8. | P. | 13. | R. |
    | 4. | P. | 9. | R. | 14. | R. |
    | 5. | R. | 10. | R. | 15. | R. |

Multiple Choice Questions

1. b. stress
2. b. the parasympathetic nervous system
3. c. role ambiguity
4. a. angry and frustrated
5. c. prevent it

Investigation Activity: Stress Self-Test

Use the "Stress Self-Test" as a device to help students relate personally to the types of stress they may encounter in the workplace during their careers as medical assistants.

Role-playing: Self-test questions may become the basis for creating role-playing exercises. For example, self-test question 4 explores how students react to difficult personalities. Students alternately take the roles of difficult or demanding patients or coworkers and the medical assistants who must interact with them in an ambulatory care setting. The self-test exercise choices become their behaviors. In this manner, students play out their own personal responses and reactions to stress and stressors within the context of situations where, as medical assistants, they are called on to behave professionally. Standards of professional, stress-reducing behaviors are established experientially. If necessary, break the class into pairs and assign self-test questions to each group to complete this role-playing exercise.

ANSWERS TO WORKBOOK CASE STUDY QUESTIONS

1. Dr. Angie Esposito's burnout is promoted by the following personality traits: a greater need for achievement, more motivation to dominate and lead than peers, an intense need to achieve one's goals, and a higher need to do a job well for its own sake than do most of one's peers. Stressors in Dr. Esposito's life include the financial pressures of repaying student loans, the physical and time pressures of working double shifts to pay back the loans, and family pressures (real or perceived) to constantly achieve.

2. Liz Corbin, CMA, should not give up her goals of attending medical school and becoming a pediatrician. Liz should observe Angie's experience to learn about the stress and stressors Liz herself is likely to encounter as she works toward achieving her own goals. By avoiding or at least considering the stressors in her mentor's life, Liz can plan more effectively to achieve her goals in a way that minimizes the taxing effects of stress on her personal resources and well-being.

3. Both Angie and Liz set high but realistic goals for their lives. The higher the goal, the more effort—and potential stress—is involved. Both women can achieve fulfillment in their careers, helping many patients and benefiting the community. But both must realize that they cannot do everything on their own; it is possible to do only as much as one's resources and talents will allow. Angie's desire to help everyone is admirable but, in practice, is an unrealistic goal to achieve.

4. "Dr. Esposito, your talents and skills help many patients and their families. And I know it is truly appreciated. You are making a difference. And I enjoy the opportunity to watch and learn from your example. Once you've had some rest, you'll regain your perspective. Would you like a cup of hot tea? Or how about a short walk in the fresh air? Or maybe you'd just like some quiet time alone?"

Chapter 6

The Therapeutic Approach to the Patient with Life-Threatening Illness

OVERVIEW

Medical assisting students are presented with the challenges of providing therapeutic care to the patient with life-threatening illness in an ambulatory care setting. By examining the epidemiology of the disease, medical assisting students understand how it progresses and learn about its defining characteristics. Providing therapeutic care for patients with life-threatening illness requires medical assistants first to confront their own feelings and comfort levels with regard to these problems. Students discover that empathy, impartiality, respect, and compassion are necessary in administering to the special needs of these patients, who may be suffering intense psychological as well as physical pain. The need for effective patient education about life-threatening illness and measures that can be taken to help prevent the disease are also emphasized.

KNOWLEDGE EVALUATION OUTCOME ASSESSMENT

Students are evaluated for their understanding of performance objectives. Students should be able to identify personal strengths and weaknesses concerning their own fears and concerns about providing therapeutic care for patients with life-threatening illnesses in an ambulatory setting. Students should demonstrate an ability to discuss the epidemiology of the disease and the social issues surrounding life-threatening illnesses openly and frankly. Students recognize the need to establish therapeutic communication with patients with life-threatening illness that is professional, empathetic, nonjudgmental, and respectful. Gaining an awareness of the importance of health promotion and disease prevention, medical assistants recognize their role in the community as educators of the public.

SUPPLEMENTARY RESOURCES

Medical Assisting Videos: Appropriate content is available on Delmar's Medical Assisting Videos, 2nd ed., for the following topics:

Tape 1:   Communication Skills
Tape 5:   Infection Control and Universal Precautions
           Apply Principles of Aseptic Technique and Infection Control
           Standard Precautions
           Infections in the Office
Tape 8:   Taking a Patient History
           Introduction to Health Promotion, Disease Prevention, and
           Self-Responsibility
Tape 12:   OSHA Regulations for Needles and "Sharps"
           Accidental Needlesticks

ANSWERS TO TEXT REVIEW QUESTIONS

1. c. be supportive and free of prejudice
2. e. only b and c
3. c. the family
4. d. all of the above
5. d. all of the above
6. b. is heightened and considered more difficult
7. d. all of the above
8. e. only a and d
9. d. only a and b
10. d. all of the above

ANSWERS TO TEXT CRITICAL THINKING QUESTIONS

1. The other chapter that discusses end-of-life legal documents is Chapter 7, Legal Considerations.
2. Answers will vary, but discussions should include topics such as who is involved with the health care decisions, how pain is managed, what the greatest fears are. Do you make a living will or a physician's directive? What would you want it to say?
3. Students' answers will vary. The instructor can help students face their fears, if those fears are known, and identify some of those fears for discussion without revealing students' names or confidences.
4. Common psychological reactions persons might have when learning they have a life-threatening illness include shock, denial, numbness, anger, guilt, rage, sadness, hopelessness, helplessness, and withdrawal.
5. Other chapters of this text that discuss life-threatening illnesses include Chapters 7, 8, and 21.
6. To keep from burnout when caring for patients with life-threatening illness, medical assistants can make certain there are play, laughter, close friends, and confidants in their lives. They should try to remember that sensitive and therapeutic care given to persons with a life-threatening illness will be truly appreciated and that medical assistants have had a role in making patients' lives a little easier. Observing all techniques in Chapter 5, Coping Skills for the Medical Assistant, is a must.
7. Advantages of physician directives include (1) patients with a life-threatening illness have some control over their care; (2) allows decisions to be made before emotions are so heavily involved. Disadvantages of physician directives include (1) no matter how carefully written and planned, patients may still have difficulty in having their choices honored; (2) people do not like to discuss life-threatening illness and choices that might have to be made.
8. Answers will vary, but a point to be remembered is that dealing with the psychological suffering is often more difficult that the physical manifestations of suffering. From this discussion should come a list of support agencies available.
9. Answers will vary here also. Students' privacy should be protected, but a good discussion may occur relating to how one chooses types of employment and ambulatory care settings in which to work. The instructor should be prepared to offer some of the positive points of working in settings that care for persons with life-threatening illnesses as opposed to working in settings where there are almost no life-threatening illnesses.
10. Answers will vary according to the location and size of the city. Local hospitals, social services, hospice agencies, and volunteer groups will provide the best resources.

ANSWERS TO WORKBOOK EXERCISES AND ACTIVITIES

Vocabulary Builder

Key terms are inserted into the paragraph in the following order:

acquired immunodeficiency syndrome (AIDS)
human immunodeficiency virus (HIV)
retroviruses
ribonucleic acid (RNA)
opportunistic infections
pathogens
hemophilia
libido
dementia
psychomotor retardation
living will
physician's directive

Learning Review

1. (1) Living will or physician directive
    (2) Durable power of attorney for health care
    (3) Pain management
    (4) Alternative methods of treatment
    (5) Finances
    (6) Emotional needs of the patient and family
2. Students will provide answers based on their own personal comfort levels.

Multiple Choice Questions

1. b. 1991
2. a. pain and loss of independence
3. e. all of the above

4. b. denial
5. d. all of the above

Investigation Activity

Use the investigation activity to help students become more open and frank in their research and discussions on the subject of life-threatening illnesses. By identifying community resources and contacting organizations and hotlines, students are drawn into an active awareness of the need to advocate for increased patient education and the practice of preventive measures by the general public. By discussing brochures and materials supplied by organizations in the classroom setting, students become more comfortable about, and prepared for, discussing such materials with patients in an ambulatory care setting. Ask students to role-play both a patient asking for information about life-threatening illnesses and a medical assistant explaining to a patient in lay terms about the disease and preventive measures to protect against it. Have students role-play the textbook and workbook "Case Study" scenarios to increase their confidence in situations involving caring for patients with life-threatening illnesses.

Invite a representative from a community-based organization or a health care professional who works closely with patients in crisis to speak to the class and answer questions about their situation; detail public health and prevention measures; talk about how patients, their families, and significant others live with the disease day to day; and help students cope with feelings they may have about caring for patients with life-threatening illnesses.

ANSWERS TO WORKBOOK CASE STUDY QUESTIONS

Case 1

1. "We are following the standard precautions that all health care professionals use in medical emergencies like this one to reduce the risk of infection to everyone present. Using standard precautions doesn't mean that Mr. Carrera has a life-threatening illness or any other infectious illness. Have you been hurt in any way? Let's wash your hands and replace that soiled shirt with a clean gown. The physician will be here to examine you and answer any questions you have as soon as Mr. Carrera's emergency situation has been attended to."
2. The medical assistant reassures the coworker by explaining the use of standard precautions, establishes that the coworker has not also been hurt in the accident, makes sure that the emergency patient's blood is removed from contact with the coworker's body, and advises the coworker that a physician will examine him and address any further questions or concerns he may have.

Case 2

1. "Mrs. O'Keefe, I'm sorry, but I can't breach patient confidentiality by discussing the treatment of other patients with you. I can assure you, however, that like any professional ambulatory care setting this office employs all necessary measures to help keep patients safe and minimize the risk of spreading infectious illnesses. The risk to you and your baby of contracting AIDS or other infectious illnesses while at the medical office is minimal. I'll tell Dr. King about your concerns, so she can answer any specific questions you may have."
2. Ellen protects patients' rights to privacy while still reassuring Mary O'Keefe about the safety of the medical office. She treats Mrs. O'Keefe's concerns seriously and refers her to Dr. King for more information.

Chapter 7

Legal Considerations

OVERVIEW

Medical assisting students are introduced to the law as it affects the health care profession and ambulatory care setting. The concepts of professional negligence, malpractice, informed consent, and effective risk management are presented. In today's litigious society, the potential for lawsuits in medical settings has increased. Medical assistants learn their role as legal agents of their physician–employers and the contractual relationships that occur between physicians and their patients. Students recognize the need for all health care professionals to act professionally within the boundaries of their scope of practice, or duty of care, and in accordance with the laws and regulations of the state in which they are employed. The importance of the medical record as a legal document chronicling the care a patient receives is introduced as well as the need for obtaining a patient's informed consent. The legal responsibilities of health care professionals in treating victims of abuse, in performing emergency procedures under the Good Samaritan laws, in honoring physicians' directives, and in complying with the Americans with Disabilities Act are discussed. Public duties and the legal release of confidential information from a patient's medical record are covered. Medical assisting students discover that their profession holds legal responsibilities to their physician–employers, the patients, and the health and welfare of the community at large.

PROFICIENCY EVALUATION OUTCOME ASSESSMENT

Students are evaluated for their understanding of performance objectives. Students should be able to understand their role in relation to the medical practice acts that regulate the practice of medicine. In recognizing that their actions carry legal import, students gain a respect for the seriousness of the medical assisting profession and the responsibilities attached to working in an ambulatory care setting and to providing care to patients. Legal concepts often deal with highly controversial societal issues, such as abuse, AIDS, drug screening, and physicians' directives. Students learn about their legal responsibilities in these sensitive areas and are encouraged to explore their own feelings and their role as patient and community educators.

SUPPLEMENTARY RESOURCES

Medical Assisting Videos: Appropriate content is available on Delmar's Medical Assisting Videos, 2nd ed., Tape 2, for the following topics:

Apply Legal Concepts to Practice
Legal Aspects and Confidentiality of Medical Records
Practice Risk Management to Prevent Professional Liability
Perform within Ethical Boundaries

ANSWERS TO TEXT REVIEW QUESTIONS

1. b. implied
2. d. discovery of a surgical instrument inside the patient's body
3. a. spoken statements that damage an individual's reputation
4. b. *respondeat superior*
5. b. reasonable, attentive, diligent care comparable to other physicians of the same specialty in the same or similar community
6. c. direct physicians based on a patient's wishes in life-threatening circumstances
7. a. is a court order requesting data and/or an appearance in court
8. d. duty, derelict, direct cause, damage
9. d. all of the above
10. a. include battery, defamation of character, invasion of privacy

ANSWERS TO TEXT CRITICAL THINKING QUESTIONS

1. Dr. King may officially withdraw from Chris's care in a formal letter to her parents stating that the parents are not following the recommended treatment plan for their 6-year-old son. The legal term for this situation is *noncompliance*.
2. It is quite probable that Audrey's error is malpractice. She used the incorrect solution, which caused damage to the patient's eyes. Much depends on the damage, the way in which the physician and the staff handled the error, and the patient. Following such an error there should be at least a discussion within the staff about correct procedures and how to avoid another error. Audrey could also lose her employment status.
3. Medical assistants are called to a standard of care that dictates they shall perform procedures only within their legal scope of practice and ability. They must never practice medicine or advise a patient. For example, the medical assistant would never agree to take radiographs unless training, education, and any required certification or licensure have been obtained in that field.
4. A consent form should always be obtained when surgery is to be performed. A preprinted consent form is likely to be used—one that has already been approved by the physician, who may also complete a part of the form regarding the surgery to be performed. The form should include all the aspects of informed consent and include a place for the physician's signature.
5. When a medical assistant speaking with a patient over the telephone repeats the patient's name and patients in the reception room hear the name, the patient's right to privacy has been violated. If a patient is to undergo a procedure, such as a sigmoidoscopy, and the physician brings an intern to observe, the patient's right to privacy has been violated unless the patient has given permission for the intern to observe.
6. Federal laws are changing all the time; however, HIV testing cannot be performed without the patient's written consent. The results cannot be shared with anyone without the patient's consent. AIDS is a reportable disease and must be reported to the health department or agency in your state receiving such data. Drug screening may be required for employment; the results are shared only with the patient and the employer.
7. Physicians and medical assistants have a public duty to the community they serve. It is suggested that there is a moral responsibility for health care professionals to protect the health of the community.
8. Good Samaritan laws vary from state to state and are often vague and confusing. They are designed to encourage health professionals to render aid in emergency situations that occur outside the professional office or hospital setting. One must always remember *never* to perform any procedure outside the scope of experience, training, or ability.
9. Three types of abuse are child abuse, domestic violence, and elder abuse. The medical assistant must notify the physician when suspicions of child abuse surface. If the physician concurs, either the physician or the medical assistant must report suspected abuse to the proper authorities. A child can be detained by the physician, if necessary, or police can be notified to do the same.
10. In the case of Lenore McDonell, the results of the physical examination can only be available to an employer once the job has been offered and then only any job restrictions the patient might require can be revealed. According to the ADA, job qualifications and specific standards of employment must be the same for all applicants. Disabled persons cannot be screened using different standards for employment.

ANSWERS TO WORKBOOK EXERCISES AND ACTIVITIES

Vocabulary Builder

1. P.	6. S.	11. T.	16. E.	21. V.
2. F.	7. H.	12. A.	17. Y.	22. N.
3. K.	8. R.	13. I.	18. X.	23. Q.
4. G.	9. B.	14. J.	19. D.	24. L.
5. W.	10. C.	15. O.	20. M.	25. U.

Learning Review

1. A. CM; the physician performs an illegal act by removing narcotics from a locked medicine cabinet and treating patients while under the influence of chemical substances.
    B. CV; the woman is suing for damages for pain and suffering caused to her personally as a result of the insurer's refusal to provide coverage for a requested treatment.
    C. CM; embezzling is a serious criminal offense that carries penalties of incarceration or a fine. Our society does not condone stealing.

2. A. E.   F. I.
    B. E.   G. X; this contract is not valid.
    C. I.   H. E.
    D. E.   I. I.
    E. E.   J. E.

3. A. The office manager should refer Jim Marshall directly to Dr. Winston Lewis to discuss the situation. A physician-patient conference should be scheduled so that both parties can meet to discuss whether the relationship should be continued. If both Winston and Jim feel comfortable in continuing the physician-patient relationship, then a letter confirming the decision made at the conference meeting should be drafted for the patient's medical record and an appointment scheduled. If the parties do not feel comfortable in continuing the relationship, then a letter confirming that decision should be issued as a final confirmation of either the patient's or physician's withdrawal.
    B. Dr. James Whitney can suggest that George Taylor obtain a durable power of attorney for health care decisions so that George can better direct the treatment provided for his father, Lenny Taylor. James can also explain George's option to have his father declared legally incompetent to handle his affairs or direct his health care. James retains the option of reinstating Lenny as a patient under these conditions or the doctor can recommend a gerontologist in the area to George and/or a social services agency that can help George get competent assistance in dealing with his father's situation.
    C. Dr. Mark Woo supplies Rhoda Au's new physician with a copy of her complete medical record under his care. Mark has no obligation to address the patient's feelings regarding his attitude toward his own ethnic heritage. He may reiterate that the treatment plan recommended is medically accurate and competent based on the confirmed diagnosis of the patient's condition.

4. The 4 Ds of negligence are
    (1) Duty of care.
    (2) Dereliction of the duty of care.
    (3) Direct cause of dereliction of the duty of care.
    (4) Damage.

5. Eleven strategies for risk management in an ambulatory care setting that will lessen the potential for litigation are
    (1) Protect patients from falling from an examination table, wheelchair, or stretcher.
    (2) Check for faulty electrocautery and have repairs made by qualified technicians.
    (3) Check patient information by correctly identifying the patient before performing a procedure or administering medication.
    (4) Never leave a patient unattended.
    (5) Be watchful of patients with special needs, such as the elderly, pediatric patients, and patients suffering from dementia or emotional problems.
    (6) Properly label, identify, and handle all specimens.
    (7) Obtain proper consent forms.
    (8) Follow all policies and procedures of the physician-employer.
    (9) Do not misrepresent your qualifications.
    (10) Document fully only facts, and do not alter medical records.
    (11) Admit errors.

6. The four things the patient must know in order to give informed consent are
    (1) The nature of the procedure and how it is to be performed.
    (2) Any possible risks involved as well as expected outcomes of the procedure.
    (3) Any other methods of treatment and those risks.
    (4) Risks if no treatment is given.

7. A. *Battery* is the unprivileged touching of one person by another. *Defamation of character* consists of injury to another person's character, reputation, or name through spoken or written words. *Invasion of privacy* is the unauthorized publicity of confidential personal information or exposure to public view.
    B. *Res ipsa loquitur* means "the thing speaks for itself." *Respondeat superior* means "let the master answer."

8. Student issues will vary according to their own comfort levels and individual preferences. This exercise can be discussed in class as a springboard to understanding the difficult and sensitive nature of living wills and their importance as legal documents in the patient's permanent medical record that must be respected. Students' individual answers must be kept confidential.

Multiple Choice Questions

1. d.   battery
2. d.   ADA
3. a.   Good Samaritan Laws
4. e.   all of the above
5. f.   malpractice

Investigation Activities

Activity 1

Use this investigation activity to help students recognize their legal responsibilities to patients who may be victims of abuse. By exploring the community resources and the kinds of functions volunteers can perform to reach out to these individuals, medical assisting students gain invaluable insight into the sensitivity of abuse situations. They discover how to handle themselves professionally and the importance of honoring their legal responsibilities to abuse victims. Students recognize the importance of providing professional, impartial care while maintaining a sense of compassion and empathy. As a class, a discussion of the medical assistant's role in patient and community education can be explored. Representatives of local organizations or agencies can be invited to class to answer student's questions and provide information about state and federal laws concerning child, elderly, and spousal abuse.

Activity 2

This activity provides students with a hands-on example of how laws and regulations affect their profession and the manner in which medical assistants perform their jobs on a daily basis. The medical practice acts and the need for behavior within the boundaries of the scope of practice set and regulated by individual states is clearly presented and explored by students. Note that the medical practice acts of individual states may or may not clearly identify the medical assistant's scope of practice.

ANSWERS TO WORKBOOK CASE STUDY QUESTIONS

Case 1

Bruce Goldman, CMA, the legal agent of Dr. Ray Reynolds, performs an invasive procedure over the direct protestation of the patient. The medical assistant could have avoided the error by properly identifying the patient to confirm that the physician's order for a venipuncture procedure to obtain a CBC was performed on the correct patient. Instead of taking Wanda Slawson's direction to the elderly woman in examination room 1 literally, Bruce should have checked the name on the patient file against a positive identification of the patient actually waiting in examination room 1.

Case 2

The medical assistant must use keen skills when interpreting nonverbal communication and must factor in the relationship of the mother and daughter in order to ascertain that proper consent for the flu shot has been given. The medical assistant correctly withdraws on a first attempt to administer the shot. Even after the daughter insists on administration, the medical assistant again asks the patient directly. Abigail Johnson gives her implied consent when she rolls up her sleeve and allows the injection to be given without withdrawing physically. The patient's verbal message allows her to reserve a note of reluctance in her consent.

Case 3

The physician, Elizabeth King, commits slander when she makes a malicious and potentially false remark about a patient's character that is overheard by the other patients waiting in the reception area. This error could have been prevented if the physician had not verbalized her feelings regarding the patient's behavior in a public setting. Elizabeth also makes the mistake of revealing private patient information when she says in front of persons not directly related to the patient's care that the patient is pregnant with a third child.

Case 4

Wanda Slawson, CMA, the legal agent of Dr. Angie Esposito, commits the error when she shouts personal information about the patient's condition that is overheard by others who are not direct participants in the patient's care. Even though the patient has waived her right to a certified sign language interpreter as provided under ADA, Wanda does not have the right to communicate with the patient in an inappropriate manner that jeopardizes the patient's right of confidentiality. This error could have been avoided had the medical assistant been more accommodating to and sensitive about the communication needs of the deaf patient.

Case 5

Bruce Goldman, CMA, the legal agent of Dr. James Whitney, reveals confidential information regarding a patient's status to someone not directly related to that patient's care. Also, it is illegal to reveal the results of drug screening tests to individuals or organizations not authorized to receive those results. This error could have been avoided by respecting the patient's legal right to confidentiality.

Chapter 8

Ethical Considerations

OVERVIEW

Medical assisting students are introduced to the concept of medical ethics. In the field of medicine, technological advances are making possible medical treatments and situations that often challenge deeply held societal beliefs and values. Health professionals and patients confront bioethical dilemmas that directly affect patients' lives and involve decisions about quality of life. Medical assisting students explore the field of medical ethics, including ethical issues across the lifespan, and bioethical dilemmas, such as the allocation of scarce medical resources and HIV/AIDS. Students learn that in order to face the ethical challenges raised in the ambulatory care setting, they must examine their own morals and values to strengthen their personal codes of ethics. Moreover, respect for the morals and values of patients and coworkers must be observed by medical assistants. Students learn that the proper maintenance of patient charts is an important way that medical assistants can safeguard the patient's ethical and legal right to confidentiality. Always, students are reminded that medical assistants must practice only within the scope of their training and certification.

PROFICIENCY EVALUATION OUTCOME ASSESSMENT

Students are evaluated for their understanding of performance objectives. Students recognize that a career in the medical assisting profession involves exhibiting high personal standards of ethical behavior and developing an understanding of the medical and bioethical issues common to the ambulatory care setting. Students identify the AAMA Code of Ethics and the AMA Principles of Medical Ethics as guidelines of ethical behavior for medical assistants and physicians. Students learn that the preparation and maintenance of medical records and the patient's right to confidentiality are important ethical responsibilities medical assistants must respect and safeguard. Students are advised of the ethical and professional responsibility to perform only those duties within their training and scope of practice.

SUPPLEMENTARY RESOURCES

Medical Assisting Videos: Appropriate content is available on Delmar's Medical Assisting Videos, 2nd ed., Tape 2, for the following topics:

> Legal Aspects and Confidentiality of Medical Records
> Use Appropriate Guidelines When Releasing Records
> Perform Within Ethical Boundaries

ANSWERS TO TEXT REVIEW QUESTIONS

1. a. what is right and wrong
2. d. ethical issues that deal with life and health care
3. a. is concerned with principles of ethical and moral conduct

4. b. report it to the proper authorities
5. b. it is unethical for the physician not to provide treatment
6. d. all of the above
7. d. all of the above
8. c. patient testimonials
9. d. all of the above
10. e. all of the above

ANSWERS TO TEXT CRITICAL THINKING QUESTIONS

1. Answers will vary, but ethics can be defined as what is right or wrong, a set of morals or values often identified in a code. Bioethics is the same except that it deals with "life" issues and the dilemmas faced by health care professionals and consumers of health care.
2. The AAMA Code of Ethics is designed for medical assistants. The AMA Principles of Medical Ethics is written for physicians. Both describe standards of conduct. Both are developed primarily for patients' benefit. The AAMA Code of Ethics Creed indicates dedication and loyalty to the physician-employer. The AMA Principles specifically call on physicians to expose physicians who are deficient in character or in competence; the AAMA Creed calls on medical assistants to have compassion, courage, and faith.
3. Ethical behavior in this situation suggests that the physician who observes a colleague put a patient in jeopardy while under the influence of alcohol should approach that colleague, identify the problem, and ask the physician to cease. If further risks are placed on patients, the offending physician should be reported to the state's licensing board and the state AMA.
4. It is ethical for a physician to charge expenses related to a medical seminar to the business. The continuing education available in the seminar is considered a necessary and appropriate business expense.
5. The physician has a right to choose whom to serve and may refuse any additional Medicaid patients. The physician or the medical assistant must be prepared to refer patients turned away to another clinic or facility that may be able to take more Medicaid patients. Unless managed care or legislation requires each physician to accept a percentage of Medicaid patients, nothing illegal or unethical has been committed.
6. There should be no discussion between employees regarding a patient's status that is not absolutely necessary. Such a remark from the medical assistant is inappropriate and unprofessional. The receptionist might respond, "That is a comment I prefer not to hear; our responsibility is to care for this person as a patient."
7. Reporting on insurance claims procedures not rendered is illegal and causes the medical assistant to commit fraud. The medical chart must clearly match the services provided to the patient. If the chart is merely incomplete and the services were rendered, the physician should be gently reminded to be more thorough in charting so proper insurance billing can occur.
8. It is ethical and legal for a physician or any health professional to refuse to perform a legal abortion. The federal guidelines indicate that health professionals cannot be asked to perform abortions against their will.
9. It is possible that a medical assistant might lose employment if he or she refuses to assist the physician with artificial insemination. It is not a procedure protected by law, such as abortion. It would be best for a medical assistant with these feelings to seek employment where artificial inseminations are not performed. The medical assistant has a right to refuse, but should understand the possible ramifications of this action.
10. Answers will vary. Encourage students to be accepting of each other's views and sensitive to the personal nature of their sharing.

ANSWERS TO WORKBOOK EXERCISES AND ACTIVITIES

Vocabulary Builder

A. Students will choose ethical issues relevant to *infants or children, adults, and senior adults* from Figure 8–1 of the textbook. Individual solutions to the ethical issues will vary.
B. Six important bioethical issues are
   (1) Allocation of scarce medical resources.
   (2) Abortion and fetal tissue research.
   (3) Genetic engineering/manipulation.
   (4) Dying and death.
   (5) HIV and AIDS.
   (6) Artificial insemination/surrogacy.
C. A *surrogate* is someone who substitutes for another. In medicine, *surrogacy* refers to the male's donation of sperm for artificial insemination of a female or to the use of a woman's eggs and womb to carry a child for another woman. Surrogacy challenges the traditional roles of pregnancy and motherhood in our society and the importance of

the biological parents in the raising of children. The AMA is not supportive of surrogacy as a viable alternative to parenthood.

D.   *Genetic engineering* is the science of identifying genes that predispose individuals to certain illnesses and diseases and manipulating or altering those genes to prevent or lessen the disease or illness. A medical benefit is the prevention or cure of disease and the prolonging of the lifespan. A danger is the risk of "playing God" in manipulating genes before implantation of a fetus in the womb through in vitro fertilization. Students will identify their personal opinions regarding the risks versus the benefits of genetic engineering.

Learning Review

1. A. 2
   B. 4
   C. 3
   D. 3
   E. 1
   F. 5
   G. 1
   H. 2
   I. 4
   J. 1

2. A. Ethical; the physician-employers of the group practice are encouraging participation in activities contributing to an improved community.
   B. Ethical; the physician is involved in the study, application, and advancement of scientific knowledge.
   C. Unethical; the physician is required by law to report suspected abuse of children immediately to the appropriate authorities. The rule of physician-patient confidentiality does not apply to situations of suspected abuse.
   D. Ethical; once a physician has formally withdrawn from providing care to a patient, that physician is under no legal or ethical obligation, except in emergency situations, to resume care of that patient.
   E. Unethical; the physician must respect the patient's right to confidentiality and report the laboratory results only to the patient herself and not to the patient's husband.
   F. Ethical; the physician provides competent medical service with compassion and a respect for human dignity.
   G. Ethical; Dr. Winston Lewis refuses to refer patients to a physician-specialist who practices unethical behavior by sending patients to a laboratory in which he has a financial stake.

3. The correct responses are B, C, D, and F.

4. A. *Public domain* means "information over which the individual right of ownership does not apply."
   B. Student answers will vary. Suitable examples are
   Birth: On 1/1/97, Jane Jones gave birth to a 7 lb. 5 oz. baby boy, John Jones Jr., at Memorial Hospital; parents and baby are doing fine.
   Death: On 1/1/97, John Jones died at Memorial Hospital from complications after a long bout with liver disease; he is survived by his wife, Jane Jones. Funeral arrangements will be announced shortly.
   Accident: Jane Jones, a local physician, suffered severe wounds when her car skidded off an icy highway last night. She remains at Memorial Hospital in critical condition.
   Police Record: John Jones was taken into custody by police last night after he was treated and released from Memorial Hospital for gunshot wounds sustained when he held up a local convenience store 2 weeks ago.

5. Three instances where health professionals are allowed or required by law to reveal confidential patient information are when
   (1) A patient threatens another person and there is reason to believe that the threat may be carried out.
   (2) A reportable injury or illness is sustained, such as knife and gunshot wounds, wounds inflicted by suspected abusers, and communicable diseases (AIDS, influenza, and sexually transmitted diseases).
   (3) Information that may have been subpoenaed for testimony in a court of law.

6. Ethical practices are noted in choices A, C, and D.

Multiple Choice Questions

1. c. Oregon
2. a. a breach of confidentiality
3. d. a and b only
4. c. abortion
5. f. all but a

Investigation Activity

By answering the multiple choice questions as honestly as possible, students are encouraged to begin an exploration of the highly charged emotions and issues involved in bioethical dilemmas. The exercise helps students identify their own positions on these issues and identify points of view that others may hold on individual subjects of concern and/or controversy. The students learn that it is often difficult to remain neutral about bioethical dilemmas. However, they also learn that it is essential for impartial, nonjudgmental, and professional behavior to be the hallmarks of the medical assistant in the ambulatory care setting. Students learn to achieve a balance between respecting and strengthening their own personal codes of morals and values and also respecting the personal ethical codes of their patients and coworkers.

   Instructors are encouraged to use the multiple choice questions as a springboard for class discussion of sensitive bioethical dilemmas and appropriate behaviors for medical assistants in medical settings in various situations.

Role-playing: Role-playing exercises can be performed where one student takes the role of the medical assistant and another of the patient or coworker as they explore the differing points of view raised by bioethical issues and the effects these issues have on the treatment patients request and receive. Students recognize experientially the ethical responsibilities that go hand in hand with a career in the medical assisting profession.

ANSWERS TO WORKBOOK CASE STUDY QUESTIONS

1. The bioethical dilemma that exists in Lourdes's situation is the decision to become pregnant after diagnosis of and treatment for breast cancer. The students' personal opinions on the ethical nature of the patient's decision to become pregnant will vary.

2. Society advocates a two-parent household with married, heterosexual parents. As the patient is a single woman, the issue of whether she should or will marry her boyfriend before becoming a mother is a sensitive one. Our society reveres motherhood and the patient's maternal feelings have strong roots in societal expectations for women to bear children. The health care team is likely to be sympathetic to the patient's desires to become pregnant, as the societal pull toward motherhood, is a great one. Although the health care team will consider Lourdes's feelings with empathy, they will focus proper concern and consideration for the medical necessity of protecting the health of both mother and baby. The issue of whether the patient's decision is an ethical one—whether it is right for the patient to potentially endanger her own health or to have a child she may not live to raise to adulthood—is an issue the health care team must face in regard to both their personal and medical codes of ethics.

3. Elizabeth will consider the specifics of Lourdes's prognosis and balance this against what is currently known about pregnancy after breast cancer to render a medically responsible opinion about the patient's desire to become pregnant. The physician may advise the patient to seek counseling from a qualified psychoanalyst to be sure that the decision to become pregnant and all of its ramifications are properly explored and considered. The physician will assemble a team of health care specialists, including the patient's surgeon and radiologist, to develop a treatment plan. The physician may investigate to see whether studies are being conducted regarding pregnancy after breast cancer in which the patient may participate or from which the patient might benefit. The physician will explore the patient's support system, particularly the commitment of the patient's boyfriend to the relationship, to ensure that should the patient become pregnant, both the patient and child will have financial and emotional support from her partner, family, friends, and coworkers, in the event of a recurrence of the cancer.

4. The medical assistant can contribute by expressing empathy and concern for the patient's situation. The medical assistant can also help the patient and physician by assisting in research related to the bioethical issue of pregnancy after breast cancer to gather information on this subject and identify potential resources of interest and support.

   Health care professionals will work with the patient as a team devoted to arriving at a prudent and responsible course of treatment that seriously considers the patient's desire to become pregnant.

Chapter

9

Emergency Procedures and First Aid

OVERVIEW

Medical assisting students are introduced to various types of potential emergency situations. Even though medical assistants may not encounter every emergency in an ambulatory setting, students learn that, as responsible health care professionals, medical assistants must develop a functional base of knowledge about emergency situations. In obtaining this knowledge, medical assistants possess the information necessary to triage and manage emergency situations with confidence, speed, accuracy, and understanding until the physician takes over care or emergency medical service personnel arrive. All students are reminded that health care professionals must provide emergency care only within the scope of their training and knowledge. Health care professionals will provide emergency care under the direction of the physician-employer as outlined in the facility's emergency policies and procedures manual. Students are encouraged to enroll in Red Cross or American Heart Association first aid and CPR programs and to update their skills in refresher courses every two years.

PROFICIENCY EVALUATION OUTCOME ASSESSMENT

Students are evaluated for their understanding of proficiency objectives. Students should be able to identify strategies for recognizing emergency situations. Students learn to triage emergency situations both in person and over the telephone. Students recognize the legal and health considerations of providing emergency care, including the need to follow the guidelines of standard precautions in emergency situations. Students also recognize the necessity of providing emergency care only within the scope of their training and knowledge. Students gain a respect for the serious nature of emergency situations and the need to provide competent professional care to emergency victims with the speed, accuracy, and efficiency that will safeguard health and potentially save lives. Students explore their own feelings and responses to potential emergency victims and situations. Students can identify broad categories of emergencies, including shock; wounds; burns; musculoskeletal injuries; heat- and cold-related illnesses; poisons; sudden illnesses, such as syncope, seizures, diabetic coma or insulin shock, and hemorrhage; CVA; and heart attack. Students also describe proper emergency concerns, care, and treatment for each.

Students can identify and name steps for performing numerous emergency procedures:

Procedure 9-1   Control of bleeding
Procedure 9-2   Applying an Arm Splint
Procedure 9-3   Heimlich Maneuver for a Conscious Adult
Procedure 9-4   Heimlich Maneuver for an Unconscious Adult or Child
Procedure 9-5   Heimlich Maneuver for a Conscious Child
Procedure 9-6   Back Blows and Chest Thrusts for a Conscious Infant Who Is Choking
Procedure 9-7   Back Blows and Chest Thrusts for an Unconscious Infant
Procedure 9-8   Rescue Breathing for Adults
Procedure 9-9   Rescue Breathing for Children
Procedure 9-10   Rescue Breathing for Infants
Procedure 9-11   CPR for Adults
Procedure 9-12   CPR for Children
Procedure 9-13   CPR for Infants

SUPPLEMENTARY RESOURCES

Medical Assisting Videos: Appropriate content is available on Delmar's Medical Assisting Videos, 2nd ed., for the following topics:

Tape 2: Triage Skills
Tape 5: Standard Precautions
Infections in the Office
Tape 10: Recognize Emergencies
Workplace Hazards and Material Safety Data Sheets
Emergency Use of Oxygen in the Office
Introduction to Airway Obstruction
Abdominal Thrust (Heimlich maneuver)
Obstructed Airway in an Unconscious Patient
Diabetic Emergencies
Bandaging

ANSWERS TO TEXT REVIEW QUESTIONS

1. c. require that all individuals providing assistance act within the scope of their knowledge and training
2. b. affect only the top layer of skin
3. b. compound fracture
4. c. tilt the patient's head forward
5. d. myocardial infarction

ANSWERS TO TEXT CRITICAL THINKING QUESTIONS

1. Most Good Samaritan laws provide some legal protection to those who provide emergency care to ill or injured persons. However, when medical assistants or other individuals give care during an emergency, they must act as reasonable and prudent individuals and provide care only within the scope of their abilities. A primary principle of first aid is to prevent further injury.

   While Good Samaritan laws give some measure of protection against being sued for giving emergency aid, they generally protect off-duty health care professionals. Also, conditions of the law vary from state to state. As part of establishing emergency care guidelines, every ambulatory care setting should understand the explicit and implicit intent of the Good Samaritan law in its state.

2. The ABCs are Airway, Breathing, and Circulation. To assess whether the patient is breathing and to determine if there is an open airway, watch the patient and notice whether the chest rises and falls with breathing. Listen for air entering and leaving the nose and mouth and feel for moving air. If the individual is not breathing, first open the airway either by tilting the head and lifting the chin or by the jaw-thrust maneuver, which involves placing both thumbs on the patient's cheekbones and index and middle fingers on both sides of the lower jaw.

   If the patient still does not breathe after the airway has been opened, rescue breathing must be performed.

   To assess circulation, check for the presence of a pulse on the side of the neck. If no pulse is present, the patient is in cardiac arrest and must be given cardiopulmonary resuscitation (CPR).

3. Every health care facility should have a crash tray or cart, with a carefully controlled inventory of supplies and equipment. These first aid supplies should be kept in an accessible place, and the inventory should be routinely monitored to ensure that all supplies are replaced and all medications are up to date.

   Whether a tray or cart is used by the facility, supplies should be customized to the facility and the type of emergencies frequently encountered. Only physicians can order medications or treatment.

   Common supplies found on most trays and/or carts include the following:

General Supplies
- Adhesive tape
- Alcohol wipes
- Bandage scissors
- Bandage strips
- Blood pressure cuff
- Catheter tip-syringe

- Defibrillator
- Gloves
- Hot/cold packs
- IV tubing
- Needles and syringes
  for injection

- Orange juice for diabetics
- Personal protective equipment (PPE)
- Spirits of ammonia
- Sterile dressings
- Stethoscope
- Tourniquet

Emergency Medications
- Activated charcoal
- Aramine

- Glucogen
- Insulin

- Sodium bicarbonate
- Spirits of ammonia

- Atropine
- Dextrose
- Diphenhydramine
- Epinephrine
- 50% instant glucose

- Lidocaine
- Nitroglycerin tablets
- Phenobarbital and diazepam (controlled substances; must be kept in a locked cabinet)

- Sterile water
- Syrup of ipecac
- Verapamil
- Xylocaine and Marcaine

Respiratory Supplies
- Airways of all sizes for nasal and oral use
- Ambu bag
- Oxygen mask and tubing
- Oxygen tank

4. When a severe injury occurs, shock is likely to develop. Shock is basically a condition in which the circulatory system is not providing enough blood to all parts of the body, causing the body's organs to fail to function properly.

 There are eight major types of shock: respiratory, neurogenic, cardiogenic, hemorrhagic, anaphylactic, metabolic, psychogenic, and septic. Shock is always life-threatening. The body's attempt to compensate for a massive injury or illness, especially those involving severe bleeding, often leads to other problems.

 During shock:
 - The heart becomes unable to pump blood properly.
 - Consequently, the body does not get enough oxygen, which is carried by the blood.
 - The body tries to compensate by sending blood to critical organs and reducing the flow of blood to arms, legs, and skin.

5. Bandages, which are nonsterile, are placed over dressings. They hold the dressing in place and are made to conform to the area to be covered. Sometimes the dressing and bandage are combined, as in a commercial bandage such as Band-Aid brand. Roller bandages, such as those made of elastic, can be placed over a dressing and used to control bleeding or swelling.

 Kling gauze, a type of gauze that stretches and clings as it is applied, and roller bandages, long strips of soft material wound on itself, are other types of bandage materials.

 Bandages and their applications can take many shapes and forms, depending on the injury and the injury site.
 1. Open or closed spiral bandages are useful for injuries to the arms or legs.
 2. A figure-of-eight bandage will hold a dressing on a wound on the hand or wrist, knee, or ankle.
 3. Fingers, toes, arms, and legs can be bandaged using a tubular gauze bandage.
 4. Commercial arm slings are used to support injured or fractured arms.

6. First-degree burns are superficial burns that involve only the top layer of skin. Although the area of the burn is often painful, first-degree burns usually heal in a week or so with no permanent scarring.

 In a second-degree burn, the skin is red and blisters are present. The healing process is slower and some scarring may occur. Second-degree burns affect the top layers of the skin.

 Third-degree burns are the most serious, affecting or destroying all layers of skin, plus the fat, muscles, bones, and nerves under the skin. These burns look charred or brown. There may be great pain or, if nerve endings are destroyed, the burn may be painless. Victims of third-degree burns must receive immediate medical attention both for the burn and for shock.

7. Poisons can enter the body in four ways:
 1. Ingestion. Ingested poisons enter the body by swallowing. Swallowed poisons include medications, plant material, household chemicals, contaminated foods, and drugs.
 2. Inhalation. Poisons are inhaled into the body in poorly ventilated areas. Such poisons include cleaning fluids, paints, chemical cleaners, and carbon monoxide.
 3. Absorption. Poisons absorbed through the skin include plant materials such as poison oak and ivy, lawn care products such as chemical pesticides, and other chemical powders or liquids.
 4. Injection. Drug abuse is the most common cause of injected poisonings. Stinging insects inject poisons into the body that can be extremely dangerous and lead to anaphylactic shock in allergic individuals.

8. *Hemorrhage* is a synonym for *severe bleeding*. The different sources of the bleeding determine the seriousness of the hemorrhage.

 External bleeding includes capillary, venous, and arterial bleeding. Capillary bleeding, often from cuts and scratches, usually clots without first aid measures. Bleeding from a vein, which is characterized by dark red blood that flows steadily, needs to be controlled quickly to prevent loss of excessive amounts of blood. Bleeding from an artery produces bright red blood that spurts from the wound; this is the most serious type of bleeding and occurs when an artery is punctured or severed. Like venous bleeding, arterial bleeding requires immediate emergency care because serious loss of blood and profound irreversible shock can quickly ensue. Epistaxis, or nosebleed, may be the result of breathing dry air for a long period of time, may result from injury or blowing the nose too hard, may be caused by high altitude, or may be caused by hypertension (high blood pressure) and can result in hemorrhage.

 Internal bleeding may be minor or serious, depending on the cause of the injury. A contusion, or bruise, may result in minor internal bleeding. A sharp blow may induce severe internal bleeding. Because there is no blood flow, it is important to recognize other symptoms of internal bleeding. Symptoms are similar to those of shock and include a rapid, weak pulse; shallow breathing; cold, clammy skin; dilated pupils; dizziness; faintness; thirst; restlessness; and a feeling of anxiety. There may be pain, tenderness, or swelling at the injury site. If internal bleeding is suspected, ask another staff member to call EMS; stay with the patient until they arrive, and take measures to prevent shock. Monitor vital signs.

9. Breathing, or respiratory emergencies, occur for a variety of reasons, including choking, shock, allergies, and other illnesses or injuries such as drowning and electrical shock. When an individual stops breathing, artificial or rescue breathing must be performed quickly—without a constant supply of oxygen, brain damage or death will occur.

   When the breathing problem is accompanied by cardiac arrest, the rescue breathing must be accompanied by chest compressions. This is known as CPR.

   A common cause of breathing difficulty results from choking. If an individual signals distress from choking, assist the patient in coughing up the object. If the patient cannot cough up the object and the breathing airway is becoming completely blocked, act immediately. It is clear that the airway is becoming blocked when the patient cannot cough or speak and the patient uses the universal sign for choking.

   Have someone call an ambulance while you perform abdominal thrusts, known as the Heimlich maneuver. Patients can be taught to give themselves abdominal thrusts if they are alone and choking.

10. It is essential that every medical assistant take first aid and CPR courses and frequent refresher courses. Although many emergencies may never be seen in the ambulatory care setting, medical assistants should be familiar with various emergency situations and know how to give or obtain aid for the patient in distress.

ANSWERS TO WORKBOOK EXERCISES, EMERGENCY PROCEDURES, AND ACTIVITY

Vocabulary Builder

A.
A. EP	G. EP	M. EC
B. EP	H. EC	N. ES
C. EC	I. ES	O. EC
D. EC	J. EC	P. EQ
E. EC	K. EP	Q. EC
F. EQ	L. EP	R. EP

B.
1. O	7. N	13. A
2. F	8. G	14. D
3. Q	9. I	15. L
4. E	10. P	16. B
5. H	11. J	17. R
6. M	12. C	18. K

Learning Review

1. Five things a medical assistant must do to triage, or assess, a patient's situation are the following.
   (1) If the patient is conscious, ask for personal identification and identification of next of kin.
   (2) Try to obtain information about symptoms being experienced.
   (3) Check for a universal emergency medical identification symbol and accompanying identification card describing any serious or life-threatening health problems of the patient.
   (4) Quickly observe the patient's general appearance, including skin color and dilation of pupils.
   (5) Check pulse.
2. A. Urgency of condition: 2. The patient suffers an open wound to the leg caused by gunshot and is experiencing symptoms of hemorrhagic shock. Some injury exists to the right arm, possibly a closed fracture and/or wound. The health care team will control the patient's bleeding and address the shock symptoms by assisting the patient to lie down; checking to make sure the patient can breathe easily (loosen tight clothing); using blankets, if necessary, to maintain a normal body temperature for the patient; reassuring the patient; checking vital signs; and not offering the patient anything by mouth. Then the health care team will assess the nature of the injury to the right arm. If a fracture is suspected, a splint will be applied to immobilize the site of injury, reduce pain, and prevent further injury.
   B. Urgency of condition: 1. The debilitating chest pains the elderly man is experiencing could likely indicate heart attack, requiring immediate medical attention. The health care team will perform an immediate electrocardiogram (ECG) to reveal the electrical activity of the heart and determine if the patient is suffering a myocardial infarction. If heart function appears within normal levels for this patient, then the health care team will address other possible diagnoses such as the hiatal hernia, which can produce pain similar to the pain of heart attack.
   C. Urgency of condition: 4. The young woman is likely suffering a sprain to the right knee and/or ankle. She also has minor abrasions to the right hand and knee. The health care team will take an X-ray to determine that no

fracture exists. If the diagnosis of a sprain is confirmed, the RICE procedure will be applied. The abrasions will be cleaned and an antiseptic ointment applied, followed by a dressing and bandage. The sprain will be wrapped in a compression bandage and the patient will be instructed to rest, apply cold compresses, and elevate the leg whenever possible for the first 24 to 48 hours. The physician may want the patient to be measured for crutches and taught how to use the appropriate gait.

D. Urgency of condition: 5. The man suffers a minor injury created by the lodging of a foreign body in the ear. The health care team will remove the foreign body and examine the ear for any injuries that require further treatment. The ear may be irrigated following removal of the foreign object to ensure that no small particles remain.

E. Urgency of condition: 3. The young woman suffers a serious eye injury caused by a blow to the eye and contact of the eye with a sharp foreign object. The health care team will examine the eye for the presence of any fragments that may have penetrated and assess potential damage to the cornea before beginning emergency treatment.

3. Five infection control measures that can greatly reduce the risk of transmitting infectious disease when providing emergency care are
   (1) Always wash hands thoroughly before (if possible) and after every procedure.
   (2) Use protective clothing and other protective equipment during the procedure.
   (3) During the procedure, avoid contact with blood and body fluids, if possible.
   (4) Do not touch nose, mouth, or eyes with gloved hands.
   (5) Carefully handle and safely dispose of soiled gloves and other objects.

4. A. Lidocaine is a local anesthetic and an antiarrhythmic agent administered intravenously during an episode of cardiac arrhythmia.
   B. Verapamil is a calcium channel blocker (antianginal, antiarrhythmic) used in the treatment of angina pectoris, hypertension, and certain cardiac arrhythmias.
   C. Atropine is an antispasmodic and cholinergic blocking agent prescribed to treat certain ophthalmologic disorders such as corneal ulcer and uveitis (inflammation of the iris), to treat certain arrhythmias, to counteract the effects of certain poisons, and occasionally in the treatment of urinary tract infections.
   D. Insulin is a hormone naturally secreted by the islets of Langerhans; it is administered to patients with diabetes mellitus to normalize insulin levels in the body.
   E. Nitroglycerin is a coronary artery vasodilator used to prevent and treat symptoms of angina pectoris.
   F. Marcaine is an epidural anesthetic administered by injection, which is used during or after surgery; for control of chronic, unremitting cancer pain; and for pain relief during childbirth.
   G. Diphenhydramine is an antihistamine used to treat allergic disorders; it is given by injection to treat anaphylactic shock.
   H. Diazepam is an anticonvulsant and muscle relaxant used for emergency treatment of epileptic seizures and prescribed to treat anxiety and insomnia.

5. A. Cardiogenic.
   B. Septic.
   C. Psychogenic.
   D. Anaphylactic.
   E. Respiratory.
   F. Metabolic.
   G. Neurogenic.
   H. Hemorrhagic.

6. Rest, Ice, Compression, and Elevation.

7. A. 1. B   4. E
      2. D   5. C
      3. A

   B. *Incision.* Incisions may require sutures. The wound must be cleaned with antiseptic soap, thoroughly rinsed, and a dressing applied.
      Puncture. The patient should be assessed for internal bleeding. Deep wounds carry the risk of infection; the patient should be advised to watch for signs of infection, such as pain, swelling, redness, throbbing, and warmth.
      Laceration. If there is no severe bleeding, which is itself a cleansing mechanism, these wounds may need to be soaked to remove debris. Severe bleeding must be controlled immediately. Lacerations with severe bleeding are likely to require suturing.
      Avulsion. After bleeding is controlled, the wound is cleaned. If there is a skin flap, reposition it. Apply a dressing, then bandage as necessary. If pieces of the body have been severed, save the body part, keep it moist, and transport it with the patient.
      Abrasion. Abrasions can be serious if they cover a large area of the body and are painful owing to the involvement of nerve endings. Administer first aid by cleaning the area carefully with antiseptic soap and water, apply an antiseptic ointment if prescribed by the physician, and cover with a dressing.

8. Three sources other than heat that can cause burns are

(1) Chemical burns. To stop the burning process, the chemical must be removed. Have someone call EMS while flushing the eyes or skin with cool water. Remove any clothing contaminated by the chemicals unless the clothing has adhered to body tissues. If clothing clings to the skin, it can be cut with scissors.

(2) Electrical burns. Never go near a patient injured by electricity unless the power has been shut off. Victims may be suffering from two burns: one where the power entered the body and one where it exited. Often burns are minor. The possibility of shock, breathing difficulties, and other serious conditions are greater. CPR is often required.

(3) Solar radiation. Sunburn is generally minor. However, severe sunburns can be covered with cool, wet clean sheets to relieve pain and lessen exposure to microorganisms. Advise patients to use sunscreen and avoid the sun between 10 a.m. and 2 p.m. Carefully observe the patient for signs and symptoms of heat exhaustion.

9. Five assessment techniques to determine the seriousness of musculoskeletal injuries are:
   (1) Note the extent of bruising and swelling.
   (2) Pain is a signal of injury.
   (3) There may be noticeable deformity to the bone or joint.
   (4) Use of the injured area is limited.
   (5) Talk to the patient to determine the cause of the injury and the sound and sensation experienced at the time of injury.

10. A. *Frostbite.* Individuals with frostbite require immediate medical attention. Warm the area of injury by wrapping clothing or blankets around the affected body part. Take care with the frozen area. Transport the patient as soon as possible to emergency care facilities where the frozen tissue can be rewarmed properly, preventing further tissue damage.

   B. *Allergic reaction.* Severe reactions can induce anaphylactic shock; patients should seek immediate emergency treatment. Epinephrine is used, and subsequently, antihistamines are also prescribed. Attempt to allay patient apprehension and monitor vital signs while waiting for EMS personnel to arrive.

   C. *Heat exhaustion.* The individual should be removed from the heat immediately. Apply cool, wet towels and have the patient slowly drink cool water. The physician will advise the patient not to resume his or her activity in the heat.

   D. *Faintness.* As a preventive measure, have the person lie down or sit down with the head level with the knees. Spirits of ammonia may be used to revive a person who faints; hold the crushed ampule of ammonia at least 6 inches away from the patient's nose and eyes, moving it back and forth to avoid irritating the eyes and mucous membranes. If a patient faints, lower him or her to a flat surface, loosen any clothing, and check the breathing and any life-threatening emergencies. Elevate the legs if there is no back or head injury.

   E. *Insulin shock or reaction.* If the patient is conscious, give sugar or any food containing sugar, such as fruit juice, candy, or cookies. This is a serious emergency requiring immediate EMS assistance and transport of the patient to a hospital. The physician will prescribe glucose before transport.

   F. *CVA.* If a patient is suspected of cerebral vascular accident or stroke, call EMS, loosen tight clothing, check vital signs, and keep the patient comfortable. Immediate emergency care is critical. For ischemic stroke, caused by a clot that blocks blood flow, rapid transport to the hospital is essential; a clot-dissolving drug must be given within 3 hours of onset of symptoms.

   G. *Seizure.* Do not restrain patient or force anything between the teeth. Protect patient from injury, cushion patient's head, and roll the patient to the side if any fluid is in the mouth. After the seizure subsides, calm and comfort the patient. Call EMS if there are repeated seizures during the same time frame or if the patient is diabetic, pregnant, injured, or does not regain consciousness after the incident.

   H. *Internal bleeding.* Symptoms are similar to shock. Ask another person to call EMS; until they arrive, stay with the patient and take measures to prevent shock. Monitor vital signs.

11. A. Inhalation.
    B. Injection.
    C. Absorption.
    D. Ingestion.
    E. Absorption.
    F. Inhalation.

12. Students' answers for sections A and B will vary according to their own comfort levels.

Emergency Procedures

Procedure 1

1. The health care team will wash hands, put on gloves and a gown, and apply eye and mask protection. Blood-contaminated patient clothing will be removed.
2. Control bleeding (Procedure 9-1).
   A. (1) Elevate the arm above heart level.
      (2) Press adjacent artery against bone.

B. The health care team will use a constriction band. The band is applied tightly enough to stem the rapid loss of blood but loosely enough to allow a small amount of blood to flow. This allows a blood supply to the remainder of the extremity, unlike a tourniquet, which cuts off all blood flow. A pulse should be felt distally to the constriction band. Tourniquet application as a last resort to control hemorrhaging from an extremity often resulted in the death of the limb, necessitating amputation.

3. A. Apply an arm splint (Procedure 9-2). As the patient is prone to fractures, a splint is applied in case a fracture has occurred. The procedure is necessary to immobilize the arm, reduce pain, and prevent further injury until an X-ray can be obtained. A thin piece of rigid board or cardboard and a roller gauze bandage are required.

B. After splinting, check circulation (note color and temperature of skin, check pulse) to ascertain that the splint is not too tightly applied.

4. The health care team will properly dispose of all waste in biohazard containers, cleanse and disinfect the work area, correctly remove and dispose of PPE, and wash hands.

5. Documentation will include the date, the extent and nature of the patient's emergency condition, the emergency procedures performed, any medications prescribed by the physician with dosage instructions, and a protocol for follow-up care. Documentation is initiated by the physician or emergency care provider.

Procedure 2

1. The medical assistant initiates rescue breathing for infants (Procedure 9-10).
   (1) Wash hands, if possible.
   (2) Tilt back the patient's head without hyperextending.
   (3) The medical assistant seals her lips tightly around the infant's nose and mouth.
   (4) Two slow breaths are given. Ellen breathes into the infant until its chest rises.

2. The medical assistant will give one slow breath every 3 seconds for 1 minute. She will recheck the infant's pulse every minute. This sequence of rescue breathing will be followed as long as a pulse is present but the infant is not breathing.

3. A. Dr. Elizabeth King initiates back blows and thrusts for a conscious infant who is choking (Procedure 9-6).
   B. (1) With the infant placed face down on Dr. King's forearm, she gives five back blows between the infant's shoulder blades with the heel of her hand.
   (2) Dr. King positions the infant face up on her forearm.
   (3) Five chest thrusts are given on about the center of the breastbone.
   (4) The infant's mouth is swept for the object.
   C. Dr. King will continue this procedure until the infant begins to breathe on its own.

4. A. (1) Call emergency medical services (EMS).
   (2) Take the mother to a private area and attend to her needs. The medical assistant will watch for signs of faintness or psychogenic shock and will attempt to reassure and calm the mother.
   B. Dr. King administers back blows and thrusts for an unconscious infant (Procedure 9-7). The procedure will be repeated until breaths go in and as long as the infant retains a pulse. If the infant loses pulse, Dr. King will begin CPR for infants (Procedure 9-13).

5. The physician will give the infant a thorough physical examination and carefully assess that no further injury has been caused by the emergency. The physician will examine the mother to determine any emergency stress-related condition and to provide counseling and advice regarding unexpected choking hazards for infants. The health care team will cleanse the work area in compliance with standard precautions, properly dispose of waste materials, correctly remove PPE, and wash hands.

6. A. Documentation will include the date; the extent and nature of the infant's emergency condition, the emergency procedures performed and the total length of time (from recognition of the emergency to successful resolution, including the amount of time the infant remained unconscious), results of the physical examination, and instructions for follow-up care. Documentation is initiated by the physician or emergency care provider.
   B. Documentation will include the date, a cross-reference to the infant's chart for information regarding the infant's emergency condition, the mother's physical symptoms of stress and any procedures performed or medications (including dosages) prescribed, and any instructions for follow-up care. Documentation is initiated by the physician or emergency care provider.

Procedure 3

1. Bruce asks someone to call EMS.

2. Bruce initiates rescue breathing for adults (Procedure 9-8). He follows these steps:
   (1) Tilt back patient's head and lift chin. The medical assistant keeps the airway open, pinches the nose, seals his mouth over the patient's, and gives two slow breaths into the patient's lungs.
   (2) The medical assistant checks for pulse on the carotid artery for 15 seconds.

3. A. The medical assistant initiates cardiopulmonary resuscitation (CPR) for adults (Procedure 9-11).
   B. The medical assistant positions his shoulders over his hands and compresses the patient's chest 15 times after locating the area on the patient's abdomen 2 inches below the xiphoid process and above the umbilicus.
   C. Two slow breaths are given, holding the nose.

D. The medical assistant will perform three more sets of 15 compressions and two breaths before checking the patient's pulse.

4. The medical assistant will not discontinue CPR unless or until
   (1) Another trained person can take over.
   (2) EMS arrives and takes over care of the patient.
   (3) He is too physically exhausted and is not able to continue.
   (4) The environment becomes unsafe for any reason.

5. A. The medical assistant will clean and disinfect the area of the emergency. He will gather any contaminated materials in a sturdy plastic bag and dispose of it in the senior center's biohazard waste container. He will remove any of his own clothing that may have been contaminated by body fluids from the emergency patient. He will wash his hands and then his face with antiseptic soap. As soon as possible, he should brush his teeth and gargle with antiseptic mouthwash.
   B. Supplies and equipment include gloves, resuscitation mouthpiece, and biohazard waste container.

Multiple Choice Questions

1. b. psychogenic	4. c. colles	
2. b. electrical	5. b. heart attack	
3. b. full thickness		

Investigation Activity

Educating patients about methods for proper and effective emergency preparedness is one way medical assistants can act to safeguard patient health and prevent possible injuries and illnesses. New and established patients can be given emergency information sheets to be completed for their families. Medical assistants can take an active role in explaining the importance of emergency data in responding to and treating emergency situations with speed, accuracy, and efficiency. Class discussion regarding information supplied by emergency resources such as the poison control center and local hospital emergency room can give patients perspective on the nature and scope of potential emergency situations. Students also learn strategies for prevention and for emergency care. Materials can be assessed for (1) methods to improve safety conditions in the home or workplace, (2) strategies for patient education, and (3) increasing the medical assistant's own knowledge of emergency situations and methods for obtaining the best source of emergency assistance and treatment.

ANSWERS TO WORKBOOK CASE STUDY QUESTIONS

1. The medical assistant establishes the identity of the caller and of the emergency victim. She determines the location of the emergency victims. She gains a description of the nature of the emergency. Once the existence of a true emergency is confirmed, the medical assistant alerts someone else in the office to call EMS and direct them to the victim's residence. The medical assistant speaks to the patient in a calming, reassuring, and professional tone.

2. The medical assistant will ask if the child is touching a source of electrical power and whether the power is turned on. If no power source is functioning, the mother can initiate emergency treatment. The medical assistant will ask questions to determine whether the patient is breathing, has a pulse, and/or exhibits symptoms of shock. If the child has no pulse or breathing, the medical assistant will ask the mother if she is qualified to perform CPR or if anyone is immediately accessible who may be qualified. CPR should be initiated by a qualified individual. If there is a pulse but no breathing, rescue breathing should be initiated; instructions can be given to the mother over the telephone. If the child is breathing and has a pulse, then the symptoms of shock should be identified and emergency procedures initiated—making sure the child can breathe as easily as possible (loosening clothing, etc.), elevating the child's legs, maintaining a normal body temperature, and reassuring the child. The breathing difficulty is the primary emergency condition of the child; however, if the child is breathing and has a pulse the mother should observe for the extent and severity of burns.

3. The medical assistant will give EMS personnel the name of the primary care physician and the telephone number of the practice. She will determine the name of the hospital or emergency facility the child is transported to. The medical assistant will stay on the line until it is determined that the emergency situation is under control and as long as the need remains for a person to comfort and attend to the needs of the mother. The medical assistant will document the emergency in the child's chart, cross-referenced to the mother's chart, and will submit the documentation to the physician for review. The physician will follow up with the emergency care providers and the O'Keefe family to determine the outcome of the emergency and to participate with other members of the health care team in establishing any necessary treatment plan. Copies of reports from the emergency care facility will be requested for the medical record.

10 Creating the Facility Environment

OVERVIEW

Medical assisting students are encouraged to analyze the physical environment of the ambulatory care setting to determine its effectiveness and efficient use of space as well as its user-friendliness for patients. Students become consciously aware of the patient's subliminal but forceful emotional response to the physical environment of the medical facility. A professional, welcoming attitude from the medical receptionist and medical assistant reinforces the positive impact of a comfortingly designed reception area. The patient's positive reaction to the medical assistant and the physical environment of the medical facility will enhance the patient's positive experience of treatment and strengthen the relationship between the patient and the health care team. Students learn the importance of compliance with the Americans with Disabilities Act (ADA) to create equal access to health care for all patients.

PROFICIENCY EVALUATION OUTCOME ASSESSMENT

Students are evaluated for their understanding of performance objectives. Students should recognize the importance of the medical receptionist and medical assistant as the first and last contacts patients have with the medical practice and the health care team. A positive, helpful attitude will enhance the patient's perceptions of the physician and the quality of treatment received from the health care team. Students should be able to describe a welcoming reception area and outline strategies for making all aspects of the physical environment less intimidating to patients. Students also recognize the need to uphold the dignity of the patient and strive to equalize the sense of disproportion that sometimes exists between health care professionals and patients. In compliance with ADA, students learn ways to accommodate the special needs of the physically challenged. The importance of providing equal access to care for all patients is stressed.

SUPPLEMENTARY RESOURCES

Medical Assisting Videos: Appropriate content is available on Delmar's Medical Assisting Videos, 2nd ed, for the following topics:

Tape 1: Communication Skills
Tape 2: Confidentiality in the Reception Area
Tape 3: Triage Skills

ANSWERS TO TEXT REVIEW QUESTIONS

1. d. live and silk plants
2. a. to give them as much control as possible
3. c. strongly contrasting patterns
4. b. providing access and opportunity for physically challenged individuals
5. c. greet patients in a friendly, warm manner

6. d. b and c above
7. c. 15 or more
8. b. May need to be entertained by the receptionist.

ANSWERS TO TEXT CRITICAL THINKING QUESTIONS

1. An interior designer or space planner will create an atmosphere of warmth and welcome while exhibiting safety and efficiency in planning for a medical office. Colors may be in pastels, lighting will be excellent, corridors and doorways will be accessible to persons with disabilities, and signage will be clear to all. There is a tendency to use live plants and fish in an aquarium as much as possible. If affordable, these should be professionally managed. Seating will be comfortable, afford security, and allow ease of movement. Patients prefer seating that does not force them to look at other patients. The receptionist should be visible, and there should be a feeling of openness to the desk area while affording privacy for confidentiality. A designer or space planner ideally works with every person in the office, determines the best way to perform the daily activities, and always keeps the patients' needs in mind.
2. Answers will vary depending on students' experiences. Their first impressions will always be most revealing.
3. Answers will vary. It is best if students do not name their physician's office when sharing information in class.
4. For a receptionist or administrative medical assistant to always have a pleasant, warm, and genuinely friendly and caring attitude, even on days when personal difficulties may interfere, it is necessary to know how to leave personal problems behind when beginning work. Have a confidant or someone who listens to your concerns so that you do not unburden yourself to other staff members, remember that the patient is not the cause of your difficulties, be professional at all times, be in control of yourself, and take mini-breaks if necessary to remain calm and pleasant.
5. These situations will vary, but tips for students to remember are
   Remain calm. The patient's anger will only be escalated if you return the anger.
   Lower your voice, apologize (even if the problem is not your fault), and ask what you can do or how you can help. When there is an exceptionally long wait, always offer the patient an alternative if it seems medically appropriate—return at a later time, reschedule, or see another physician. It is also very helpful to keep waiting patients up to date on their wait—what is happening, when they can expect to see their physician, how much longer the wait will be.
6. Children aged 4 to 6 can benefit from some books that might be read to them or picture books they could enjoy themselves. Some facilities have a television that could be used for good quality children's stories.
7. Consider getting some samples of work interior designers have done in medical settings. Explore costs and whether the first consultation is free. Find out exactly what an interior designer can do for you in the project you have in mind.

ANSWERS TO WORKBOOK EXERCISES AND ACTIVITIES

Vocabulary Builder

A. The purpose of the ADA is to provide a clear and comprehensive national mandate to end discrimination against individuals with disabilities and to bring them into the economic and social mainstream of life.
B. Accessibility is a major consideration in creating the facility environment because it is essential that health care professionals set the example by providing fully accessible, barrier-free environments to physically challenged individuals. It is important to provide equal access to health care for all patients in all settings.
C. Four ways an ambulatory care setting can accommodate the physically challenged are
   (1) Doors and hallways that accommodate wheelchairs.
   (2) A bathroom facility for handicapped individuals.
   (3) Braille signage for the visually impaired.
   (4) Elevators if the facility is on more than one level.

Learning Review

1. *Reception area:* Reception windows or desks can make the patient feel cut off from health care professionals. A poorly lit room may suggest that the physician is hiding poor housekeeping, haphazard maintenance, or a rundown physical plant. The reception area should be properly illuminated and free of clutter, with clear access to the medical receptionist.
   Corridors: Exposed medical equipment, including dials, hoses, and nozzles, can frighten or intimidate patients. Distasteful odors from necessary antiseptics can create discomfort. Clearly marked directions help patients gain confidence in a confusing labyrinth of hallways. Equipment should be positioned to minimize any intimidating or overwhelming patient impressions or should be stored or placed out of the way of general traffic.
   Examination rooms: Lack of privacy is an issue in the examination room. Mirrors and private spaces are helpful in preserving the patient's sense of autonomy and well-being. Medical equipment and supplies should be positioned to minimize any perception that is threatening or frightening or, if possible, kept out of sight in cabinets or closets. The proper use of color in examination rooms can minimize a harsh or intimidating impression for patients. The

proper respect and empathy of health care professionals can do much to mitigate the sense of unequalness or fear a patient may experience in the examining room.

2.   A.   The physician and medical assistant can leave the room to allow the patient to disrobe in privacy. A specific area designed to hold the patient's personal belongings can be reassuring and empowering. The physician can perform the examination so that only one specific area of the patient's body is exposed at any particular time; the patient will not need to appear fully disrobed.

    B.   It might help to create separate waiting areas for men and women to accommodate those who are embarrassed by waiting for treatment while only partially clothed and wearing a hospital gown. Private dressing rooms, lockers, and bathroom facilities can help to create an atmosphere of privacy and discretion. Patients who are very sick, or who feel their privacy is invaded when other patients can see them and potentially guess the nature of their illness and treatment, should be given a solitary place in which to wait for treatment. Medical professionals need to be sensitive to the lack of privacy and sense of invasion these patients may experience and strive to uphold each patient's dignity, autonomy, and sense of self.

    C.   The medical assistant needs to be respectful of the partially disrobed state of the patient while the Holter monitor is placed on him. The patient could be given the option of dressing before instructions regarding the diary are given. Should the patient have questions about completing the diary—for example, questions about bowel habits or sexual activities—that he feels uncomfortable asking the female medical assistant, the physician should be called to the examination room. The patient should also have the option of discussing the test with the physician in the physician's office where both the physician and the patient will be fully clothed and seated on an equal level.

3.   A.   Patients who are very ill need not be left to wait in the reception area, but can be immediately escorted to an examination room. Should a patient become ill in the reception area, the medical receptionist should assist this patient to a bathroom facility or other appropriate place as quickly and professionally as possible. If necessary, a physician or other health care professional should be summoned to examine the patient for a potential emergency situation.

    B.   The medical receptionist can use active listening skills to confirm the patient's message. The medical receptionist should offer the patient the option of discussing an alternative payment plan, according to the policy of the individual medical practice. The receptionist should maintain a professional and courteous attitude and avoid arguing with the patient. If necessary, the patient may be referred to the practice's office manager.

    C.   The patient should be politely escorted into the reception area. If patients are frequently losing their way, the medical receptionist should speak to the office manager about putting up clear directional signage for patients to follow.

    D.   The medical receptionist can determine the name of the patient's primary care physician to see whether a proper referral can be faxed immediately to the gastroenterologist's office. If a referral cannot be obtained, the patient should be given the available options of rescheduling a new appointment, seeing the physician anyway and paying for charges directly, or seeing the physician and establishing a payment plan for charges. The medical receptionist should politely and courteously explain in full the requirement for obtaining proper referrals for treatment and apologize for the inconvenience to the patient. If necessary, the patient should be referred to the office manager.

4.   1.   E.
    2.   C.
    3.   A.
    4.   B.
    5.   D.

5.   A.   Five activities for opening the facility are
      (1) Arrive at least 20 minutes before the first patient.
      (2) Make a visual check of each room.
      (3) Check all necessary supplies and equipment.
      (4) Retrieve patient charts.
      (5) Check the answering machine or service for messages.

    B.   Five activities for closing the facility are
      (1) Turn off all equipment.
      (2) Secure all windows and doors.
      (3) Put away supplies and make sure that sensitive materials are properly under lock and key.
      (4) Place petty cash in a safe container.
      (5) Put each room and area in readiness for the next day.

Multiple Choice Questions

1.   b.   accessibility
2.   a.   receptionist
3.   c.   promote health

4.   d.   all of the above
5.   b.   in a locked, secure cabinet

Investigation Activity

This activity allows students to think about and experiment with the design of a reception area for an ambulatory care setting. Students choose the template elements that will create the atmosphere that they feel is most efficient and comfortable for the expected patient population. Students consider the many alternatives in designing an effective reception space and discover their own preferences and predispositions. By actively determining the physical environment of the reception area, students are confronted directly with the issues of functionality and patient comfort important to enhancing the relationship between patients and health care providers.

As a class, students can collect their designs and use them as a springboard to discuss the many alternatives available in creating an effective reception space. The special requirements of certain patient populations can be considered. The class discussion should focus on arriving at a consensus of criteria necessary for reception areas based on looking at the student designs. Avoid criticisms or negative critiques of individual student ideas.

ANSWERS TO WORKBOOK CASE STUDY QUESTIONS

1. The hearing impaired patient needs to have visual contact with the health care team in order to communicate effectively. The physical environment should have proper lighting, and individuals should take care not to stand in front of bright lighting fixtures or window blinds. The hearing impaired patient will need to use telecommunication devices such as the TDD or the government-funded relay services to communicate by telephone with the medical practice. Employees should be trained in the use of TDDs and relay services. The deaf or hearing impaired patient should be given written instructions. Health care professionals should be sure that any hearing impaired person clearly understands treatment options and is capable of giving proper informed consent before administering any procedure.

2. The sensitivity or insensitivity of the medical assistant can make a direct impact on the hearing impaired person's ability to understand and participate in treatment decisions. Insensitivity can foster a negative or paranoid attitude on the part of the patient. If the medical assistant constantly turns or walks away, grows impatient, or simply refuses or neglects to fully explain procedures, the patient's care is compromised.

3. The medical assistant will need to exhibit extra empathy and care in dealing with the elderly person who denies a hearing loss. Patience and concern for the patient's dignity will enhance the potential for successful communication. Written instructions should be given to this patient. If the elderly patient has a family member or friend who regularly assists in care, the medical assistant may ask permission to discuss the treatment with that person by telephone to ensure that all instructions are properly understood and will be followed by the patient in the home.

Chapter 11

Computers in the Ambulatory Care Setting

OVERVIEW

As the Information Age progresses and computers become an integral part of the work-place, the role of the medical assistant will continue to expand, reflecting the growing reliance of the ambulatory care setting on the capabilities of computers. Medical assist-ing students must learn what tasks computers can perform easily in the medical office. The basics of computer hardware and software configurations, operation, and mainte-nance are discussed. The study of ergonomics is explored, along with strategies for avoid-ing computer-related injuries such as back strain, eye strain, and damage to the wrist. The need for medical assistants to follow guidelines preserving the confidentiality of com-puterized patient records, including the release of computerized information, is stressed. Medical assisting students are encouraged to consider their role as information managers, using computers to perform tasks and access services, resources, and information that will assist themselves and their physician–employers and enhance patient care.

PROFICIENCY EVALUATION OUTCOME ASSESSMENT

Students are evaluated for their understanding of performance objectives. Students gain an appreciation for the ways in which computers are streamlining administrative tasks in the ambulatory care setting. Students discover how computers are influencing the course of medicine by contributing to the performance of state-of-the-art clinical procedures and other modern medical advances. Students identify types of computer hardware and distinguish between systems and applications software. Students identify the categories of applications software and describe the uses of each within the context of the ambulato-ry care setting. Students apply the principles of database management and recognize the potential of computers for locating resources and information for physicians and patients. Students explore ergonomics and apply ergonomic theories to creating optimum work-stations and minimizing computer-related injuries. Students recognize the medical assis-tant's growing role as an information manager and understand the need for preserving patient confidentiality in computer applications of patient data.

SUPPLEMENTARY RESOURCES

Medical Assisting Videos: Appropriate content is available on Delmar's Medical Assisting Videos, 2nd ed., for the following topics:

Tape 2   Control of and Access to the Computerized Medical Record
Tape 3   Use Basic Office Equipment
          Apply Computer Concepts for Office Procedures
          Computerized Medical Records
          Billing Cycle and Collections
          Manage Physician's Professional and Hospital Schedule
Tape 4   Computerized Management of Reimbursement Systems

ANSWERS TO TEXT REVIEW QUESTIONS

1. c. are widely used in today's health care facility
2. a. is the brain of the computer system
3. d. consists of the manuals and documents that define how programs operate
4. b. financial analysis
5. d. all of the above
6. a. are a collection of bytes
7. b. allow users to carry a text file into another applications program
8. c. tax and other financial reporting
9. a. they are the smallest unit of data a computer can process
10. d. expect the computer system to be 100% operational immediately

ANSWERS TO TEXT CRITICAL THINKING QUESTIONS

1. For a busy ambulatory care setting, the value of computerized operations has an impact on most office functions. The wish list could include
   • Patient scheduling: appointment scheduling, cancellations, appointment reminders.
   • Word processing: correspondence, medical transcription, patient education brochures.
   • Clinical matters: research reports, treatment plans, medical records.
   • Accounting: accounts payable, payroll, profit and loss statements, monthly statements, charge slips.
   • Billing, collecting, and insurance: accounts receivable, aging accounts receivable, collections letters, electronic transmission of claim forms, patient billing, insurance claim processing.
   • Practice management: inventories, employee records such as vacation and sick time, ordering, referrals.
2. Computerizing the ambulatory care setting must be a well thought out, methodical process if the transition from manual to computerized systems is to be a smooth one. The office manager or the medical assistant in charge of the process should
   • Recognize the needs of the medical practice; this starts with the wish list in critical thinking question 1.
   • Network with others in the industry and ask the advice of other ambulatory care centers who have survived the manual-to-computer transition.
   • Talk to staff members and gather information and advice from those who are computer knowledgeable and initiate training programs for staff members who need to develop basic computer skills.
   • Select a down period for installation of the computer hardware to avoid disrupting patients and staff.
   • Allow adequate time for the transition and input of data.
3. The four main types of computers and a possible function of each:
   (1) Supercomputer: the fastest and most powerful of computers. Often used in medical research.
   (2) Mainframe computer: with great processing ability, it is valuable for large volumes of repetitive calculations. Often used in government programs like Medicare and Medicaid.
   (3) Minicomputers: today, these computers challenge older mainframes by quickly processing a large volume of data. Often used in health care facilities for decentralized processing of insurance claims and analysis of statistical data.
   (4) Microcomputers: the smallest of the four types and most widely used in today's ambulatory care setting for a range of functions. Includes the personal computer (PC), handheld, laptop, and notebook systems.
4. The four components of a computer system consist of hardware, software, data, and documentation. Hardware includes all the physical equipment such as the CPU, printer, keyboard, and monitor. Computer software is the set of programmed instructions that controls the computer operations. Documentation consists of the instructions for using hardware and software applications referenced by computer users. Data are the raw information input into the computer system.
5. The six functions used in establishing and manipulating a file typically are
   (1) Creating.   (4) Saving.
   (2) Formatting.   (5) Printing.
   (3) Editing.   (6) Storing for future retrieval.
6. The major categories of applications software include
   (1) Word processing, used to create textual documents.
   (2) Spreadsheets, used for calculations and financial forecasts.
   (3) Database management, used for collection and retrieval of information pertaining to individual records.
   (4) Graphics, used in presentations, for producing artwork and for creating different types of charts.
   (5) Communications, used for coordinating data transmission between computer systems.
7. To research a medical topic on the computer, you would first need to know what information retrieval systems you have at your disposal, either on the job or at a nearby research library. If your ambulatory care center is not electronically connected to the Internet, you may need to use a university or hospital library. Often, these will

permit community residents to conduct research; most subscribe to the MEDLARS (Medical Literature Analysis and Retrieval Systems) database, which permits users to conduct literature reviews on any of twenty on-line bibliographies.

An on-line service available on an individual subscription basis for use on personal computers is called MEDLINE; this has more than six million references to journal articles relevant to health care professionals.

8. Patient confidentiality is essential in all medical computing environments. Both legal and ethical aspects of patient confidentiality must be considered. Some specific examples include never mentioning a patient's name or condition to anyone outside of the ambulatory care setting; making sure that all files, patient charts, computer databases, etc., are closed and secured when you are not working on them; and respecting that information regarding the treatment and progress of a patient is privileged information.

9. Ergonomics is the study of work environments and its purpose is to effectively design work areas that both increase productivity and ensure worker safety and satisfaction. Ten suggestions to prevent computer injury on the job could include any of the points listed in Table 11–3 found in the textbook.

ANSWERS TO WORKBOOK EXERCISES AND ACTIVITIES

Vocabulary Builder

A. 1. G.   5. I.   9. J.
    2. A.   6. B.   10. H.
    3. D.   7. F.   11. K.
    4. E.   8. C.

B. 1. J.   9. T.   17. X.
    2. E.   10. Q.   18. P.
    3. O.   11. H.   19. I.
    4. V.   12. S.   20. U.
    5. M.   13. C.   21. G.
    6. R.   14. L.   22. D.
    7. B.   15. N.   23. W.
    8. K.   16. A.   24. F.

Learning Review

1. A. PM.   H. A.
   B. C.   I. WP.
   C. BCI.   J. C.
   D. S.   K. A.
   E. PM.   L. WP
   F. A.   M. WP.
   G. BCI.   N. C.

2. Five steps medical assistants should take in the care and handling of computer components are
   (1) Make sure all hardware, including monitor, printer, and central processing unit, are turned off at the end of the day.
   (2) Store all diskettes in appropriate storage containers.
   (3) Cover all computer system hardware with dust covers as required.
   (4) Avoid eating or drinking near the computer. Spilled food or drink can cause damage to the keyboard or computer components.
   (5) Never attempt repairs to a computer system without first unplugging all of its components.

3. A. Editing.   D. File creation.
   B. Printing.   E. Saving.
   C. Formatting.   F. Retrieval.

4. 1. F.   4. B.
   2. D.   5. A.
   3. E.   6. C.

5. A. Also called the cell address, this is the unique intersection of a specific row and column in a worksheet. It is identified by the letters and numbers of the coordinates of the intersection, such as C8 or AA5520.
   B. Worksheets consist of empty rows and columns that form spreadsheets similar to the accountant's columnar pad. Worksheets can be formatted to fit the specific needs of an individual document containing text and numerical values, such as an inventory list or a work schedule.
   C. Values are numbers and can be displayed in decimal format, currency format with a dollar sign, or as a percentage.
   D. Labels denote text entries such as column headings.

Spreadsheet software is particularly useful for
(1) Expense sheets.
(2) Tax reporting and other financial reporting.
(3) Medical billing packages.

6. A. (1) Bits.
(2) Bytes.
(3) Fields.
(4) Records.
B. Ten fields of patient information are

(1) Name.
(2) Address.
(3) Work phone.
(4) Home phone.
(5) Insurance.
(6) Gender.
(7) Social security number.
(8) Date of birth.
(9) Occupation.
(10) Place of employment.

7. A. The Electronics Communications Privacy Act of 1986
B. The Code of Fair Information Practice

8. A. Authorized personnel.
B. Identified in the record.
C. Authorized computer programs requiring the medical data.
D. Three security measure are
(1) Passwords.
(2) Encryption (encoding) of information.
(3) Scannable badges or other user identification.

Multiple Choice Questions

1. b. data output
2. a. application software
3. d. formatting
4. c. carpal tunnel syndrome
5. b. firewall

Investigation Activity

Instructors can use this activity to help students become excited about the potential of computers. Students gain exposure to the wide range of programs, services, and resources available to computer users. Any fear or feelings of intimidation about computer use is replaced with a sense of curiosity, interest, and eagerness to learn. If possible, instructors should bring a selection of computer magazines to class to pass among the students. Discuss how information in computer periodicals can be used by administrative medical assistants to improve or enhance the use of computers in the ambulatory care setting.

The school's research librarian can be invited to class to advise students on computerized research techniques and to outline database and on-line resources relevant to the medical assisting profession. If the necessary equipment is available, a database search on MEDLINE or MEDLARS can be demonstrated to show students exactly how such searches are performed. Have the class come up with a topic for research and then work with the librarian to gather information. Possible research topics could include (1) finding the names, addresses, and phone numbers of national health organizations, such as the American Cancer Society, to create a patient education brochure; (2) locating information on physical therapy for sports injuries to the knee; and (3) gathering data on the benefits of low-fat diets in reducing the risk of heart disease.

ANSWERS TO WORKBOOK CASE STUDY QUESTIONS

1. The co-office manager, Shirley Brooks, CMA, will perform benchmarks, or comparisons, to assess the patient insurance databases of other ambulatory care settings. By networking with other office managers who have systems in place, Shirley can evaluate what system might work best for the needs of the offices of Drs. Lewis and King. Shirley will come up with a list of information the database may contain and determine whether any of this information can be imported from the existing patient information database already in place. Shirley will research the kinds of database programs available and decide whether a new database program will work best or whether existing database software can be used for the creation of the new database. Shirley will check the medical practice's hardware and software to make sure the new program will run efficiently on the existing system or whether additional memory, workstations, or other items are needed.

2. The patient insurance database will need to include the patient's name and address; whether the patient is insured; whether the patient has more than one insurance policy; the names, addresses, and telephone numbers of insurers; if insurance is supplemented by government forms of insurance such as Medicare or Medicaid; whether the patient's

insurance requires co-payments or deductibles; what services, procedures, and medications are covered by which insurance policy; whether the patient is the primary insured and the names of other family members who are covered under the policy; whether the patient assigns benefits directly to the provider; and whether the patient is covered by Worker's Compensation.

3. The office manager will present the physician-employers with a written proposal detailing what software or hardware will be needed to implement the database, what staff power will be necessary, and what information the database will contain. The report will include a cost and time analysis of implementation as well. If approved by the physician-employer, the office manager will execute the written proposal to implement the patient insurance database.

Chapter

12

Telephone Techniques

OVERVIEW

The telephone is the mainstay of an ambulatory care setting. When medical assistants take incoming calls and make outgoing calls, they represent their health care setting to the outside world. It is crucial that medical assisting students learn to communicate with others in a caring, professional, and competent manner. The difficult and important task of telephone communication demands excellent administrative, clinical, and interpersonal skills. Students recognize the importance of respecting and upholding patient confidentiality and of practicing within the scope of their training and expertise.

PROFICIENCY EVALUATION OUTCOME ASSESSMENT

Students are evaluated for their understanding of basic telephone techniques, procedures, etiquette, technology, and triage. Students should exhibit an ability to communicate effectively with others and respond appropriately to a wide variety of situations common to the ambulatory care setting. Students will demonstrate the ability to convey concern and empathy in communicating with patients, to exhibit competence in screening and performing telephone triage, and to act within the limits of their professional expertise and authority. As effective communicators in the modern health care profession, medical assisting students understand the importance and uses of various communication tools, including pagers, answering services, automated routing units (ARUs), e-mail, and fax machines.

Procedure 12-1   Telephone Techniques
Procedure 12-2   Handling Problem Calls
Procedure 12-3   Placing Outgoing Calls

SUPPLEMENTARY RESOURCES

Medical Assisting Videos: Appropriate content is available on Delmar's Medical Assisting Videos, 2nd ed., for the following topics:

Tape 1   Communication Skills
Tape 2   Complete Medical Records
          Confidentiality on the Telephone
Tape 3   Use Basic Office Equipment
          Triage Skills

ANSWERS TO TEXT REVIEW QUESTIONS

1. a. using the hold button sparingly
2. a. volume, enunciation, pronunciation, and control of speed
3. c. are used to avoid clipping off the office name
4. d. getting the caller's name and telephone number is not necessary

5. d. a patient requests test results
6. a. is the act of evaluating the urgency of a medical situation and prioritizing treatment
7. b. listen calmly to the upset person
8. b. should always be documented
9. c. use a recorded voice that identifies departments or services the caller can access by pressing a specified number
10. c. capable only of one-way transmission

ANSWERS TO TEXT CRITICAL THINKING QUESTIONS

1. It is acceptable to put callers on hold when you have asked for and received permission to do so. Place a caller on hold after you know who and why the person is calling and when it is not an emergency.
2. Methods to improve how you sound on the telephone are
    - Use same tone and volume as if speaking to someone in the same room.
    - Enunciate.
    - Use proper pronunciations.
    - Speak at a normal rate of speed, neither fast nor slow.
    - Use good posture.
    - Show enthusiasm.
    - Smile. When you smile, a pleasant tone will come through in your voice. The act of smiling will subconsciously affect your mood and enhance your ability to communicate therapeutically and professionally with patients and others.
3. Some calls that should be referred to the physician will include (students may list any six)
    - Requests for test results.
    - Medical emergencies and medical treatment.
    - Other physicians.
    - Requests for medication (other than standard refills).
    - Requests for patient information from third party.
    - Requests for referrals.
    - Complaints.
    - Patients who refuse to provide information to anyone else.
4. In a medical office, all patient complaints should be viewed as potential malpractice suits and are best handled by the physician or office manager.
5. Triage is the act of evaluating the urgency of a medical situation.
6. Questions that could be asked to evaluate the urgency of a call include (student may list any six)
    - What happened?
    - Who is the patient (name and age)?
    - Is the patient breathing?
    - Is the patient bleeding? How much? From where?
    - Is the patient conscious?
    - What is the patient's temperature?
    - *If the patient ingested something:* How much was taken? Are there poison or overdose instructions on the bottle?
7. The eight elements necessary to a proper telephone message include
    - Date and time call is received.
    - Caller's name and phone number.
    - Nature and urgency of the call.
    - Who the call is for.
    - When the caller can be reached.
    - Action to be taken (e.g., caller will call back, returned your call, and please call back).
    - Message, if any.
    - Name or initials of person taking message.
8. When taking a message, it is proper to give callers an approximate time when they might expect to receive a call back. For example, if the person called is away for two weeks and will not be returning calls, the caller should be told not to expect a call back before the person's return.
9. When giving the physician a message from or about a patient, the patient's chart should always be provided with the message.
10. To properly transfer a call to someone else in your office, tell the caller to whom you are transferring the call and why. Call the party to whom you are transferring the call and tell the party the caller's name and reason for the call; give as much detail as the caller has already provided.
11. To handle an angry caller:
    - *Listen* to what the person is upset about.
    - Remain calm.

- Let the caller have his or her say, do not interrupt.
- Ask questions during pauses.
- Lower your voice, both pitch and volume.
- Empathize with the caller by using the words *I understand*.
- If the person becomes abusive, tell him or her that you will hang up and do so immediately.
- Report all angry calls to the physician or office manager at once.

12. When speaking with a hearing–impaired individual:
    - Speak more slowly than normal.
    - Speak more clearly than normal.
    - Speak slightly louder than normal.

ANSWERS TO WORKBOOK EXERCISES AND ACTIVITIES

Vocabulary Builder

1. A. Key terms are inserted in the paragraph in the following order: etiquette, enunciate, posture, diaphragm, jargon, obfuscation, slang, fluent, empathy, screen, triage, confidentiality, ethical, and Good Samaritan laws.

   B. 1. C.   4. F.
     2. A.   5. E.
     3. D.   6. B.

Learning Review

1. A. The medical assistant greets the caller politely, identifying herself and the office: "*Good morning. This is administrative medical assistant Karen Ritter at Inner City Health Care. How can I help you today?*"

   B. The medical assistant provides the patient with an approximate time she can expect a return telephone call from the physician and provides information in a reassuring and confidence-building tone: "*I'm sorry, but Dr. King is not available at this time. She is on rounds at the hospital and won't be able to speak with you until 4:30 this afternoon. I know she will want to hear your concerns about the medication you are taking; let me verify the phone number where Dr. King can reach you. She'll call you as soon as possible this afternoon.*"

   C. The medical assistant will ask the caller's permission before placing the call on hold: "*Mr. Schwartz, I have another call coming in that I must take. Could I put you on hold for one minute or is there a number where I can reach you in about ten minutes? Thank you for your patience and cooperation; your appointment is important to us.*"

   D. The medical assistant will direct the caller to the appropriate person or department: "*Mrs. Hansen, our office manager, Walter Seals, is the person who handles all insurance questions. If you hold please, I will transfer your call to him so we can help resolve this situation.*"

2. A. Four reasons a potential patient contacts the office are
    (1) The caller is ill or in pain.
    (2) A family member is ill or in pain.
    (3) The caller or a family member has been referred to the office by another physician to treat or evaluate a problem.
    (4) The person is selecting a physician and may have many questions about the ambulatory care setting.

   B. Nine pieces of information to record in the appointment book are the patient's

    (1) Name.   (6) Insurance carrier or HMO.
    (2) Address.   (7) Name of insured (self, spouse, other).
    (3) Daytime telephone number. (8) Name of referral source.
    (4) Age.   (9) Reason for appointment.
    (5) Employer.

3. A. MA. Calls will come from both patients and insurance carriers. If the call is from an insurance company or HMO, the patient's chart must be consulted for a signed "release of information" form before giving patient information.

   B. MA. Scheduling requires coordination. Appointment times involve the availability of the physician, staff, and patient and the hours of the facility where the appointment is made.

   C. P. The physician, when present, should be interrupted and notified of all emergency calls. Physician-employers will create emergency policy and procedure manuals for employees to follow should emergency situations arise.

   D. MA. Medical assistants may take the call from a pharmacy, patient, or family member requesting a prescription refill. However, they may not authorize a refill or tell the pharmacy or patient that a prescription will be refilled without the physician's approval. A message and the patient's chart are given to the physician regarding the approval for refill.

   E. P. All patient complaints should be viewed as potential malpractice suits. Patients who complain about the office or the quality of care are best referred to the physician.

F. MA. An information sheet with the practice hours, location, financial policies, and the nature of the practice's services should be kept near the telephone for easy access when providing details to callers.

G. P. The physician may need to make changes in medication or treatment, or the patient may need to be seen right away. These decisions are beyond the scope of practice of the medical assistant.

H. P. Prescribing medications is beyond the scope of practice of the medical assistant.

I. P. Medical assistants may not give medical advice without risking practicing medicine without a license.

J. MA. The medical office will have policies regarding the scheduling of salespeople, such as pharmaceutical representatives.

4. A. "Hello, you have reached the medical practice of Drs. Lewis and King. Our offices are open daily between the hours of 8:30 A.M. and 6:00 P.M., with extended hours on Tuesdays and Thursdays until 8:30 P.M. Currently, the offices are closed. If this is not an emergency situation and you would like to leave a message, please do so when you hear the tone, and we will return your call promptly. If this is an emergency, please hang up and dial 555-1234 for immediate assistance."

B. Message #1. To: Marilyn Johnson. From: Anna Preciado. Telephone: 555-6622. Message: Won't be in today, have the flu. Joe Guerrero said he may be able to sub. Dr. Lewis has several patients scheduled for clinical testing in the afternoon. Initials: EA. Attachments: information sheet or appointment book with Dr. Lewis's clinical testing schedule. Joe's telephone number.

Message #2. To: Dr. Lewis. From: Dr. Kwiczola. Telephone: 555-7181. Message: New psychiatric patient with symptoms of fatigue, anxiety, palpitations, and weight loss may be experiencing hyperthyroidism. Would like to consult with you. Dr. K. is in between 2 P.M. and 7 P.M. Assistant's name is Heidi. Initials: EA. Attachments: none.

Message #3. To: Shirley Brooks. From: Martin Gordon. Telephone: Ellen will insert the telephone number after researching the patient information database. Message: Patient of Dr. Lewis's has question about out-of-pocket maximum. Initials: EA. Attachments: none.

Message #4. To: Dr. Lewis. From: Charles Williams. Telephone: 555-6124(h) or 555-8215(o). Message: One of Holter monitor leads came off approx. 11 P.M. Patient put back on. Worried about whether we will have to redo the test. At office number after 9 A.M. Initials: EA. Attachments: patient chart.

5. It is crucial that medical assistants understand and comply with the legal and ethical principles and restrictions that govern issues of patient confidentiality. The following list specifies with whom and under what conditions a medical assistant may discuss a patient with another person.

Person	Yes	No	Yes, w/Signed Release
Patient's spouse or family	☐	☒	☐
Patient's employer	☐	☒	☐
Patient's attorney	☐	☐	☒
Another health care provider	☒	☐	☐
Insurance carrier or HMO	☐	☐	☒
Referring physician's office	☒	☐	☐
Credit bureaus and/or collection agencies	☐	☒	☐
Members of the office staff, as necessary for patient care	☒	☐	☐
Patient's insurance carrier	☐	☐	☒
Other patients	☐	☒	☐
People outside the office (friends, family, acquaintances of the medical assistant)	☐	☒	☐
Patient's parent or legal guardian, except concerning issues of birth control, abortion, or sexually transmitted diseases	☒	☐	☐

6. Four paging system options are

(1) Voice alerts. The voice message is automatically heard by the person being paged. Anyone in the vicinity will hear the message.

(2) Beep alerts. The pager emits a beeping sound or silent vibration that notifies the person being paged to call one designated telephone number to obtain the message.

(3) Alphanumeric digital message display. The message can include an entire typed message via a computer modem or through an operator who will input the message and transmit it to the receiver.

(4) Numeric digital message display. The callback telephone number, selected by the person initiating the page, is displayed on a small screen.

Multiple Choice Questions

1. c. enunciation
2. c. triage
3. a. confidentiality

4. a. ARU
5. c. 20–30 seconds

Investigation Activity

Use the activity to help students develop proper telephone techniques and become comfortable performing telephone procedures. Role-playing gives students practical experience to increase their confidence in handling a variety of telephone calls. By taping the scenarios, students have the opportunity to hear how they sound to others on the telephone and gain insights that can help them improve their telephone technique. Although responses will vary depending on the caller's prompts, students' should communicate in a professional, articulate, and caring manner.

After performing the activity, students should discuss as a class how they felt about facing tough telephone situations and share strategies for dealing with specific problems or challenges. Students learn that while they can control their own behavior and actions, they cannot control the behavior and actions of others. In the medical profession, where the health and well-being of patients may be at stake, professionalism and efficiency in performing telephone triage for effective communication are essential.

ANSWERS TO WORKBOOK CASE STUDY QUESTIONS

1. Desirable caller options might include to schedule or change an appointment, for emergencies, for billing or insurance information, for clinical testing, to speak with the medical receptionist, to speak with an office manager, for office hours and location, for prescription refills, and to speak with a physician.

2. Instructions can be given in the outgoing message for the caller to choose an option that will connect him or her directly to a medical assistant, bypassing the complete option menu.

3. ARUs boost efficiency by routing calls directly to the appropriate person when the caller chooses a menu option. By including voice mailboxes in the system, individual physicians and staff members can receive their messages instantly and completely—without the extra time and effort to transcribe and route messages manually.

4. An information sheet can be prepared explaining how the system functions, along with instructions for its use. For patients, accessibility in emergency situations must be stressed in the information sheet to reassure patients that the new system will not impede their ability to reach a physician when needed. For physicians and staff members, the sheets will include internal extensions and routing features.

Chapter 13

Patient Scheduling

OVERVIEW

The medical assisting student discovers the importance of effective and efficient patient scheduling to the successful management of the ambulatory care setting. Students are exposed to the many scheduling methods and systems, along with information on the advantages and disadvantages of each in regard to specific scheduling criteria—such as patient population, the nature of the practice, and physician preferences. The function of the patient appointment schedule as a legal document of patient flow is emphasized. Students learn to properly document appointment changes, no-shows, and cancellations. Finally, the importance of maintaining positive patient relationships and focusing on patient needs throughout the scheduling process is presented as a critical element of the medical assistant's duties.

PROFICIENCY EVALUATION OUTCOME ASSESSMENT

Students are evaluated for their understanding of performance objectives. Students assess various scheduling tools and systems and demonstrate the ability to choose the most appropriate system for individual facilities and situations. Students establish appointment matrixes and prepare daily appointment sheets, daily worksheets, and patient reminders. The importance of triage in determining how patients are scheduled is explored and emphasized. Legal requirements of scheduling are presented. Patient informational brochures are introduced as scheduling tools for patient education. Students gain insight into the interpersonal skills necessary for effective scheduling and recognize the importance of maintaining good patient relationships to the success of medical practice management.

Procedure 13-1   Checking in Patients
Procedure 13-2   Cancellation Procedures
Procedure 13-3   Establishing the Appointment Matrix

SUPPLEMENTARY RESOURCES

Medical Assisting Videos: Appropriate content is available on Delmar's Medical Assisting Videos, 2nd ed., Tape 3, for the following topics:

Perform Administrative Duties
Manage Physician's Professional and Hospital Schedule
Triage Skills

ANSWERS TO TEXT REVIEW QUESTIONS

1. d. a current and accurate record and saved as documentation
2. b. is assessing the urgency of a call and need for appointment
3. c. can provide a valuable service and should be scheduled for short visits
4. a. gives two or more patients the same appointment time
5. b. schedules appointments at set times throughout the workday
6. b. provide a permanent record for legal risk management and quality management
7. d. all of the above
8. c. be flexible
9. d. both b and c

ANSWERS TO TEXT CRITICAL THINKING QUESTIONS

1. When an appointment is canceled or a patient is a no-show, the cancellation should be indicated in the appointment book and in the patient's chart, and the appointment rescheduled, if possible. This allows the physician to check back with the patient to make certain quality care is given.

2. Stream appointment system: patients are seen through the day, each patient having a specific appointment time.
   Cluster appointment system: patients with similar complaints are scheduled consecutively in blocks of time.
   Modified-wave appointment system: multiple patients are booked at the beginning of the hour, with additional patients booked at 10- to 20-minute intervals throughout the hour. One variation uses minor, major, and work-in slots.

Group questions: Guidelines for possible responses to the questions are presented. However, these are only suggestions; there are other possibilities. Determination of a correct student answer should be based on the plausibility of the answer. The purpose is to promote discussion and critical thinking about how the student would handle an actual situation in the physician's office.

3. There is no one best system of scheduling because each medical office has different staffing requirements and physical setups that affect the flow of patients. In addition, the type of practice and the services it performs places different requirements on how patients are processed. The bottom line is that a system of attending to patients needs to ensure that patients are seen and treated in as timely a fashion as possible.

4. *Problem:* Lenore does not appear to be involved in assisting with her care as she has high blood pressure but does not keep her appointments.
   Solution: Note the cancellation in the appointment book and patient chart. An appropriate staff member needs to speak with the patient, or the physician should write her a letter to discuss the importance of treating her problem and having her cooperation in this effort. If she is unwilling to do so, care should be terminated (with appropriate notice) or transferred to another physician with whom the patient might participate.

5. *Problem:* Dr. Lewis is behind schedule and cannot see all of the patients who are scheduled.
   Solution: Inform the patients of the problem and see if they are willing to reschedule. Accommodate them as much as possible to reassure them that they have chosen a practice that cares about them. Personalize this contact as much as possible to establish a link, so patients feel motivated to continue care at this office.

6. *Problem:* Patients are not being seen in a timely fashion.
   Solution: It appears that there are sufficient examination rooms to use the double-booking system. However, there is only one medical assistant. Look at what appointments are being double-booked. Are there double-bookings procedures that can be handled simultaneously? If not, it would be better to choose a scheduling system that allows patients to be seen at their scheduled times.

7. *Problem:* A patient states the need to be seen immediately. Is this an emergency?
   Solution: The first and foremost step is to triage the situation. What are the patient's complaints and symptoms? Is this a true medical emergency or just an urgent matter? Does the situation require a referral to the emergency room or could the patient be seen in the office? If the patient can be seen in the office, is the condition one that Dr. King's staff could attend to or does it require Dr. King herself? A true emergency could be referred to the emergency room or be seen at 10:40 in the office. If it were an urgent but not stat matter that could wait until after lunch, the patient could be worked in during the afternoon.

8. *Problem:* Dr. Whitney is running behind schedule and has a surgery that cannot be changed. Two patients are waiting in the reception area.
   Solution: The first step would be to explain to the waiting patients that Dr. Whitney is running behind schedule, then offer the option of rescheduling (be sure to offer the patients the next possible appointment that is convenient for them.) If Dr. Whitney is willing, patients may be seen through the lunch hour. If both appointments are 15 to 30 minutes in duration and if Dr. Whitney finishes at 12:10 as expected, both patients could be seen. However, if afternoon patients begin at 1:00 and these two appointments take 30 to 45 minutes, someone will need to be rescheduled. Tact and diplomacy will need to be employed in this situation.

9 and 10. A variety of answers is possible. Correctness of students' answers depends on whether the answers are well thought out and are logical. There is no one right answer. This is a good opportunity to look at the variety of choices the students make and, without being judgmental, discuss the various answers to provide students with decision-making skills that will help them make these choices in an actual office setting.

ANSWERS TO WORKBOOK EXERCISES AND ACTIVITIES

Vocabulary Review

1. Open hours.
2. Double booking.
3. No-show.
4. Clustering.
5. Wave.
6. New patient.
7. Established patient.
8. Practice-based.
9. Triage.
10. Stream.
11. Modified wave.
12. Slack time.
13. Matrix.

Learning Review

1.

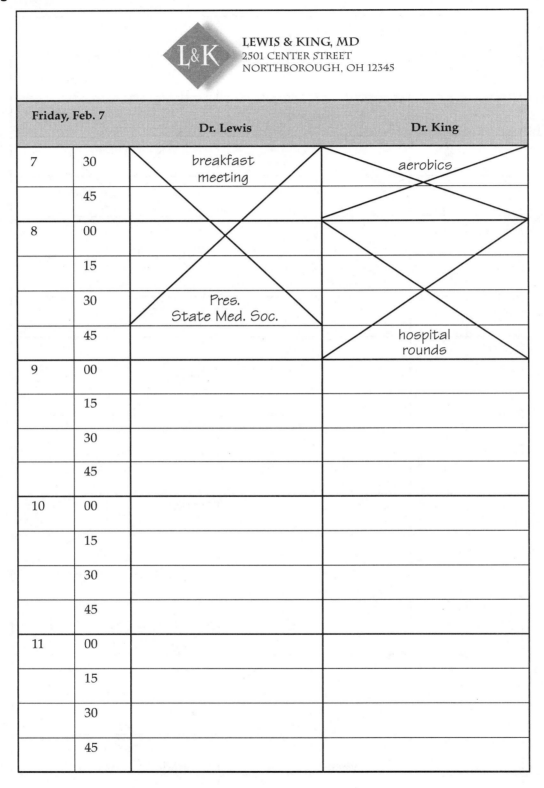

LEWIS & KING, MD
2501 CENTER STREET
NORTHBOROUGH, OH 12345

Friday, Feb. 7		Dr. Lewis	Dr. King
7	30	breakfast meeting	aerobics
	45		
8	00		
	15		
	30	Pres. State Med. Soc.	
	45		hospital rounds
9	00		
	15		
	30		
	45		
10	00		
	15		
	30		
	45		
11	00		
	15		
	30		
	45		

12	00		
	15		
	30		AMWA
	45		
1	00	lunch in	
	15		luncheon
	30	office	
	45		
2	00		
	15		
	30		
	45		Staff
3	00		Marilyn Johnson / Shirley Brooks
	15		Meeting
	30	Golf	
	45		Planned Parenthood Lecture
4	00	Dr. Wilson	
	15		
	30		Planned Parenthood Lecture
	45		
5	00		

2. A. For a manual appointment book, cancellations and no-shows should be documented in red pen on both the daily appointment sheet and the patient chart.

    For a computerized appointment system, a permanent record exists on the hard drive, disk, or annotated computer printout. Printouts of daily appointment sheets should be documented in red pen. Appropriate documentation should also be included in the patient chart.

    B. Two primary goals are a smooth flow of patients with a minimal amount of patient waiting time and flexibility to accommodate acutely ill, stat, or emergency, appointments; walk-ins; cancellations; and no-shows.

    C. 1.   45 minutes.   4.   45 minutes.
        2.   15 minutes.   5.   15 minutes.
        3.   30 minutes.   6.   15 minutes.

    D. Students will schedule appointments for Drs. Lewis and King according to the open time slots revealed in the appointment matrix established in Figure 13-1. Dr. King's patient appointments total 3½ hours out of 4½ hours of scheduling time available to patients. Dr. Lewis's patient and other appointments total 6 hours of scheduling time and will completely book his available time.

3. The daily patient appointment sheet for Dr. Lewis will include all *seven patient* appointments. The order of patients will vary in students' answers according to the scheduling slots they have used for each patient in exercise 2D (see *Workbook* Figure 13-1). Correct information for "patient name," "time allotted," and "reason for visit" columns of the appointment sheet are listed below in alphabetical order by the patient.

Helen Armstrong	1 hour	PE; mild edema, right leg
Martin Gordon	30 minutes	prostate cancer, follow-up
Veronica Hallett	15 minutes	dermatitis, follow-up
Mark Johnson	15 minutes	lower back pain, recheck
Rowena Lawrence	1 hour	PE/lab work; hoarseness and bloody sputum
Anne Ortiz	45 minutes	stomach problems
Charles Williams	1 hour	PE/Holter monitor; chest pain

4. The order of patient appointments in Dr. King's daily worksheet will vary in students' answers according to the time slots they have used for each patient in exercise 2D (see *Workbook* Figure 13-1). Information for appointments entered into the schedule to establish Dr. King's appointment matrix appears below, followed by Dr. King's patient appointments—presented here in alphabetical order by patient name.

Friday, February 7

7:30	aerobics	½ hour	
8:00	hospital rounds	1 hour	
12:30	AMWA luncheon	1 hour	
2:45	Staff meeting/office managers	½ hour	
3:45	community lecture/ Planned Parenthood		
	Lourdes Austen	1 hour	PE, lab work, consult pregnancy after breast cancer
	Herb Fowler	15 minutes	ankle sprain, recheck
	Abigail Johnson	½ hour	hypertension, diabetes mellitus, angina, routine follow-up
	Susan Marshall	1 hour	PE, ECG; stress, heart palpitations
	Margaret Thomas	45 minutes	B12 injection, routine follow-up; Parkinson's disease

5. A. Six variables in scheduling appointments are (1) the urgency of the need for an appointment; (2) whether the appointment has a referral from another physician; (3) recording methods for new and established patients; (4) implementation of check-in, cancellation, and rescheduling policies; (5) use of reminder systems; and (6) accommodating visits from medical supply and pharmaceutical company representatives.

    B. Patient flow data assist in estimating how many patients to schedule and establishing realistic time frames for particular problems or procedures.

6. A. The five steps of scheduling a specific appointment for a patient are (1) ask the patient what day and time would be most convenient for them and make the appointment for the first available time stated; (2) provide the patient with a choice of possible appointment times; (3) confirm that the patient clearly understands the date and time of the appointment—repeat the date and time to ensure you agreed to the same information; (4) spell the patient's name back if confidentiality is ensured; and (5) provide or mail an appointment reminder to the patient.

    B. The program will search a database of appointments, find an open time slot, and allocate an appointment time according to the medical assistant's instructions. Instructions can include finding an open appointment with a specific time length, on a specific day, or within a specified time frame. Once the appointment time is confirmed with the patient, patient data are keyed in and the appointment is automatically scheduled.

7. A. Student answers will vary according to the appointment matrix and schedule they have established for Dr. King in workbook Figure 13-1. Students will consider available time in Dr. King's schedule and will triage patient urgency in determining suggestions for working in the emergency patient. Dr. King should have one hour of available time for scheduling patient appointments that can be considered in this rescheduling process.

B. Mark Johnson's appointment is noted on Dr. Lewis's schedule (see *Workbook* Figure 13-1) with a red X. Mark's no-show will also be documented in the patient's chart. It is important to accurately document patient no-shows and cancellations to thoroughly record the physician's care and treatment of the patient. If the patient develops complications and claims the physician was unavailable, the appointment sheet and chart will document the patient's failure to show. If the patient routinely cancels or fails to show, the physician will review the record and assess the patient's cooperation with the treatment plan. If necessary, the physician will formally terminate services to the patient and explain the reason for discontinuing care.

C. (1) Martin's name is marked through on the appointment schedule (see *Workbook* Figure 13-1) with a single line in red pen.

    (2) A. "Mr. Martin Gordon" is entered on the first line of the card. The space for Friday is completed by entering the date "February 21," two weeks from the patient's original appointment date. Students' answers for appointment time will vary according to the appointment slot they had originally assigned for Martin in Dr. Lewis's schedule for Friday, February 7.

    B. Patients are telephoned in the afternoon to remind them of an appointment the next day. Confidential information should not be left on answering machines or recording devices without the patient's prior permission to do so.

8. A. Seven scheduling systems are open hours, double booking, clustering, wave, modified wave, stream, and practice-based.

    B. (1) The open hours scheduling system works well in hospital emergency rooms, as it allows for a steady flow of walk-in patients, triaged according to urgency of need for care or seen on a first-come, first-served basis.

        (2) The wave scheduling system would work well for a laboratory where several patients are scheduled in the first half of each hour and seen throughout the hour. This system easily accommodates no-shows, late arrivals, and walk-ins.

        (3) The double-booking method is effective for a two-physician group practice. Patients can be given the same appointment time but are scheduled to see different physicians.

        (4) The urgent care center with emergency and clinic facilities would choose a practice-based scheduling system. This system would combine a number of scheduling methods to achieve the most efficient and effective balance of scheduling for the various types of services the facility provides to patients.

Multiple Choice Questions

1. a. Medical Manager
2. a. flexibility
3. c. group appointments

4. b. three
5. b. efficient patient flow

Investigation Activity

Use the investigation activity to encourage medical assisting students to view the ambulatory care setting's scheduling policies and procedures from the patient's perspective. The student reinforces the knowledge that health care is a patient-centered profession; consumers have the right to choose their health care providers. Therapeutic care and respect for the patient are high priorities in patient scheduling and build trustworthy and lasting relationships between patients, their physicians, and other staff in the ambulatory care setting.

By analyzing patient information brochures, students discover which brochures are most effective in promoting smooth patient flow and efficient scheduling. Students explore the scheduling needs and requirements of a number of medical facilities that focus on providing different health care services, treat different patient populations, and employ a variety of health care professionals in a wide array of specialties. Students consider ways in which the brochures enhance the administrative functions of scheduling through patient education and a clear statement—for both employees and patients—of a facility's scheduling practices and policies.

ANSWERS TO WORKBOOK CASE STUDY QUESTIONS

1. Ellen will offer Martin the opportunity to wait to be the first patient seen by Dr. Winston Lewis after the emergency with Lenore is resolved. Ellen will give Martin a reasonable time frame for the expected waiting period. If Martin is unwilling or unable to wait, then Ellen will give Martin first priority to reschedule the first available appointment that is mutually convenient. Ellen will take Martin's depression into account when rescheduling his appointment, taking time to listen with compassion to Martin's concerns and feelings. Providing therapeutic communication to Martin at this time is critical to promoting his health and well-being while he fights a life-threatening illness.

2. Ellen will try to reach Hope by telephone to alert her to the emergency situation and reschedule Hope's appointment. If Hope is already on her way to the office, Ellen will give her the option of rescheduling the next available appointment that is mutually convenient. If Hope insists on seeing Dr. Lewis that day, Ellen can consider contacting nonemergency patients with afternoon appointments to see if they are willing to reschedule.

3. As Jim is experiencing chest pains, Ellen should make every attempt to preserve his appointment time. The patient's medical condition is more important to the decision to hold his appointment time than his aggressive and impatient manner—and the fact that Jim would be very unhappy at the prospect of being rescheduled.

4. Patient triage is essential to effective rescheduling. Martin's serious condition and depression make him an important patient to reschedule with care. As a new patient in good general health, Hope is not a priority for scheduling from a standpoint of medical urgency. However, the medical assistant will need to display sensitivity and responsiveness to this new patient in order to preserve her positive impression of the physician and the medical practice. Jim's potentially serious medical condition makes him a priority to be seen according to his scheduled appointment time, if possible. If Ellen needs to contact Jim regarding rescheduling, she will need to display diplomacy and professionalism in dealing with a potentially difficult patient and schedule an appointment at the earliest mutually convenient time.

Chapter

14

Medical Records Management

OVERVIEW

Medical assisting students must possess the skills required for sorting, filing, retrieving, and maintaining information effectively. With the need for thorough and proper documentation, a majority of interaction on the patient's behalf is concerned with proper information processing. The role of medical assistants in medical records management is an important one, ensuring that records are complete, up-to-date, and easily accessible to physicians and other members of the health care team. An awareness of computer applications is helpful to upgrading the organization and utilization of files in the medical office, particularly in regard to storage and archiving of files and records. Legal and ethical concerns related to medical records management must also be considered.

PROFICIENCY EVALUATION OUTCOME ASSESSMENT

Students are evaluated for their understanding of performance objectives. The legal and ethical ramifications of accurately documenting and filing information in patient records is recognized by the student, including rules of confidentiality and the crucial rule that, under the law, an action not documented is an action not performed. Students demonstrate the ability to recall and apply basic filing rules; to distinguish between alphabetic, numeric, and subject filing systems; and to cross-reference files within systems. Steps for filing medical documentation in patient files are mastered, as well as procedures for filing general correspondence. Students distinguish between POMR and SOMR methods of recordkeeping and understand the components of the SOAP approach to progress notes used by many physicians. Computer applications and archive requirements are also discussed.

Procedure 14-1 Steps for Manual Filing with a Numeric System
Procedure 14-2 Steps for Manual Filing with a Subject Filing System

SUPPLEMENTARY RESOURCES

Medical Assisting Videos: Appropriate content is available on Delmar's Medical Assisting Videos, 2nd ed., for the following topics:

Tape 2 Legal Aspects and Confidentiality of Medical Records
Access to Medical Records
Control of and Access to the Computerized Medical Record
Use Appropriate Guidelines When Releasing Medical Records
Document Accurately
Complete Medical Records

Tape 3 Perform Administrative Duties
Use Basic Office Equipment
Prepare and Maintain Medical Records
Apply Computer Concepts for Office Procedures

ANSWERS TO TEXT REVIEW QUESTIONS

1. c. purging
2. b. tickler file
3. b. out guide
4. a. O'Keefe John Porter II
5. c. the one that is customized to the needs of the office
6. b. vertical, open-shelf lateral, and movable file units
7. b. both b and c
8. d. Wardenbloomberg
9. b. index using a social security number
10. d. inspect, index, code, sort, file

ANSWERS TO TEXT CRITICAL THINKING QUESTIONS

1. Two key issues involving the management of a patient's medical record could include
    *   Legal issues. If it is not in writing, it did not happen. Malpractice suits could result from a delay in diagnosis due to lost or misfiled records.
    *   Efficient records. Ensure that the practice provides the best care for patients and ensures patient confidence in the care provided.
2. Considerations for choosing a medical office filing system could include any of the following two:
    *   The type of practice.
    *   The number of patients seen in the practice.
    *   The number of personnel accessing and maintaining the files.
    *   The objectives for maintaining the files.
    *   Confidentiality.
    *   Training considerations for those managing the files.
3. Alpha-Z utilizes the first three letters of the last name and uses thirteen colors, colored letters on white backgrounds and colored backgrounds with white letters. Tab-Alpha uses the first two letters of the last name and uses a different color for each letter.
4. It is important to have an alphabetic card file in a numeric filing system, because there must be a method of linking the file number to the person given that number and linking the person to the number assigned. If only a number is referenced, any information that comes into the office without a number, such as correspondence, could not be properly filed.
5. Answers will vary. Determine whether
    *   The divisions are applicable to communicable diseases.
    *   There are five useful divisions for the subject.
6. The correct filing order would be:
    a. Beckwood, Alabama.
    b. Little Rock.
    c. Minneapolis.
    d. Shreveport.
7. Establish consistent procedures for locating missing files.
    *   Check all of the items within the file.
    *   Check other files with similar labels.
    *   Check the folders filed before and after the proper location of the misplaced file.
    *   Check the physician's desk or other file trays at other stations throughout the office.
    *   If using a color-coding system, look for folders with the same color-coding as the misplaced file.
    *   If using a numeric system, look for possible transposition combinations of numbers.
8. While many patient charts are still maintained by manual methods, ambulatory care settings use computers and scanners in medical records management to establish databases, store inactive patient files, and exchange information through e-mail. Databases are especially useful because they allow easy retrieval of information by different sortings, for example, a patient list might be organized and retrieved by patient name, zip code, city, or state. Databases can be utilized in many ways, for example, to retrieve information about patients in a particular locality, patients on a particular drug, or for general mailing lists and address labels. Purchased biomedical databases provide a library of health care information and permit users to search available literature on any number of topics.

    When used for archival storage of patient records, computers can eliminate the bulky storage associated with traditional records while providing quick access to files. Often patient records can be copied with a laser beam onto optical disks, eliminating the need to key in all information. They can also be scanned to create a computer file from the paper file.
9. Answers will vary depending on the name.

10. Answers will vary depending on state; however, the time is usually 3 to 6 years. Activity can be triggered when a negligent act is discovered, which might be much later in the process of patient care.
11. Keep in mind the following: (1) available floor space for records and their accessibility, (2) the number of records to be stored, (3) whether the records need to be closed and locked when not in use, and (4) the kind of filing system used.
12. Everyone believes they understand the alphabet that is the basis to all filing systems. However, mistakes are made so easily. Then a file is out of place. It takes concentration and much practice to file accurately, efficiently, and speedily.

ANSWERS TO WORKBOOK EXERCISES AND ACTIVITIES

Vocabulary Builder

1. tickler file
2. SOAP
3. purging
4. indexing
5. out guide
6. inspection
7. key unit
8. identification label
9. cut
10. accession record
11. nonconsecutive filing
12. release mark
13. units
14. cross-reference
15. Problem-Oriented Medical Record (POMR)
16. guides
17. coding
18. shingling
19. consecutive or serial filing
20. color-coding
21. captions
22. Source-Oriented Medical Record (SOMR)

Learning Review

1. A. 1. unit 1 Levine-Dwyer unit 2 Jackson unit 3 Hugh
      2. unit 1 Poole-Petit unit 2 Leslie unit 3 Jane
   B. 1 unit 1 Wildasin unit 2 Keith unit 3 Sr.
      2. unit 1 Maggart unit 2 Gerald unit 3 III
   C. 1. unit 1 Udolf unit 2 Louise unit 3 Dr.
      2. unit 1 Rajah unit 2 Valerie unit 3 Professor
   D. 1. unit 1 Martin unit 2 Lindsay unit 3 Adair
      2. unit 1 Johnson unit 2 Abigail unit 3 Sue
   E. 1. unit 1 O'Keefe unit 2 Mary unit 3 Jane unit 4 Mrs. John
      2. unit 1 Fowler unit 2 Nora unit 3 Patrice unit 4 Mrs. Herb
   F. 1. unit 1 de la Hoya unit 2 Joseph unit 3 Jack
      2. unit 1 van deVeer unit 2 Maurice unit 3 John

2. A. 1. Larry Paul Samuels
      2. Larry Peter Sanders
      3. Lawrence Paul Sanders
   C. 1. Lynn Elaine Brenner
      2. Lynn Ellen Brenner
      3. Lynn Eloise Brenner
   B. 1. James Edward Reed
      2. James Edward Reed Jr.
      3. James Edward Reed Sr.
   D. 1. Patrick Sam Saint
      2. Paul Sam Saint
      3. Patrick Sam St. Bartz

3. A. unit 1 Riverview unit 2 One unit 3 Locksmith
   B. unit 1 24 unit 2 Office unit 3 Cleaning
   C. unit 1 Target unit 2 Specimen unit 3 Laboratory
   D. unit 1 10 unit 2 Dollar unit 3 Filing unit 4 Cabinets
   E. unit 1 Janoff's unit 2 Office unit 3 Supplies unit 4 2Go
   F. unit 1 Richmond unit 2 Therapy unit 3 Group unit 4 The
   G. unit 1 Laboratory unit 2 Kits unit 3 4 unit 4 Analysis
   H. unit 1 Ace unit 2 Prosthetics unit 3 Inc
   I. unit 1 1 unit 2 Metropolitan unit 3 Hospital

4. A. 1
   B. 3
   C. 1
   D. 2
   E. 2
   F. 1
   G. 1

Multiple Choice Questions

1. b. last
2. d. tab–alpha system
3. a. consecutive or serial

4. d. accession record file
5. a. date stamp and initials

Investigation Activity

Use this activity to encourage students to memorize filing rules and to develop the skill of applying filing rules quickly and accurately. By volunteering to do some filing for a campus organization, department, or library, students see different filing systems at work. They also see the effect a filing system can have on the efficiency, or inefficiency, of a professional workplace environment. Students learn that filing is a task of real importance and consequence to the ambulatory care setting, ensuring that patient records are kept accurate, up-to-date, and easily accessible to physicians and other members of the health care team.

ANSWERS TO WORKBOOK CASE STUDY QUESTIONS

1. Accurate, up-to-date, and complete documentation is important for legal reasons. The standard in court is that if there is no written record of a temperature, a visit, a history or physical, a laboratory report, and so forth, it did not happen. To be prepared in the event of medical litigation, all medical treatment must be documented.
2. POMR is an effective recordkeeping system for a family practice office because it works well in settings where physicians see patients for a variety of problems over a long span of time.
3. Color-coded filing systems minimize filing errors.
4. An effective, easy-to-use, and easy-to-access filing system is integral to the smooth operation and efficiency of the ambulatory care setting. Records must be located quickly and contain accurate, up-to-the-minute information in order to provide the highest quality care to patients. An inaccurate filing system creates inefficiencies in administrative processes and could lead to errors in treatment and diagnosis (potentially opening up the practice to the risk of litigation) if key documents are lost or misfiled.

Chapter 15

Written Communications

OVERVIEW

It is essential for medical assisting students to understand that written correspondence in the ambulatory care setting relates necessary information to patients, referring physicians, and other health care organizations. Students need to master written communication skills because correspondence makes a statement about the professional standards of the medical office. It is imperative for medical assisting students to understand that all written correspondence serves as a legal record in the event of any kind of litigation.

PROFICIENCY EVALUATION OUTCOME ASSESSMENT

Students are evaluated for their understanding of performance objectives. Students should demonstrate the ability to compose clear and concise correspondence with attention to format, content, word choice, tone, spelling, grammar, and adherence to office (or other preordained) style. Students will display the ability to recognize proofreader's symbols and apply them to their own (and others') written correspondence. Medical assisting students demonstrate their skill as efficacious communicators and health care professionals by understanding business letter components, supplies, and procedures for mailing for written correspondence (including new technologies for written correspondence, such as fax machines and modems). Students' comprehension of medical transcription is also established.

Procedure 15-1	Preparing and Composing Business Correspondence Using All Components
Procedure 15-2	Addressing Envelopes According to United States Postal Regulations
Procedure 15-3	Folding Letters for Standard Envelopes
Procedure 15-4	Preparing Outgoing Mail According to United States Postal Regulations
Procedure 15-5	Preparing, Sending, and Receiving a Fax

SUPPLEMENTARY RESOURCES

Medical Assisting Videos: Appropriate content is available on Delmar's Medical Assisting Videos, 2nd ed., for the following topics:

Tape 1	Communication Skills
Tape 2	Legal Aspects and Confidentiality of Medical Records
	Access to Medical Records
	Use Appropriate Guidelines When Releasing Records
Tape 3	Perform Administrative Duties
	Use Basic Office Equipment
	Prepare and Maintain Medical Records
	Triage Skills

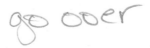

ANSWERS TO TEXT REVIEW QUESTIONS

1. c. read long documents a section at a time
2. d. with individualized addressing when possible
3. a. full block
4. a. letters containing laboratory and/or diagnostic results
5. a. on line 15 or two to three lines below the letterhead
6. d. never use a letterhead page as a second page
7. b. look in the envelope to make certain that all contents have been removed
8. b. first class
9. d. a and c only
10. a. privacy disclaimers

ANSWERS TO TEXT CRITICAL THINKING QUESTIONS

1. The five tips for more effective communication include
    1. Identify topics.
    2. Use clear and concise language.
    3. Establish tone of voice.
    4. Follow office style.
    5. Encourage response.

    The student's letter should incorporate these tips; the student should annotate the letter, pointing out how the tips were used.
2. This could involve the whole class if desired. While the word choices are infinite, use some of those medical words found in Chapter 16. Consult the textbook glossary for a complete listing of key vocabulary terms.
3. The four major letter styles are
    - Full Block: all elements start at the left margin.
    - Modified Block, Standard: all elements start at the left margin except the date, complimentary closing, and keyed signature.
    - Modified Block, Indented: same elements as standard modified block except the subject line and paragraphs are indented.
    - Simplified: no salutation or complimentary closing, and subject line and keyed signature are all upper case.

    The sample letters should be evaluated to see if the students followed the elements of each style.
4. Component parts of a business letter include
    - Date line: usually keyed on line 15 or two to three lines below the letterhead.
    - Inside address: name and complete address of the person to whom the letter is being written, keyed flush with left margin.
    - Salutation: formal or informal introductory greeting, keyed flush with the left margin on the second line below the inside address.
    - Subject line: if used, a brief reference to the subject of the letter is keyed on the second line below the salutation. It may be flush with the left margin, indented five spaces, or centered.
    - Body of letter: begins on second line below salutation or below the subject line if one is used.
    - Complimentary closing: begins on second line below the body of the letter. The style (formal or informal) should match the salutation.
    - Keyed signature: begins four to six lines below the complimentary closing.
    - Reference initials: two lines below the keyed signature and flush with the left margin.
    - Enclosure notation: if included, this appears one or two lines below the keyed reference initials.
    - Carbon copy notation: if included, this appears one or two lines below the reference initials or enclosure notation.
    - Postscripts: two lines below last of either reference initials, enclosure notation, or carbon copy notation.
5. Student's answers will vary. However, they may include any of the following
    - Clearly identifying topics
    - Using clear and concise language
    - Establishing tone of voice, formal or informal
    - Follow office style
    - Encourage response
    - letter placement suggestions provided
6. The instructor should provide students with one or more letters that need revision and correction. Have students rewrite, rekey, and proofread the letter before sharing it with other students.
7. Organize small groups to share the rewritten letter from #6. Students should compare and evaluate changes made to the letter, commenting on readability, format, and correct word usage.
8. Have students address envelopes and then evaluate the results against the information in Procedure 15-2.

9. The fax cover sheet should include the names of sender and receiver and the number of pages being sent and whether this total includes the cover sheet. A statement on the cover sheet should include a notice that the fax is confidential material, intended for use only by the designated recipient. Once the cover sheet meets these specifications, the student should determine whether the fax and the situation meet the Fax Security System. If it does, the student can fax the document.

10. A copy of any written communication should be maintained in the patient chart or in office files should it need to be referenced at a later date. E-mail should be included in your office's confidentiality policy. Confidentiality must be considered if the office sends or receives clinical e-mail from a computer that can be used by more than one person. A privacy disclaimer should establish boundaries and ground rules for e-mail messages. Clinical e-mail should be printed and filed in the patient chart along with any reply. A written agreement of understanding should be designed for signature by patients before clinical e-mail is implemented in the office.

ANSWERS TO WORKBOOK EXERCISES AND ACTIVITIES

Vocabulary Builder

Key vocabulary terms are inserted into the passage in the following order: full block letter, standard modified block letter, indented modified block letter, simplified letter, keyed, bond paper, watermark, ZIP+4, optical character reader (OCR), medical transcription, voice recognition technology (VRT).

Learning Review

A. Full block letter style.
B. Proofreading corrections to the letter appear below.
C. Students will transcribe the letter correctly and prepare it in the standard modified block style. Students' completed letters should contain no errors.

Multiple Choice Questions

1. b. full block
2. a. 20 pound stock
3. c. minutes
4. d. certified mail
5. c. financial

Investigation Activity

Use this exercise to help students recognize their strengths and shortcomings in written communications. Compare students' findings to your own assessment of their performance. Self-tests give students a heightened awareness of their abilities and may help them overcome obstacles, especially ones that may be self-imposed.

After students have completed the self-survey, encourage them to discuss their findings with the class. Suggest ways to improve critical areas of weakness such as spelling, grammar, and vocabulary—especially medical terminology. The important role written correspondence plays in the health care environment is reinforced. Students learn strategies for becoming effective written communicators and discover the value of practice as a method of improving writing skills.

ANSWERS TO WORKBOOK CASE STUDY QUESTIONS

1. Bias-free language is important in respecting the diversity of patients and coworkers. Bias-free language with regard to ethnicity, age, gender, sexual orientation, disability, physical condition, or race exhibits an awareness of and sensitivity to an individual's identity. The use of bias-free language will reflect positively on the medical practice.
2. Students' responses will vary. Some examples include
   • Avoiding words that end in "man"; for example, instead of workmanship use well-crafted.
   • Staying away from words with potentially pejorative overtones, such as fat/skinny or handicapped.
   • Choosing adjectives and adverbs with an awareness of gender-biased usage; for example, nurturing may be considered a feminine word by some people and strong a masculine word.

16 Transcription

OVERVIEW

Medical assisting students are introduced to the medical transcriptionist's attributes, employment opportunities, and membership benefits in AAMT. The benefits of the profession along with the types of work environment are presented. Students are shown the proper ways to make corrections within the transcription and are shown the different types of reports used in the medical office. Medical assisting students recognize the importance of understanding ethical and legal issues as they apply to medical transcription in the ambulatory health setting.

PROFICIENCY EVALUATION OUTCOME ASSESSMENT

Students are evaluated for their understanding of performance objectives. Students will describe the attributes of the medical transcriptionist along with the benefits of membership in AAMT. Students should demonstrate the proper ways to make corrections within the medical record transcription and be able to differentiate between the many different reports used in the medical office. In this chapter, students gain insight into the ethical and legal issues that apply to medical transcription.

SUPPLEMENTARY RESOURCES

Medical Assisting Videos: Appropriate content is available on Delmar's Medical Assisting Videos, 2nd ed., for the following topics:

Tape 1	Professionalism and Communication Skills	
	Display Professionalism	
	Communication Skills	
Tape 2	Legal and Ethical Issues	
	Legal Aspects and Confidentiality of Medical Records	
	Access to Medical Records	
	Complete Medical Records	
Tape 3	Administrative Skills	
Tape 9	Introduction to Body Mechanics	
	Body Mechanics	

ANSWERS TO TEXT REVIEW QUESTIONS

1. c. anyone not working as an MT and currently enrolled in a nine-month or two-semester student-instructor related course
2. a. minimum keyboarding speed of 60 words per minute
3. b. freelance MT
4. c. MTCC
5. d. straight, flat keyboards
6. a. line length of document
7. c. flag the document
8. b. HPI
9. d. both a and b
10. a. cannot restructure reports and emphasize critical information

ANSWERS TO TEXT CRITICAL THINKING QUESTIONS

1. The personal attributes of a medical transcriptionist include
   - The MT enjoys words which is necessary in the profession because physicians create new terms as descriptions and new techniques, procedures, and medications are continually being developed.
   - The MT must be a good listener and understand different accents and languages. This skill is helpful in transcribing the dictation of foreign-speaking physicians.
   - The MT must be self-disciplined, detail-oriented, and independent. Often MTs work in solitary surroundings and have no one else to ask questions or discuss possible solutions with. The turnaround time must be met, so sticking to the task and seeing that it is done correctly is vital.
   - MTs must have integrity and understand medical confidentiality. Discussing a patient's medical record with someone outside of the office environment could lead to litigation.
   - The MT's acquired skills include keyboarding and knowledge medical terminology, anatomy and physiology, medications, and surgical procedures necessary to complete the medical documents correctly and in a timely manner.
2. Answers to this question will vary.
3. Design configurations will vary; ergonomic considerations may include, but are not limited to
   - Prevention of carpal tunnel and other repetitive motion injuries by wearing specialized computer gloves, or use of a wrist rest or split keyboard.
   - Prevention of eye strain could include: wearing tinted glasses to reduce glare; placing the monitor away from windows or using drapes, blinds, or an antiglare screen; selecting a color monitor that is restful to the eye; taking frequent short breaks; and blinking more often.
   - Prevent ear infections by cleaning and maintaining earphones properly and by not allowing others to use them.
   - Do exercises such as rolling the shoulders or head to prevent neck and back strain. Adjust the chair height; use a lumbar cushion, rolled-up towel or small, thin, firm pillow for the back. Use a footrest if short-legged.
4. QA means quality assurance, which measures documents to ensure they are accurate, complete, consistent in health care documentation, and prepared in a timely manner. Health care documentation is critical for insurance reimbursement.
5. If a medical record were to be requested as court evidence and the record appeared to have been tampered with or could not be read, the physician would not have documentation to support the question. It is important that the physician date and sign any alteration to the medical chart. This signifies that what was stated was correct at that time.
6. STAT means immediately or within 12 hours. These reports may be required before a surgical procedure to confirm diagnosis.

   Current reports must be turned around within 24 hours. Follow-up may be based on information contained within these reports.

   Old reports must be turned around within 72 hours.
7. JCAHO requires each hospital to submit a list of abbreviations and symbols used by that specific hospital for approval. This list serves as protection in case of litigation. Many abbreviations have more than one meaning; that is, CVA could mean cardiovascular accident or cerebrovascular accident.

ANSWERS TO WORKBOOK EXERCISES AND ACTIVITIES

Vocabulary Builder

1. American Association for Medical Transcription (AAMT): the national association for medical transcriptionists started in 1978. Certification can be obtained through successful completion of the certification exam administered by the Medical Transcriptionist Certification Program through AAMT.
2. Breach of confidentiality: the medical transcriptionist is expected to treat the patient's medical information as private and not for publication. A breach of confidentiality is the unauthorized release of confidential information.
3. Consultation report: a report generated when one physician requests the services of another physician in the care and treatment of a patient. Contents may contain all the elements of an H&P, any supporting laboratory data, diagnosis, and suggested course of treatment.
4. Continuous speech recognition: the process of direct conversion of spoken documentation into a written text (electronic) version using a computer equipped with voice recognition software.
5. Editing: the process of reviewing the transcribed document for accuracy and clarity.
6. Flag: a way to alert the dictator that something needs to be corrected or resolved. This may be done by using a color-coded approach or may simply consist of a sticky note attached or use of a preprinted flag attachment.
7. Home-based MTs: medical transcriptionists who work out of the home.
8. Index counter: measures the length of dictation on a cassette and is useful when scanning cassettes or finding correct dictation location.

9. Turnaround time: indicates the specific time period in which a document in expected to be completed. STAT means immediately, current means turnaround should be within 24 hours, and old means turnaround should be within 72 hours.

10. Split keyboard: a slanted keyboard to accommodate the natural position of the hands, in an attempt to decrease carpal tunnel syndrome and other repetitive motion injuries.

Learning Review

A. 1. Subscription to *Journal of the American Association for Medical Transcription (JAAMT)*.
   2. Networking opportunities.
   3. *AAMT Desk Companion* (updated annually).
   4. Information on state-of-the-art technology.
   5. Continuing education.
   6. Access to professional assistance.
   7. Membership help desk.
   8. Discounts on AAMT programs, products, and services.
   9. Professional development opportunities.
   10. Peer recognition.
   11. Insurance programs.
   12. Discounted travel services and car rental.
   13. No-fee credit card.

B. 1. Personal attributes
   a. Innate ability to listen to others closely.
   b. Skill for hearing and understanding different accents and languages.
   c. Enjoys detective work.
   d. Self-disciplined, detail-oriented, independent, and is usually a perfectionist.
   e. Dedicated to professional development.
   f. Committed to learning.
   g. Not afraid to ask questions.
   h. Possesses integrity.
   i. Understands the importance of confidentiality.
   2. Acquired skills developed
   a. Excellent keyboarding skills.
   b. Ability to operate a variety of software programs.
   c. Excellent language skills.
   d. Above average spelling skill.
   e. Has knowledge of anatomy and physiology; has knowledge of medical terminology.

C. 1. Medical terminology, 30%.
   2. English language and use, 25%.
   3. Anatomy and physiology, 20%.
   4. Disease processes, 15%.
   5. Health care record, 5%.
   6. Professional development, 5%.

D. 1. Index counter: measures the length of dictation on the cassette. It is useful when scanning cassettes or finding the correct dictation location.
   2. Speed control feature: allows you to increase or decrease the speed at which the words are spoken.
   3. Tone feature: similar to treble/bass on a radio; it mutes or accentuates consonants for nasal tones or a stuttering style of dictation.
   4. Earphones: plug into the transcriber and allow you to hear what has been dictated.
   5. Foot pedal: frees your hands for use on the keyboard. Push the center of the foot pedal to play, release to stop, fast-forward is on the left, and rewind is on the right.

E. Paragraph corrections:
   Her past medical history is **positive** for the usual childhood diseases and the births of **two** children following normal pregnancies. **S**he has a negative **past surgical** history. **S**he has no allergies **t**o medications and takes **T**ylenol for occasional **headaches**. She is married and has **two** children, ages 3 **years** and 12 months. She does not smoke or drink.

F. Two examples of each type of turnaround time report and the time of turnaround:
   STAT: 1. Radiology   immediately
             2. Pathology reports
             3. Laboratory reports

CURRENT:	1. H&P	within 24 hours
	2. Consultations	
	3. Operative reports	
OLD:	1. Discharge summaries	within 72 hours
	2. Emergency department notes	

Multiple Choice Questions

1. c. 1978
2. a. experience in the medical field
3. b. 2

4. b. 3
5. d. STAT

Investigation Activity

Educating medical assisting students about the many different ways transcription services can be offered is one way to show them the versatility of the profession. Class discussions on what was found in the investigation can give students insight into the profession. Students can learn the requirements of the job as well as the strategies used by transcription companies to provide services to medical offices.

ANSWERS TO WORKBOOK CASE STUDY QUESTIONS

All information transcribed is confidential information. Telling your neighbor her test results would be a breach of confidentiality and sharing the information would be unethical on your part. If you speak to your neighbor, encourage her to contact her physician, who will give her information about her test results.

Chapter 17

Daily Financial Practices

OVERVIEW

Medical assistants are presented with the principles and practices of bookkeeping and accounting that guide the daily financial activities of an ambulatory care setting. These principles and corresponding practices are essential to creating and maintaining a financially sound environment for patients and staff. Students learn the importance of communicating financial policies to patients, developing good work habits, and keeping accurate and current records. Students explore the range of tasks involved in managing patient accounts, purchasing office equipment and supplies, handling banking activities, and establishing a petty cash system.

PROFICIENCY EVALUATION OUTCOME ASSESSMENT

Students are evaluated for their knowledge of performance objectives. Students should understand basic bookkeeping and accounting principles and terms as well as the advantages and disadvantages of both manual and computerized systems of financial management. Students demonstrate knowledge of petty cash systems as well as banking procedures, including the ability to prepare bank deposits, write and record checks, and reconcile bank statements. Students show an understanding of purchasing procedures and tasks, including generating purchase orders, tracking purchased supplies and equipment, and preparing purchase orders for payment. Students should possess the work habits essential to creating and maintaining accurate and current financial records. The importance of informing patients of financial policies and procedures is stressed; students demonstrate the ability to communicate effectively with patients on these topics.

Procedure 17-1 Preparation for Posting a Day Sheet
Procedure 17-2 Recording Charges and Payments Requiring a Charge Slip (Patient Visits)
Procedure 17-3 Receiving a Payment on Account Requiring a Receipt
Procedure 17-4 Recording Payments Received Through the Mail
Procedure 17-5 Balancing Day Sheets
Procedure 17-6 Preparing a Deposit
Procedure 17-7 Reconciling a Bank Statement
Procedure 17-8 Balancing Petty Cash

SUPPLEMENTARY RESOURCES

Medical Assisting Videos: Appropriate content is available on Delmar's Medical Assisting Videos, 2nd ed., for the following topics:

Tape 3 Use Manual Bookkeeping Systems
Billing Cycle and Collections
Electronic Banking
Tape 4 Charge Slip

ANSWERS TO TEXT REVIEW QUESTIONS

1. b. the fee typically charged by a physician for certain procedures
2. d. a credit arrangement that can be used with discretion
3. c. to post individual transactions
4. c. being meticulous about aligning columns
5. b. the manual and computer systems may need to run concurrently for a few months
6. c. only a and c are correct
7. c. that records financial transactions into a bookkeeping or accounting system
8. a. always accept third party checks
9. c. voucher check
10. c. to permit employees to order items for personal use
11. d. only b and c are correct
12. d. in the checkbook, check off each check listed on the statement and verify the amount against the check stub

ANSWERS TO TEXTBOOK CRITICAL THINKING QUESTIONS

1. The three functions of a charge slip are (1) provides patients with a record of their account activity for the day; (2) generally eliminates the need for separate insurance forms; and (3) provides the office with a copy of that day's services, which will be filed in the individual's chart. Charge slips can be customized by including the applicable CPT codes and diagnosis codes for the most common services of that particular medical practice. The charge slip is also printed with the name, address, and telephone number of the practice.

2. The pegboard system of bookkeeping is efficient and time-saving because information is entered on all forms at the same time. It is impossible to enter incorrect information on one of the forms caused by copying errors or omission. A complete pegboard system consists of the day sheets, ledger cards, charge slips, and receipt forms.

3. Ledger cards are necessary to maintain a record of services provided, charges, and payments for each individual seen in the medical office. Ledger cards help track patient accounts because they show activities for each individual patient within one family and also show the total running balance for the entire family account.

4. The running tapes of a calculator will be an invaluable time-saver if the initial balance is incorrect and mistakes in calculations need to be found.

5. The five sections of a day sheet and function of each are as follows:
   - Section 1 is where the individual transactions are posted, using the ledger card and charge slips or receipt forms. The information here includes the date, patient name, description of transaction or service, charges, credits, and previous and current balances. This is the write-it-once portion of the day sheet.
   - Section 2 is the deposit portion (some companies make this part detachable to be used as an actual deposit slip). If the transaction includes a payment, the payment amount will be listed under the appropriate right-hand column showing the method of payment after the ledger portion is posted.
   - Section 3 is for business analysis. These columns might be used for recording payments or charges to be credited to different physicians; they are often used as a breakdown for types of service (i.e., office exam, hospital visit, surgery, etc.). Because the use of this area will vary from practice to practice, the office manager will explain how it should be handled.
   - Section 4 is where the transactions are totaled and balanced at the end of the day (see Procedure 17-5, Balancing Day Sheets, in Chapter 17 of the textbook).
   - Section 5 is used to verify the daily balances and to balance and track cumulative accounts receivable figures. The total accounts receivable figure shows how much is owed to the practice by all patients to date, allowing the physician or administrator to see the total outstanding balance at a glance without having to add hundreds of individual balances.

6. The following steps help prepare a new day sheet: (1) At the start of the day, a new day sheet and strip of charge slips are placed on the pegboard. (2) Information at the top of the day sheet (date and page number) is filled in. (3) Balances forwarded from the previous sheet are entered in Section 4, "Previous Page" columns A–D and the "Previous Day's Total" and "Accts. Rec. 1st of Month" in the Accounts Receivable Control and Proof boxes of Section 5. Now the day sheet is ready to use.

7. When a payment is received in person, it is necessary to prepare a charge slip if services were provided that day, or a receipt form if they were not. When entering a payment received in the mail, only the ledger card and the day sheet are necessary for posting.

8. Deposits are made daily because they serve as another proof of posting and because it is unwise to leave large sums of money in the office overnight.

9. An accurate balance should be maintained in the checkbook as each check is written. The account should be reconciled monthly against the statement received from the bank. It is necessary to reconcile the account to verify that there are no errors either in the checkbook or in the bank's records.

10. Petty cash is money kept in the office for minor, sometimes unexpected, expenses, such as postage-due mail or coffee supplies. Keeping this cash on hand eliminates the need for the physician or office manager to sign checks for such items.

ANSWERS TO WORKBOOK EXERCISES AND ACTIVITIES

Vocabulary Builder

A.   1.   Petty cash voucher.
2.   Ledger card.
3.   Day sheet.
4.   Charge slip.
B.   1.   Pegboard system.
2.   Petty cash.
3.   ROA.
4.   Credit.
5.   Charge.
6.   Currency.
7.   Superbill.
8.   Disbursement.
9.   Balance.
10.   Posting.
11.   Adjustment.
12.   Write-it-once system.
13.   Accounts payable.
14.   Accounts receivable.

Learning Review

1.   A.   Seven checking account features are (1) interest paid; (2) monthly fees; (3) per check fees; (4) automated teller machine (ATM) access and fees; (5) initial deposit and balance requirements; (6) fees for checks; (7) special services extended free of charge, such as notary services, cashier's checks, traveler's checks, balance reconciliation, and small business services.
B.   The completed check should include
Date: September 15, x.
Payable to: RJ Medical Supply Company.
Amount: $323.45.
For: Blood pressure equipment.
Signature: Susan Rice, M.D.
Check stub should include
Date: September 15, x.
To: RJ Medical Supply Company.
For: Blood pressure equipment.
Total: $323.45.
Balance forward: $2610.00.
This payment: $323.45.
Balance: $2286.55.
C.   Five rules to ensure that checks are properly written and recorded are (1) make sure that the numerical and written amounts agree, (2) make sure that everything is spelled correctly, (3) make sure that the check has been signed by an individual with signature privileges, (4) follow office procedure for having the physician or office manager approve all expenditures and/or sign all outgoing checks, and (5) make sure the check is payable to the correct payor and that the current date is used.
2.   A.   Four reasons are (1) to avoid purchase of unnecessary items, (2) to avoid duplication of items purchased, (3) to prevent employees from ordering items for personal use, and (4) to provide a system for payment of only those items properly ordered and received.
B.   The completed purchase order includes the following information:
Purchase Order #1743

Bill to:	Ship to:	Vendor:
Inner City Health Care	Inner City Health Care	Mayflower Supply Co.
222 South First Avenue	222 South First Avenue	642 East Sixty-fifth Street
Carlton, MI 11666	Carlton, MI 11666	Carlton, MI 11623
(814) 555-7155	(814) 555-7155	(814) 555-9999
Req. by: Karen Ritter	Buyer: Walter Seals	Terms: net 30 days

Quantity	Item	Units	Description	Unit Price	Total
2	62145	Box	Fax paper	$8.99	$17.98
5	24598	Each	Desk calendars	$4.25	$21.25
4	72148	Case	Copier paper	$20.00	$80.00
5	26773	Box	Highlighter pens	$3.98	$19.90
4	96187	Each	Printer cartridges	$49.99	$199.96
				Subtotal:	$339.09
				Tax:	$27.13
				Freight:	Prepaid
				Balance due:	$366.22

    C. To verify that the correct items and quantities are received, the medical assistant should check the item numbers and quantities against the original purchase order. Discrepancies should be noted on the office copy of the purchase order, and the vendor should be contacted immediately. If the order is correct, the invoice received from the vendor is compared to the original purchase order to verify quantities, unit prices, and other charges. If there are discrepancies, the vendor's accounts receivable department should be contacted. Once the invoice and purchase order are reconciled, the PO number is noted on the invoice and the invoice is marked "Okay to pay" and passed along to the office's accounts payable department for payment.

3. (1) A cashier's check is used when a check must be guaranteed by a bank for the amount written. This kind of check is obtained at the bank in exchange for equivalent cash or a personal check.

    (2) A certified check is a depositor's check on which the date and amount have been certified by the bank to indicate that the check is good for the amount written.

    (3) A money order is similar to a cashier's check and may be purchased with cash at banks and through the U.S. Postal Service.

    (4) A voucher check is a check with a stub attached to record the invoice dates and services provided that are associated with the check. In the ambulatory care setting, voucher checks are commonly used for payroll and for accounts payable.

    (5) A traveler's check is used in the same way that cash is used. Because these checks require a signature when purchased and again when used, traveler's checks are a convenient and safe alternative to cash when traveling.

4. A. Information will be entered into the manual patient ledger card, according to the table below:

Date	Reference	Description	Charges	Credits	Balance
1/26	Mary O'Keefe	Total OB care 59400	1,200.00	1,200.00	
1/26	Mary O'Keefe	Intermed. exam, new pt. 99202	30.00		1,230.00
1/26	Mary O'Keefe	Pap smear/88150	18.50		1,248.50
1/26	Mary O'Keefe	Deposit OB care		250.00	998.50
2/18	Mary O'Keefe	Insur. Pmt. 1/26: 90015		20.00	978.50
2/18	Mary O'Keefe	Adj. Cat. #1 1/26: 90015		10.00	968.50
2/25	Mary O'Keefe	CBC/85022	12.50		981.00
2/25	Mary O'Keefe	Limited exam, est. pt. 99212	15.00		996.00
2/25	Mary O'Keefe	Cash Pmt. 1/26: 94000		75.00	921.00
4/26	Mary O'Keefe	CBC/85022	12.50		933.50
4/26	Mary O'Keefe	Limited exam, est. pt. 99212	15.00		948.50
4/26	Mary O'Keefe	Diagnostic ultrasound 76805	55.00		1,003.50
4/26	Mary O'Keefe	Pap smear/88150	18.50		1,022.00

    B. Three reasons why adjustments are made are (1) to show a reduction in fee for a service granted by the physician, (2) to show a write-off to the account if the physician has agreed to accept insurance as payment in full, and (3) to correct an error in posting.

5. A. Two guidelines are (1) always work with care and accuracy and (2) keep work current or it may become overwhelming.

    B. Six habits are (1) form numerals and letters carefully with good penmanship, (2) use a consistent ink color, (3) align columns, (4) be careful when carrying decimals, (5) double-check math, and (6) correct errors neatly by crossing out incorrect figures and writing the correct figures above them.

6. According to this bank statement:
   A. There are *seven* outstanding checks.
   B. The total amount of outstanding checks equals *$1745.58.*
   C. The last deposit was made on *January 9.*
   D. The amount of the last deposit was *$1092.68.*
   E. The total amount of deposits not listed on the bank statement is *$3162.50.*
   F. The bank fees equal *$15.24.*
7. A. An endorsement of a check transfers rights to whoever holds the check. Checks are usually endorsed with a rubber endorsement stamp bearing the name of the depositor, the name of the bank, and the depositor's account number. A blank endorsement consists of a signature only; if the check is lost or stolen, someone else could endorse the check below the signature and cash it. A restrictive endorsement includes the signature as well as the words *deposit only* or *to the order of [name of the bank].*
   B. Medical assistants should inspect the check for the correct date, amount, and signature. Third-party checks should not be accepted unless they are from insurance carriers. If a check is returned for insufficient funds, the checking account should be adjusted accordingly. Office procedures should be followed for notifying the patient that the check was returned.
8. Balancing all financial information ensures that no mistakes in calculation are made, that all amounts are properly credited to patient accounts, and that all charges shown as outstanding on the day sheet agree with the outstanding balances of the individual patient accounts. If a payment is misplaced, the deposits will not agree with the patient ledgers or credits. This system of checks and balances also protects against embezzlement of funds.
9. A. AP.   D. AP.
   B. AR.   E. AR.
   C. AP.   F. AP.

Multiple Choice Questions

1. b. ledger cards
2. c. charge slip
3. a. business analysis
4. a. cashier's check
5. c. special endorsement

Investigation Activity

Use the investigation activity to encourage students to become better informed about the financial opportunities open to small businesses and individuals. By experiencing the banking relationship from the standpoint of the consumer, the student discovers the range of alternatives available and becomes more confident about the consumer's influence over the services and products received from banks and other financial institutions. All banks are not "just the same." Students who may be intimidated by financial matters or who may see financial duties in the ambulatory care setting as routine and uninspired chores begin to view the larger picture of the medical practice's financial relationship with a banking establishment.

If possible, invite a bank representative who handles small businesses, such as a medical group practice, to speak to the class and answer questions.

ANSWERS TO WORKBOOK CASE STUDY QUESTIONS

1. "Ms. Berry, I'd like to take a few minutes to review Drs. Lewis and King's policies regarding medical fees and patient accounts. I see that your insurance carrier covers 80 percent of the usual, reasonable, and customary fees for your family's medical expenses after a $100 deductible. Because you have already reached the required deductible, you generally will be responsible only for the remaining 20 percent of charges that your insurance does not cover. After every visit, we will provide you and your insurance carrier with a detailed statement of your visit, including treatment or services provided, the charges for those services, and the amount for which you are responsible. We do ask that you keep your account current. We prefer personal checks, but will accept credit card payments as well. It's important for both you and the practice that patients keep their appointments. We require 24 hours' advance notice of cancellations. Except in emergency situations, you will be charged the full office fee if proper notice is not given to the office. Do you have any questions I can answer at this time?"
2. *Usual* refers to the fee typically charged by a physician for certain procedures, *reasonable* refers to the midrange of fees charged for this procedure, and *customary* is based on the average charge for a specific procedure by all physicians practicing the same specialty in a defined geographic area.
3. Credit cards are accepted in ambulatory care settings for the convenience of the patient. According to the AMA Code of Ethics, physicians may not increase their charges for patients who use credit cards or encourage patients to use them. The patient should be informed about the issue of maintaining confidentiality and about possible intrusions on the right to privacy when paying for medical services with a credit card.

Chapter 18

Medical Insurance

OVERVIEW

Students are introduced to the important role of the medical assistant in performing duties related to medical insurance. Students gain insight into the importance of insurance and learn its terminology and various forms.

PROFICIENCY EVALUATION OUTCOME ASSESSMENT

Students are evaluated for their understanding of performance objectives. Students are able to discuss the changes occurring in health insurance today, including the growing influence of managed care on insurance issues. The difference between HCFA-1500 and the UB92 forms is explained. Students recognize the importance of the medical assistant as a patient educator on office policies and procedures and related insurance issues.

SUPPLEMENTARY RESOURCES

Medical Assisting Videos: Appropriate content is available on Delmar's Medical Assisting Videos, 2nd edition, for the following topics:

Tape 4   Types of Reimbursement
          Analyze and Use Third Party Guidelines
          Responses from Insurers
          Dealing with Frequently Asked Questions from Patients

ANSWERS TO TEXT REVIEW QUESTIONS

1. a. not see any patient that does not have proof of Medicaid coverage
2. c. HCFA–1500 form
3. b. was created in 1965
4. d. 80 percent of UCR after $100 deductible
5. c. six
6. a. often require the provider to work exclusively for that organization
7. a. was created by Title 19 of the Social Security Act
8. d. stands for Civilian Health and Medical Program for Uniformed Services

ANSWERS TO TEXT CRITICAL THINKING QUESTIONS

1. Basic insurance makes payments on a base amount before a deductible is applied. This payment is often much less than the amount billed. Major medical insurance pays after a deductible amount is met. The insurance applies a percentage or coinsurance to the billing amount.
2. A copayment is a flat fee of $5 or $10 that is collected at each office visit from the patient. Coinsurance is the percentage (60 percent, 75 percent, 80 percent, or other) that is applied to the allowed charges before payment is made.

3. Children of undivorced parents covered under both parents' medical insurance policies are primarily covered under the parent's policy whose birthday falls earlier in the calendar year.

4. The four things to keep in mind when treating a patient are:
   • Is the patient covered by insurance?
   • Is this procedure covered by insurance?
   • Is the procedure being performed by the primary care provider?
   • Is a referral required for this procedure or visit?

5. The traditional approach is to pay for treatment of illness and injury, no coverage for preventive care, and income is based on fee for service. HMOs pay for preventive care as well as illness and injury, and income is based on capitation rather than fee for service.

6. Dr. Lewis will receive direct payment from Medicare on a schedule 5 percent, higher than that for physicians who do not accept assignment. Mrs. Johnson will owe only her deductible and the 20 percent that Medicare does not pay; Dr. Lewis will write off the remainder of the charge.

7. The patient will need a preauthorization, because he lives within the catchment zone.

ANSWERS TO WORKBOOK EXERCISES AND ACTIVITIES

Vocabulary Builder

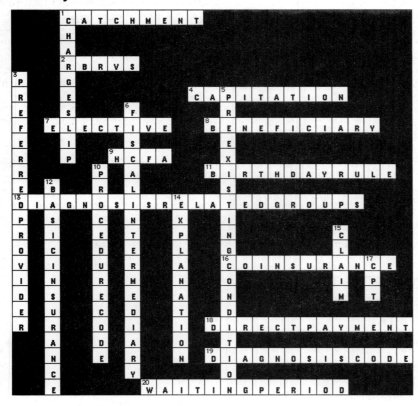

Learning Review

1. A. Is the patient covered by insurance?
   B. Is this procedure covered by the insurance?
   C. Is the primary care provider performing the procedure?
   D. Is a referral required? Is an authorization number or authorization code required?

2. A. Use PCPs or case managers.
   B. Utilize reauthorization for medical services, prospective and retrospective view of treatment plans, and significant discharge planning.
   C. Use specific treatment guidelines for high cost chronic disorders.
   D. Place emphasis on outpatient care versus hospitalization.
   E. Use a **drug formulary** or list of medications that may be prescribed without preapproval.
   F. Place emphases on health education and preventive care.

G. Place emphases on patient/family collaboration with health care providers to improve patient's compliance with treatment regimen.

H. Utilize selective contracting with all health care providers and institutions involved to achieve discounted rates.

3. A. Integrated delivery systems.

B. Health maintenance organizations.

C. Exclusive provider organizations.

D. Preferred provider organizations.

E. Physician-hospital organizations.

F. Utilization review organizations.

Multiple Choice Questions

1. d. all of the above
2. c. beneficiary
3. d. coordination of benefits

4. b. on the back of the insurance card
5. d. traditional insurance organization

Investigation Activity

Use this activity to encourage students to explore their own health care coverage and to gain further insight into the importance of being educated about one's own insurance policy's limits of coverage and allowable benefits. Students who are aware of the specifics of various types of medical insurance will be better patient educators about insurance issues and will also exhibit a higher degree of knowledge to apply when coding and processing patient claims in the ambulatory care setting.

ANSWERS TO WORKBOOK CASE STUDY QUESTIONS

1. The administrative medical assistant in the specialist's office can call the primary care physician to see whether it is possible to fax a completed referral form to the gastroenterologist's office for the follow-up appointment. However, all correct procedures outlined by the insurer must be observed. If referrals by fax are not accepted, the patient must schedule a new appointment or pay for the office visit herself.

2. The administrative medical assistant in the specialist's office could have prevented the misunderstanding by reminding Lourdes at the time she scheduled the follow-up appointment that a new referral form would be necessary. However, it is important to note that it is the patient's responsibility, not the health care provider's, to obtain proper referral forms. The medical assistant should be empathetic, compassionate, and polite to the patient and should strive to reach a resolution to the situation that follows office policies and procedures and also is as convenient as possible for the patient.

Chapter

19

Medical Insurance Coding

OVERVIEW

Medical assisting students are introduced to the important role of the medical assistant in performing duties related to medical insurance coding. Accurate coding saves time and avoids errors that may have an impact on both the physician's office and the patient. The ability is demonstrated to implement precise and accurate coding of diagnoses and procedures on insurance claim forms submitted to insurance carriers for patient treatment and care.

PROFICIENCY EVALUATION OUTCOME ASSESSMENT

Students are evaluated for their understanding of performance objectives. Students recognize the references used to perform coding of insurance claims and possess the ability to code claims efficiently and accurately. The use of computers in the claims process is described. Procedures for claims follow-up are understood.

SUPPLEMENTARY RESOURCES

Medical Assisting Videos: Appropriate content is available on Delmar's Medical Assisting Videos, 2nd edition, for the following topics:

Tape 4 Types of Reimbursement
Charge Slip
Implement Current Procedural Terminology
Common Problems in the Use of ICD-9 and CPT Manuals
Computerized Management of Reimbursement Systems

ANSWERS TO TEXT REVIEW QUESTIONS

1. b. have five digits and may have two-digit modifiers
2. c. Volume II of ICD-9-CM
3. c. procedure is an add-on to previously described procedure
4. a. uses a five-digit alphanumeric code to clarify procedures
5. d. code every disease, illness, condition, injury, and cause of injury known
6. b. HCFA-1500
7. c. monitor claims that have been sent to insurance companies for processing
8. c. refers to incidents or practices of providers, physicians, or suppliers of services and equipment that are inconsistent with accepted sound medical, business, or fiscal practices

ANSWERS TO TEXT CRITICAL THINKING QUESTIONS

1. The HCFA-1500 claim form developed by the Health Care Financing Administration is the form most commonly accepted by insurance companies.
2. ICD-9-CM, *International Classification of Diseases, 9th Revision, Clinical Modification*, is used to code a diagnosis. To code a diagnosis use Volume II first (alphabetical index), then check your answer in Volume I (numerical index).
3. CPT-9, *Current Procedural Terminology*, should be referenced when coding office visits and procedures.
4. When coding a claim:
   • Be as precise as possible.
   • Do not guess.
   • Do not code what is not there.
5. Accident-related charges should first be billed to the company handling the accident exposure. This could be Worker's Compensation or the State Industrial Fund on on-the-job injuries, auto insurance or homeowners insurance for private injuries, or business liability insurance for premises injuries.

ANSWERS TO WORKBOOK EXERCISES AND ACTIVITIES

Vocabulary Builder

1. Breach of confidentiality: unauthorized release of confidential patient information to a third party.
2. Charge slip: form used to record services supplied and charges and payments for those services; functions as billing form for insurance reimbursement.
3. Claim: demand for payment; in this case it is a demand by the beneficiary to the insurance company for payment of medical expenses incurred during the effective dates of the medical policy.
4. Current Procedural Terminology (CPT): standard codes for procedures and services. Used by most ambulatory care settings in encoding the claim form and recognized by most insurance carriers.
5. E code: ICD-9-CM codes for the external causes of injury, poisoning, or other adverse reactions that explain how the injury occurred.
6. Explanation of benefits (EOB): insurance report that is sent with claim payments explaining the reimbursement of the insurance carrier.
7. Fraud: deliberate misrepresentation of facts.
8. HCFA Common Procedure Coding System (HCPCS): standardized coding system used to process Medicare claims on a national basis.
9. Insurance abuse: incidents or misrepresentations that are inconsistent with acceptable practice of medicine, which lead to improper reimbursement treatment that is not medically necessary for a disorder.
10. International Classification of Diseases, 9th Revision, Clinical Modification (ICD-9-CM): standard diagnosis codes used to identify a patient's medical problem. Used by most ambulatory care settings in encoding the claim form and recognized by most insurance carriers.
11. Point-of-service (POS): device allowing direct communication between a medical office and the health care plan's computer.
12. Subrogation: right of an insurer to collect monies it has paid out on behalf of its insured from another party.
13. Superbill: billing the patient receives from the physician at the time of service delineating the visit, tests,
14. Uniform Bill 92 (UB92): unique billing form used extensively by acute care facilities for processing inpatient and outpatient claims.
15. U codes: ICD-9-CM codes representing either factors that influence a person's health status or legitimate reasons for contacting the health facility when the patient has no definite diagnosis or active symptoms of any disorder.

Learning Review

1. A. 1. Evaluation and Management
      2. Anesthesia
      3. Surgery
      4. Radiology, Nuclear Medicine, and Diagnostic Ultrasound
      5. Pathology and Laboratory
      6. Medicine
      7. Index
   B. 1. code: 96410   section: Medicine
      2. code: 86291   section: Pathology and Laboratory
      3. code: 12004   section: Surgery
      4. code: 93000   section: Medicine
      5. code: 75889   section: Radiology, Nuclear Medicine, and Ultrasound
      6. code: 86293   section: Pathology and Laboratory
      7. code: 01202   section: Anesthesia

2. A. Volume I, Tabular List, contains all the codes in numerical order. This volume is the second place that is referred to when coding a diagnosis.

   Volume II, Alphabetic Index, contains all possible diagnoses, including symptoms, accidents and their causes, and concurrent diagnoses. This volume also contains a table of drugs and chemicals and a list of external causes for injuries. This volume is the first place that is referred to when coding a diagnosis.

   Volume III, Procedures: Tabular List and Alphabetic Index, includes procedures used. The procedure codes of the CPT are more commonly used in the United States and are accepted by all the insurance companies. When unable to find a correct procedure code in the CPT, this volume of the ICD-9-CM contains information that can be useful in helping to identify the procedure in the CPT.

   B. Volume II; 730. 27; External causes; 278.0; Supplementary Classification of Factors Influencing Health Status and Contact with Health Services.

3. Three far-reaching effects on physicians and patients caused by insurance coding errors include, but are not limited to:

   (1) If an error is made in coding, the insurance company will downcode, paying the lesser of the two amounts in question according to the physician's fee profile.

   (2) If an incorrect code is used, that incorrectly coded diagnosis will stay with the patient and may affect future coverage for the insured.

   (3) Incorrect coding can be a problem with ruling out a diagnosis. Until a diagnosis is confirmed, code according to patient symptoms.

4. The chart is completed as follows:

1.	CPT	code 99050	PE
2.	ICD	code 977.9	incorrect medication administered may cause adverse or toxic reaction
3.	ICD	code 307.1	eating disorder characterized by severe loss and distorted body image
4.	CPT	code 32420	DP
5.	ICD	code 250.1	high levels of ketones in the body, associated diabetes mellitus
6.	CPT	code 81015	LAB
7.	ICD	code 306.8	grinding of the teeth
8.	ICD	code 136.3	parasitic infection of the lungs, an opportunistic infection seen in patients with lowered immune response, such as AIDS
9.	CPT	code 59000	DP
10.	ICD	code 075	virus that causes infectious mononucleosis
11.	CPT	code 97116	RM
12.	CPT	code 99075	LEG
13.	ICD	code V06.1	PM
14.	CPT	code 90782	MA
15.	ICD	code 760.72	harmful effects of controlled substances on fetus during pregnancy

Multiple Choice Questions

1. a. HCFA 1500
2. c. V codes
3. b. capitation
4. a. hospice care
5. b. point of service

Investigation Activity

In exploring the various types of coverage available to health care consumers, encourage students to explore the ethical issues involved in insurance issues. Some examples include: Does an insurer have the right to deny coverage for a specific treatment, drug, or surgery? who determines whether a treatment, drug, or surgery is experimental? should insurers have the right to use the results of genetic tests to determine insurance coverage for individuals? should every American have a legal right to a basic standard of medical care? and if so, who sets the standard?

ANSWERS TO WORKBOOK CASE STUDY QUESTIONS

1.	colonoscopy with biopsy, single or multiple	45380
	flex sig (colon)	211.3
	family history, malignant neoplasm GI tract	V16.0
	personal history, malignant neoplasm, breast	V10.3
	low complexity office visit	99213

Chapter 20

Billing and Collections

OVERVIEW

Medical assisting students discover the importance of maintaining healthy accounts receivable and collection ratios to the financial well-being of the ambulatory care setting. Medical assistants play an important role in the patient billing and collection practices, a role that requires excellent administrative skills as well as excellent communications skills. Students are introduced to the ethical and legal issues involved in the collection process and are reminded that respect for the patient as a health care consumer is mandatory.

PROFICIENCY EVALUATION OUTCOME ASSESSMENT

Students are evaluated on their knowledge of performance objectives. Demonstrating a knowledge of billing and collection processes and techniques, students recognize the importance of accurate documentation and compliance with all applicable laws and regulations. Students explore the ethics of debt collection and also explore the potential emotionality of telephone collection calls, emphasizing the need for professional behavior at all times. The balance of a healthy accounts receivable and cash flow for the medical practice with the equal satisfaction of patients, who are health care consumers, is recognized as the goal of the billing and collection processes.

SUPPLEMENTARY RESOURCES

Medical Assisting Videos: Appropriate content is available on Delmar's Medical Assisting Videos, 2nd ed., for the following topics:

Tape 3   Billing Cycle and Collections
Tape 4   Charge Slip
         Computerized Management of Reimbursement Systems
         Dealing with Frequently Asked Questions from Patients

ANSWERS TO TEXT REVIEW QUESTIONS

1. c. is also known as the Truth-in-Lending Act
2. d. in which accounts are divided alphabetically for billing purposes
3. a. inability to pay because of financial hardship
4. a. is a process of identifying overdue patient accounts
5. b. the medical office is still responsible for collecting even if the court finds in its favor
6. a. provides information about a patient's credit history
7. d. b and c above
8. b. those who are unwilling to pay
9. c. one who moves without a forwarding address and leaves an unpaid bill
10. d. 90 days

ANSWERS TO TEXT CRITICAL THINKING QUESTIONS

1. In the ambulatory care setting, patient billing is a critical administrative function that helps maintain a healthy, viable practice. Timeliness is essential in billing, for the ambulatory care setting depends on its accounts receivables to pay its bills in a responsible manner. Cash flow and the setting's financial status are also determined by a conscientious collection process. A patient who sees organization and competence in the billing process sees that in the medical care also.

2. Even uncomplicated patient billing should be done according to credit and collection policies established by the physician-employers of the ambulatory care setting. A formalized policy makes decision-making easier and gives the medical assistant who is responsible for billing and collections the authority to act. Some of the issues the physicians and office manager may want to address include:
   - When will payment be due from the patient?
   - What kind of payment arrangements can be made if the patient does not pay at the time of service?
   - Will a collection agency be utilized? Who decides?
   - At what point should a patient be reminded of an overdue bill?
   - How is that reminder initially managed: by telephone or letter?
   - At what point will a patient bill be considered delinquent?
   - If exceptions to office policy are to be made, who makes those exceptions?

3. Because the best opportunity for collection is at the time of service, many ambulatory care settings provide the patient with a bill and require payment at that time. This ensures prompt collection, eliminates further bookkeeping work, and provides better cash flow for the practice. It is important to note that payment at time of service will be adjusted according to the patient's insurance and the terms of that policy. If the patient is a member of an HMO and the ambulatory care center is a participating provider, the ambulatory care center is bound to the terms of the agreement with the HMO.

4. Statements to patients must be professional in appearance, neat, accurate, and inclusive of all services and charges. If the statement is to be mailed, an enclosed self-addressed envelope is a convenience for many patients and may result in a faster turnaround of payment. The charge slip (also known as superbill), statement, and insurance reporting information are often combined on one form. A well-prepared patient statement should contain not only information for the patient but information needed to process medical insurance claims.
   - Patient's name and address.
   - Patient's insurance identification number.
   - Insurance carrier.
   - Date of service.
   - Description of service.
   - Accurate procedure (CPT) and diagnosis (ICD-9-CM) codes for insurance processing.
   - Physician's signature.
   - Ambulatory care center name, address, telephone number, and possibly the fax number

5. Monthly billing, a system in which all accounts are billed at the same time, is an efficient method of billing for the smaller ambulatory care setting. One or two days are devoted to billing and mailing statements. A major disadvantage of monthly billing is that other activities may be neglected during those one or two days. Cycle billing, a system that staggers billing during the month, is a flexible system for the large practice. In cycle billing, accounts are divided alphabetically into groups and each group is billed at a different time. They can be mailed as completed or all groups can be held and mailed at one time. This is an efficient system with few disadvantages; the one disadvantage may be the billing task "never seems done."

6. Account aging is a method of identifying how long an account is overdue. A typical aging process for a private client is shown in textbook Figure 20-3.

7. The student should write three collection letters, based on textbook Figures 20-4A, B, C. Names and the patient who is presenting a problem can be drawn from Inner City Health Care Center or Drs. Lewis & King at the Northborough Family Medical Group. Although the letters can vary, the first one should gently alert the patient that the bill is three months' overdue and ask for a call or an immediate payment; the second should describe the situation the patient was presented with at the medical setting, ask for payment, and indicate that the unpaid amount can no longer be kept on the books; and the last letter should state that this is a final attempt at collection of a six-month-old bill and that the account is being assigned to a collection service.

8. The student may select a patient from one of the two ambulatory care settings used in the text or may invent their own situation. The student role-playing the medical assistant should follow legal and ethical rules for telephone collections, including
   - Identifying themselves.
   - Ascertaining that they are speaking to the correct party.
   - Avoiding making calls to a place of employment.
   - Calling only during stated hours (typically 8:00 A.M. to 9:00 P.M.).
   - Maintaining a professional tone.
   - Avoiding the use of threats or any conduct that can be construed as harassment.
   - Keeping written records of the telephone transaction.

9. The students should use the criteria described in question 8 to evaluate the professionalism of the call. Any subjective remarks regarding tone of voice, and so on, can also be noted.

10. Students may have very strong feelings about whether it is ethical to ever use collection techniques. Using some of the discussion in this chapter, and drawing on their own personal judgments, students should take a position for or against collections and defend their points of view. At the conclusion, students may list all of the points for and against collections and present them to the other small groups, comparing notes.

ANSWERS TO WORKBOOK EXERCISES AND ACTIVITIES

Vocabulary Builder

1. C.
2. A.
3. D.
4. G.
5. F.
6. B.
7. E.

Learning Review

1. Five pieces of data are the previous month's billing backlog, the number of new accounts, the number of processed accounts, the weekly number of accounts that were rebilled, and amount of time billing personnel spent on billing accounts.

2. The three most common reasons patient accounts become overdue are
   (1) Inability to pay due to temporary financial hardships.
   (2) Negligence. People may forget to make a payment or miss a payment due to a vacation, business trip, or family emergency.
   (3) Unwillingness to pay. Patients may be dissatisfied with care or treatment. These patients should be referred to the office manager or physician.

3. A. In the pegboard system, the method used to identify the age of accounts is the placement of colored strips on the ledger cards to show the age of an account—for example, a red strip may indicate one month overdue, a blue strip may indicate three months' overdue, and so on.
   Or, the ledger cards for overdue accounts may be placed behind a color-coded divider in a separate file labeled "Unpaid."
   B. Overdue notice No. 2, mailed April 1.
   C. Five criteria are past due balance, zero balance, credit balance, government agency category (such as Medicare or Medicaid), and insurance carrier.
   D. Three pieces of information included on accounts receivable reports are a listing of each overdue account, the balance overdue for each, and how long each account has been overdue.

4. The two services provided by credit bureaus are:
   (1) To provide an intercept letter. For a nominal fee, the collection agency will send a letter requesting payment before the account is formally turned over for collection.
   (2) To provide credit ratings of patients at the physician's request. This service allows a practice to monitor patients' abilities to pay their bills, as well as to trace a "skip," a patient who leaves with an outstanding balance and no forwarding address.

5. Responsible actions for collecting from estates or representatives of a deceased patient are A, C, and D.

6. Three actions to trace "skips" include
   (1) Determining if there were internal errors in addressing the envelope.
   (2) Calling the patient at the telephone number listed on the ledger card to obtain a possible forwarding telephone number or reach the patient directly if the same telephone number has been retained.
   (3) Turning the overdue account over to a collection agency.

7. Three classes of accounts are open book accounts, which may have periodic charges against them; written contracts; and single-entry accounts, which only have one charge against them.

Multiple Choice Questions

1. b. scheduling first appointment
2. a. Consumer Credit Protection Act
3. b. superbill
4. c. accounts receivable ratio
5. d. the value of the dollar owed decreases rapidly

Investigation Activity

Use this activity in coordination with the text critical thinking questions 8 and 9 to explore the delicate nature of telephone collection calls. Medical assisting students may be reluctant to speak to patients about overdue balances and feel uncomfortable about speaking with aggressive or emotionally distraught individuals. Maintaining a professional viewpoint, while remaining courteous and empathetic to the patient, can be difficult when the patient's response is emotional and often unpredictable. Patients must be respected as health care consumers; however, the medical practice has the right to demand payment for services rendered in good faith. This exercise gives students the opportunity to explore the emotions involved in telephone collection calls from both the medical assistant's and the patient's perspectives.

ANSWERS TO WORKBOOK CASE STUDY QUESTIONS

7.1	Williams, C.		SERVICE CODE	345:00	345:00	ADJ.	00 ←		00 ←	Ellen Armstrong, CMA	02882
DATE	PATIENT		SERVICE CODE	FEES CHARGE	PAID		BALANCE DUE		PREVIOUS BALANCE	NAME	RECEIPT NO.
					CREDITS						

THIS IS YOUR RECEIPT _____▲
AND/OR A STATEMENT OF YOUR ACCOUNT TO DATE _____▲

PATIENTS NAME   Charles Williams   ☒ M ☐ F
ADDRESS   123 Greenside St.
CITY Northborough   STATE OH   ZIP 12346
RELATIONSHIP self   BIRTHDATE 7/6/xxxx
SUBSCRIBER OR POLICY HOLDER   employer: High Tech Computing Group
☐ MEDICARE ☐ MEDICAID ☐ BLUE SHIELD ☐ 65-SP.
INSURANCE CARRIER   All American
AGREEMENT #   112-45-9980
GROUP #   333210

		OFFICE VISITS AND PROCEDURES					
99211	EST PT - MINIMAL OV	1		HOSPITAL VISIT	14		
99212	EST PT - BRIEF OV	2		EMERGENCY	15		
99213	EST PT - INTERMEDIATE OV	3		CONSULTATION	16		
99214	EST PT - EXTENDED OV	4	93000	EKG	17	75	
99215	EST PT - COMPREHENSIVE OV	5	93224	ELECTROCARDIOGRAPHIC MONITORING	18		
99201	NEW PT - BRIEF OV	6	93307	ECHOCARDIOGRAPHY	19		
99202	NEW PT - INTERMEDIATE OV	7	85025	CBC	20	20	
99203	NEW PT - EXTENDED OV	8	81000	URINALYSIS WITH MICROSCOPY	21	25	
99204	NEW PT - COMPLEX OV	9	36415	ROUTINE VENIPUNCTURE	22	25	
99205	NEW PT - COMPREHENSIVE OF	10	71020	RADIOLOGY EXAM-CHEST-2 VIEWS	23	200	
99238	HOSPITAL DISCHARGE	11	30300	REMOVE FOR. BODY-INTRANASAL	24		
99025	NEW PT - SURGERY PROC. PRIMARY	12			25		
	NURSING HOME VISIT	13			26		

D - OTHER SERVICES

AUTHORIZATION TO RELEASE INFORMATION: I HEREBY AUTHORIZE THE UNDERSIGNED PHYSICIAN TO RELEASE ANY INFORMATION ACQUIRED IN THE COURSE OF MY EXAMINATION OR TREATMENT.
SIGNED (PATIENT, OR PARENT IF MINOR)
X Charles Williams   DATE 7/1/XXXX

NEXT APPOINTMENT 7/8   AT 1:00   AM (PM)
RETURN _____ DAYS 1 (WEEKS) _____ MONTHS

PLACE OF SERVICE   ☒ OFFICE ☐ OTHER _____
DIAGNOSIS OR SYMPTOMS   intermittent, irregular heartbeat or palpitations, dizziness, chest pain

DOCTOR'S SIGNATURE   X Dr. Winston Lewis

L&K   **LEWIS & KING, MD**
2501 CENTER STREET
NORTHBOROUGH, OH 12345

02882

Figure 20-1

Chapter

21

Accounting Practices

OVERVIEW

Medical assisting students are instructed on the basics of accounting practices and the importance of managing finances in the ambulatory care setting. It is important for those medical assistants not directly involved in financial management to understand the need for sound financial practices in ensuring the profitability of the medical practice or facility. Students will also gain an understanding of the impact of utilization review on reimbursement procedures and the interaction between data management and computerized accounting environments.

PROFICIENCY EVALUATION OUTCOME ASSESSMENT

Students are evaluated for their knowledge of performance objectives. They should have a basic understanding of accounting practices. Students learn how the performance of accounting functions fits into an overall medical financial management system and consider accounting and bookkeeping systems, computerization, financial records, fixed and variable costs, and utilization review. Students recognize the importance of accounting and financial management to the success of the ambulatory care setting and discover the impact of financial decision making on the daily operations of a medical practice or facility.

SUPPLEMENTARY RESOURCES

Medical Assisting Videos: Appropriate content is available on Delmar's Medical Assisting Videos, 2nd ed., Tape 3, for the following topics:

> Perform Administrative Duties
> Use Manual Bookkeeping Systems
> Billing Cycle and Collection
> Electronic Banking

ANSWERS TO TEXT REVIEW QUESTIONS

1. b. pegboard
2. c. depreciation of equipment
3. b. balance sheet
4. b. W-4
5. c. is a review of a procedure or treatment before it is performed to determine whether it is needed by the patient
6. d. all of the above
7. d. b and c above
8. c. should be almost 85%
9. d. a and b above

ANSWERS TO TEXTBOOK CRITICAL THINKING QUESTIONS

1. Medical financial management is important in the daily functioning of the ambulatory care setting, for it directly affects bookkeeping and accounting procedures. It also provides financial information for key decision making.

2. Single-entry bookkeeping has been used in the physician's office for many years and includes a daily journal, patients' statements, ledgers, checks, and disbursement and expenditure records. It is a simple and inexpensive system to maintain. However, it is difficult to find errors when they occur because the system has no internal controls.

3. An on-site computer system gives the ambulatory care setting a great deal of control over bookkeeping and accounting functions. Patient confidentiality is easier to ensure and staff become thoroughly familiar with patient accounts. However, the startup costs and time may be significant; also, certain staff will need to become very adept to fully use the computer's capabilities.

   A computer service bureau offers ambulatory care settings flexibility and the option to computerize accounts without the investment in staff training and equipment. These bureaus often employ computer professionals who know how to get the most from a software program. However, the ambulatory care setting may sacrifice control and worry regarding patient confidentiality.

4. Fixed costs are those that do not vary in total as the number of patients vary. For example, annual depreciation cost of equipment is fixed because it will stay the same regardless of the number of patients who use it. Variable costs are those that vary in direct proportion to patient volume. These include expenses such as clinical supplies and laboratory procedures.

5. Financial records reflect the daily operations of the practice, providing data for use in preparing reports, making decisions, and managing the practice. Income statements show the cumulative profit and total expenses for the month. The statement is itemized to show operating expenses and employees' withholding taxes and retirement contributions. The income statement enables the practice to monitor increases and decreases easily. The balance sheet is an itemized statement of the assets, liabilities, and owner's equity. It is sometimes called the statement of financial condition or financial position. It is made possible through the double-entry system of accounting, because every transaction is recorded by two sets of entries made in a ledger or journal. Increases in assets are recorded as debits; decreases are recorded as credits. Increases in liabilities and owner's equity are recorded as credits; decreases are recorded as debits. Debit and credit entries to one or more accounts make up the system. In any recording, the total dollar amount of the debit entries must equal the total dollar amount of the credit entries. Each ledger or journal entry should have the following:
   * Date of transaction.
   * Journal or ledger account names involved.
   * Dollar amount of the charges.
   * Brief explanation of the transaction.

6. There are a few financial ratios that can help evaluate how the practice is doing. Data from the current year and previous year's financial statements can be converted into ratios to highlight different financial characteristics. Ratios should always be viewed in relationship to the total financial picture, however. Three useful ratios include the accounts receivable ratio, collection ratio, and cost ratio.

7. *Accounts Receivable Ratio.* The accounts receivable (A/R) ratio formula measures the speed in which outstanding accounts are paid. The accounts receivable ratio provides a picture of the state of collections and probable losses. The longer an account is past due, the less likely a successful collection will be made.

   Total accounts Receivable ÷ Monthly Receipts = Turnaround Time (in months)

   Example:
   $120,000 ÷ $60,000 = 2 months' Turnaround Time for payment on an account

   The goal of an efficient billing and collecting policy should be a turnaround time of 2 months or less.

   Collection Ratio. The collection ratio shows the percentage of outstanding debt collected. The goal should be a 90 percent collection ratio. Total receipts divided by total charges give the unadjusted collection ratio, but adjustments may include federal and state insurance programs (Medicare and Medicaid, Worker's Compensation), managed care adjustments, and any other adjustments as directed by the physician.

Unadjusted Total Receipts	$40,000
Managed Care Adjustments	$3,000
Medicare Adjustments	$2,000
TOTAL RECEIPTS	$45,000

   Total Charges = $52,000

   Total Receipts ÷ Total Charges = Collection Ratio after Adjustments
   $45,000 ÷ $52,000 = 86.5% Collection Ratio after Adjustments

Cost Ratio. This cost ratio formula shows the cost of a procedure or service and can help in determining, for instance, the cost-effectiveness of maintaining a laboratory in the ambulatory care setting. The ratio is:

Total Expenses ÷ Total Number of Procedures for 1 month = Cost per Procedure
$48,000 ÷ 240 = $200 per Procedure

A conclusion might be reached that the laboratory is too costly because each procedure is not billed at $200.

8. Utilization review is an analysis of the service required before it may be performed. If it is determined that the procedure is not necessary, it will not be approved for financial reimbursement to the facility.

ANSWERS TO WORKBOOK EXERCISES AND ACTIVITIES

Vocabulary Builder

1. I.	6. K.	10. C.	14. G.
2. M.	7. P.	11. H.	15. N.
3. D.	8. E.	12. A.	16. Q.
4. L.	9. O.	13. J.	17. B.
5. F.			

Learning Review

1. Three manual bookkeeping systems are single entry (B), pegboard or write-it-once (C), and double-entry (A).
2. A. Procedure codes (CPT) and diagnostic codes (ICD-9-CM).
   B. (1) Billing statements, (2) insurance forms, (3) collection letters, (4) financial statements and ratios.
3. Three ways computer service bureaus handle accounts from medical facilities are
   (1) Through the office's own terminal. On-line sharing occurs when the office is tied directly to the bureau's mainframe computer.
   (2) Through on-line servicing. The office has its own terminal that allows direct communication with the service bureau's computer.
   (3) Through off-line batch processing. The medical assistant or bookkeeper sends daily batches of data to the bureau to process.
4. Five points to consider are
   (1) Computerization will require more time than estimated.
   (2) The paper-pencil bookkeeping system will have to be maintained concurrently for a period of time.
   (3) A poorly managed paper-pencil system will not be made better by computerization.
   (4) Adequate on-site computer training for all staff is essential.
   (5) Notify patients of the move to a computer system and the changes that will occur.
5. A.
1. VC.	6. FC.	11. VC.	
2. FC.	7. FC.	12. FC.	
3. VC.	8. VC.	13. FC.	
4. VC.	9. FC.	14. VC.	
5. FC.	10. VC.	15. VC.	

   B. Calculating and reviewing costs provides data to (1) set fees, (2) market the practice, (3) determine profit, and (4) monitor the practice's performance.
6. Four items included are (1) date of transaction, (2) journal or ledger account names involved, (3) dollar amount of the charges, and (4) a brief explanation of the transaction.
7. The correct accounts receivable ratios are May = 1.3, June = 2.65, July = 4.3, August = 2.1. May has the healthiest ratio because the most efficient billing and collection policy considers a turnaround time of 2 months or less as most desirable.
8. A. The collection ratio for September is 77.8%.
   B. The collection ratio for October is 88%.
   C. October has the more desirable collection ratio because the goal for a healthy collection ratio is 90% of the outstanding debt collected.
9. A. The average cost for the mammogram procedure is $150 using the cost ratio formula.
   B. The practice makes a profit of $35 per mammogram procedure or $7,000 profit each month based on an average of 200 procedures per month.

10. A.

Office Expenses	January	February	March	Year-to-Date	Budget for Year
Office supplies	$1,200.62	$325.45	$446.26	$1,972.33	$8,000.00
Postage	$725.45	$550.90	$601.33	$1,877.68	$8,000.00
Telephone	$323.46	$425.93	$393.87	$1,143.26	$4,000.00
TOTALS	$2,249.53	$1,302.28	$1,441.46	$4,993.27	$20,000.00

B. The office is $6.73 under the quarterly office expense budget of $5,000. The office manager can use data to determine whether telephone, postage, and office supply expenses are on target or need to be managed in some other way. It is important to establish and track budgets to control spending, determine the efficiency of the expense category, and forecast future spending.

Multiple Choice Questions

1. d. equity
2. a. financial accounting
3. c. depreciation

4. b. journals
5. d. a and b

Investigation Activity

Use this investigation activity to encourage students to relate their own financial opinions, practices, and habits to the process of financial management in the ambulatory care setting. As a class, discuss how attitudes about money and finances can shape the success or failure of a professional environment. Students discover why financially responsible accounting practices are integral to the successful operation of the ambulatory care setting. A medical practice that functions under sound accounting practices fosters a high quality of patient care and efficient operation, earning the trust and respect of patients who are, in fact, health care consumers.

ANSWERS TO WORKBOOK CASE STUDY QUESTIONS

1. The physician-owners will collect financial data and compare these data to the figures established in the financial analysis and projection.
2. The physician-owners will look to see whether revenues and profits are sufficient to sustain the new staff and what resources are required to meet the increased patient load. Decisions about specific aspects of the practice's daily operations, such as maintaining the proper inventory of clinical supplies, will depend on whether the numbers are working or not. The physician-owners will look for solutions to any potential problem areas in the budget.
3. An additional clinical medical assistant means that more clinical office procedures may be performed, facility hours may be expanded, and the number of patients seen may be increased. Patient scheduling, using the double-booking method, for example, can become more sophisticated as an expanded staff can simultaneously perform different duties related to patient care.

Chapter 22

Infection Control, Medical Asepsis, and Sterilization

OVERVIEW

The principles and practices of infection control are critical to creating and maintaining a safe environment for patients, health care professionals, and visitors in an ambulatory care setting. Medical assistants who are in contact with patients and participate in medical and surgical procedures in the course of their workday must observe infection control techniques to achieve medical and surgical asepsis. Medical assisting students are presented with the underlying theories of infection control, including principles of immunity, classifications of infectious agents, and related means of transmission and symptoms. Students learn how to sanitize, disinfect, and sterilize instruments and equipment frequently used in the ambulatory care setting. Quality control and maintenance procedures are stressed as being equally important aspects of maintaining proper infection control standards.

PROFICIENCY EVALUATION OUTCOME ASSESSMENT

Students are evaluated for their knowledge of performance objectives. They will identify key glossary terms as well as understand the importance of maintaining adequate infection control in an ambulatory care setting and will demonstrate an understanding of the origin, classification, stages, transmission, and symptoms of infectious diseases. Students should acquire knowledge of the role the immune system plays in preventing and fighting disease and the role vaccines play in preventing certain infectious diseases. Students will become proficient in carrying out critical infection control procedures, including medical and surgical asepsis, instrument sterilization techniques, and instrument wrapping methods for sterilization. An understanding of quality control and maintenance of equipment is demonstrated. Students also become aware of their role as patient educators on the subject of proper infection control techniques that individuals can use to reduce or prevent the spread of infectious disease in the home, workplace, or other daily living environment.

SUPPLEMENTARY RESOURCES

Medical Assisting Videos: Appropriate content is available on Delmar's Medical Assisting Videos, 2nd ed., Tape 5, on the following topics:

Standard Precautions
Perform Medical Aseptic Procedure of Handwashing
Use Disposable Single-Contact Gloves (Putting On and Removing)

Personal Protective Equipment
Perform Medical Aseptic Procedures
Ultrasound Cleaners
Wrap and Autoclave an Article
Perform Surgical Aseptic Procedures

ANSWERS TO TEXT REVIEW QUESTIONS

1. a. hepatitis B (HBV)
2. b. CDC
3. a. reducing the transmission of HIV and hepatitis B infections
4. a. reservoir
5. b. prodromal stage
6. b. steam sterilization

ANSWERS TO TEXT CRITICAL THINKING QUESTIONS

1. Infection control in the health care setting greatly reduces the transmission of infectious diseases and ensures a clinical environment that is as safe as possible for employees, patients, and families. Infection control can be achieved through medical and surgical asepsis and by observation of all standard precautions. For instance, in the ambulatory care setting, the medical assistant, among other actions, would be sure to: (1) wash hands, (2) disinfect surfaces, (3) properly dispose of contaminated items in biohazard containers, (4) use gloves for certain procedures, and (5) sanitize instruments.

2. Each step or link in the chain of infection is necessary in order for infectious diseases to spread. Infection control is based on the fact that the transmission of infectious diseases will be prevented when any link is broken or interrupted. These links or steps include the following:
    1. *Infectious agent.* Microorganisms, which are grouped into five classifications: viruses, bacteria, fungi, parasites, and rickettsiae.
    2. *Reservoir.* The location of the infectious agent, which may include people, equipment, supplies, water, food, animals, or insects.
    3. *Portal of exit.* The method by which the infectious agent leaves the reservoir, such as through body fluids.
    4. *Means of transmission.* Ways in which microorganisms travel from the reservoir to a susceptible host, including direct contact, airborne transmission, bloodborne transmission, ingestion, and indirect contact.
    5. *Portal of entry.* Allows the infectious agent access to another person. Common entrance sites include broken skin; mucous membranes; and the respiratory, gastrointestinal, and reproductive systems.
    6. *Susceptible host.* A person who is able to contract the pathogenic organism and is not immune or resistant to the organism.

3. The five classifications of infectious agents are viruses, bacteria, fungi, parasites, and rickettsiae. The student should identify and describe four of these five.
    *   Viruses are pathogens that require a living cell for reproduction and activity. Because they live inside cells, they are protected against agents such as chemical disinfectants. To survive, viruses change characteristics over time and adapt to their environment. Viral infections have only a few pharmacological treatment agents, most of which are palliative.
    *   Bacteria are single-celled microorganisms that live in tissues rather than cells. They are identified by characteristic shapes. Three classifications of bacteria are cocci, bacilli, and spirilla. Bacteria are either pathogenic or nonpathogenic.
    *   Fungi are microorganisms that may be single celled or multicelled. Mushrooms and molds are examples of nonpathogenic fungi. Pathogenic fungi cause infections such as athlete's foot, ringworm, and candida.
    *   Parasites are organisms that live in or on another organism. These may be single celled or multicelled and include protozoa, metazoa, and ectoparasites. These organisms cause a range of infections such as malaria, trichomoniasis, pinworms, and tapeworms.
    *   Rickettsiae are intracellular parasites similar to viruses. However, they are larger than viruses and susceptible to antibiotic therapy. Examples of rickettsiae infections include Lyme disease and Rocky Mountain spotted fever.

4. Sanitization is physically cleaning and scrubbing to remove contaminated debris. Sanitization of instruments and equipment is needed to rid contaminated reusable instruments of tissue, debris, blood, secretions, excretions, and other contaminants.

5. Several materials are available for wrapping surgical instruments and other surgical and medical items before placing them in the autoclave. (1) Muslin is a reusable cloth wrap that is cost-effective. However, one cannot view the items through the wrap and must be vigilant about inspecting the cloth for holes and tears. (2) Paper sterilization wrapping squares are available in different sizes and types. Because these are disposable, a new paper must be used

each time, but the need for laundering is eliminated. Paper wraps are also opaque, so that viewing the contents is impossible. (3) Sterilization pouches or bags may be plastic or paper or a combination of both. They are inexpensive, easy to use, and no wrapping is involved. Items inside are visible. These bags are probably the preferred method for most medical offices today.

6. The following body fluids are considered to be biohazardous: blood, vaginal secretions, cerebral spinal fluid, synovial fluid, pleural fluid, peritoneal fluid, amniotic fluid, pericardial fluid, and saliva. Medical assistants can become exposed to blood and body fluids any time while taking care of their patients.

7. Needlesticks can occur by accidentally sticking oneself with a used needle after performing an invasive procedure such as injections or venipuncture. Studies have shown that a needlestick contaminated with HBV has a much greater incidence of transmission of the virus than does a needlestick that is contaminated with HIV.

8. Infectious waste is described as any items that have come into contact with patients' blood or body fluids. Infectious waste must be incinerated or subjected to sterilization, as in an autoclave, before disposal in a sanitary landfill.

9. The purpose of OSHA's standard for bloodborne pathogens is to reduce occupational-related causes of HIV and HBV infections among health care workers. It covers all employees "reasonably anticipated" to come into contact with, as a result of performing their job duties, blood and OPIM. It seeks to limit exposure to pathogens.

10. Employers must provide PPE at no cost to the employee. PPE is used to place a barrier between the employee and blood and/or OPIM that can contaminate the skin, mucous membranes, or nonintact skin. PPE consists of such items as latex gloves, masks, goggles, face shields, gowns, laboratory coats, and plastic mouthpieces used during cardiopulmonary resuscitation. PPE provides protection only if it prevents blood or OPIM from permeating through it onto clothes, eyes, skin, mouth, or other mucous membranes. The employer must be certain that PPE is available and accessible and provide an alternative type of glove if an employee is allergic to those originally provided.

Cleaning and laundering and disposal of PPE are the responsibility of the employer and the employee does not incur any expense for such. All PPE must be removed before the employee leaves his or her work site and placed in an appropriate container, which is supplied by the employer. Gloves must be worn when there is a possibility of hand contact with blood or OPIM, with mucous membranes and nonintact skin, and when performing such procedures as phlebotomy. Disposable gloves cannot be decontaminated. They must be discarded into a biohazard container used for regulated waste. Masks, face shields, and goggles must be worn if there is a possibility of splashing or splattering of blood or OPIM.

Gowns, laboratory coats, and other clothing must be worn to protect against exposure and must be left at the work site in an area set aside for their storage.

ANSWERS TO WORKBOOK EXERCISES AND ACTIVITIES

Vocabulary Builder

A. Key terms are inserted into the paragraphs in the following order: epidemiology, microorganisms, infection control, transmission, medical asepsis, surgical asepsis, contaminated, excoriated, and sanitization.

B.
1. Trichomoniasis
2. Scabies
3. Palliative
4. Infectious agent
5. Amoebic dysentery
6. Bloodborne pathogen
7. Malaria
8. Fomites
9. Pathogen

C.
1. Resistance: the ability of the immune system to resist or withstand an infectious disease.
2. Vaccine: a pharmacologic agent capable of producing artificial immunity.
3. Antibody: specific chemicals produced by B cells of the immune system in response to an antigen.
4. Immunoglobulins: antibodies produced by the cells of the immune system.
5. Immunity: ability of the body to resist specific pathogens and their toxins.
6. Disinfection: chemical destruction of most harmful microorganisms but not their spores.
7. Antigen: pathogens and agents that the body recognizes as foreign; the stimulus for antibody production.

Learning Review

1. Stages of infectious diseases are as follows.
   (1) *Incubation stage:* The interval of time between exposure to a pathogen and the first signs and symptoms of the disease. Some diseases have short incubation stages, whereas others have prolonged stages, some lasting for years.
   (2) *Prodromal stage:* Vague or undifferentiated from symptoms of other diseases. This stage is characterized by common, general complaints of illness, including malaise and fever. This stage is the interval between the earliest symptoms and the appearance of a fever or rash, which suggest that an impending disease process is occurring.
   (3) *Acute stage:* The peak of the disease process. Symptoms are fully developed during this stage and commonly can be differentiated from other specific symptoms. Various treatments are used to reduce patient discomfort and the possibilities of debilitation and adverse effects, and to promote healing and recovery. Inflammation, a common immune system response to foreign substances, occurs during this stage.

(4) *Declining stage:* Symptoms subside during this stage. Despite the patient's improvement, the infectious disease is still present.

(5) *Convalescent stage:* Recovery and recuperation occur during this stage. The patient regains strength; the goal in this stage is to return the patient to his or her original state of health.

2. DTP   Diphtheria, tetanus, pertussis   IM

    HBV   Hepatitis B virus   IM

    MMR   Measles, mumps, rubella   SC (needle free of alcohol; use only supplied diluent)

    Hib   Meningitis caused by *H. influenza* B   IM

    OPV   Polio or poliomyelitis   PO

3. A. Portal of exit; means of transmission.   G. Portal of exit.
   B. Means of transmission.   H. Reservoirs.
   C. Infectious agent.   I. Susceptible host.
   D. Portal of entry.   J. Means of transmission.
   E. Susceptible host.   K. Portal of exit.
   F. Means of transmission.   L. Means of transmission.

4. A. Five causes of susceptibility are the presence of other diseases, immunosuppression, surgical procedures, trauma, and the absence of immunity to the specific microorganism.

   B. (1) Occupation or lifestyle environment, (2) general physical condition, (3) youth or advanced age, (4) presence of underlying diseases or conditions, (5) psychological health status, (6) duration of exposure to pathogens, and (7) number and specific type of pathogen.

5. A. Cell-mediated immunity.   D. Congenital passive immunity.
   B. Humoral immunity.   E. Acquired active immunity.
   C. Artificial active immunity.   F. Passive immunity.

6. A. AIDS. *Agent:* virus (HIV); *transmission:* bloodborne, sexual contact, intrauterine, lactation; *symptoms:* opportunistic infections, lymphadenopathy, fatigue, malaise, fever.

   B. TB. *Agent:* bacteria (Mycobacterium tuberculosis bacillus); *transmission:* inhalation of infected airborne mucus droplets, and possibly ingestion; *symptoms:* productive cough, fatigue, fever, weight loss; in elderly, behavioral changes and anorexia.

   C. Gastroenteritis. *Agent:* bacteria or virus; transmission: ingestion of contaminated food or water; *symptoms:* nausea, intestinal cramps, vomiting, diarrhea, dehydration, respiratory failure, death.

   D. Hepatitis B. *Agent:* virus (hepatitis B virus); *transmission:* bloodborne, sexual contact, intrauterine; *symptoms:* fatigue, malaise, anorexia, headache, icterus, liver tenderness and enlargement, fever.

   E. Chickenpox. *Agent:* virus (varicella zoster virus); *transmission:* direct and indirect contact with respiratory droplets; *symptoms:* sudden fever, malaise, skin rash.

   F. Influenza. *Agent:* virus (A, B, or C strains); *transmission:* inhalation, aerosolized, mucus droplets; *symptoms:* acute upper/lower respiratory infection, severe cough, fever malaise, sore throat, coryza.

7. A. Three methods used to achieve medical asepsis are as follows. *Handwashing* is considered the most important infection control procedure, aiming to reduce the presence of pathogens that could be transmitted to others through direct or indirect contact. *Sanitization* is a technique that rids contaminated reusable instruments of tissue, blood, debris, and other contaminants. This method, which is done as soon as possible after a medical or surgical procedure, involves physically cleaning and scrubbing instruments using mild detergents and scrub brushes. *Disinfection* removes, through the use of chemical solutions or heat, a large number of pathogens from instruments and equipment.

   B. Entries (1) and (5) represent proper aseptic technique.

   C. (2) The medical assistant attempts to reuse a patient gown when it seems as if the previous patient did not use the protective garment. Each patient should receive a fresh gown. (3) Used materials should be considered contaminated. Bruce should take the used gauze from the patient and dispose of it properly in a biohazard waste container. Wet items should be placed in a plastic bag before disposing of them in the biohazard waste container. (4) Anna could not have prevented the accident caused when she attempts to help the potentially fainting patient and knocks sterile instruments to the floor. Regardless of the patient's inadvertent error of placing the contaminated instruments within the sterile field, the entire tray should be replaced as a safety precaution.

8. Sterile technique and surgical asepsis are terms used interchangeably. Two examples of keeping skin free of pathogens are (1) preparing the patient's skin with a surgical scrub solution before applying sterile drapes around the intended surgical site, and (2) the use of surgical handwashing technique before applying sterile gloves.

9. A. (1) CS   (5) CD
        (2) SS   (6) CD
        (3) CD   (7) SS
        (4) CS   (8) CD

   B. Gynecological instruments are sanitized separately before sterilization because of the risk of transmission of sexually transmitted diseases (STDs), HIV, and HBV.

10. Steam sterilization is the most widely used method of sterilization in the ambulatory care setting. This technique uses an autoclave, or pressure cooker, to achieve sterilization. Through conversion to steam, water reaches greater temperatures than boiling (250°–254°F versus 212°F). This high heat and at least 15 pounds of pressure eradicates all microorganisms and their spores.

11. A. The six general rules medical assistants should follow to achieve proper sterilization using an autoclave are (1) articles placed in the autoclave have been sanitized and dried; (2) articles are placed in such a way that all surfaces are adequately exposed; (3) containers are placed on their sides with lids loosely in place to avoid trapping air pockets; (4) only approved wrapping material is used; (5) timing does not begin until gauges read 15 pounds of pressure and 250°F; and (6) after the completed cycle, sterile, wrapped packs are left in the autoclave to cool and dry to prevent microorganisms from contaminating the damp wrapping.

    B. Temperature: 250–254°F and 50 pounds of pressure.
    Time for sterilization of unwrapped items: 20 minutes.
    Time for sterilization of wrapped items: 30 minutes.
    Time for sterilization of tightly wrapped items: 40 minutes.
    Frequency of draining water and cleaning autoclave: at least once a week.

Multiple Choice Questions

1. b. 250°F
2. c. indirect contact
3. a. inflammation

4. a. intact skin
5. b. immunoglobulins

Investigation Activity

Students' answers will vary according to their place of residence, personal and professional lifestyle, and general physical and emotional health history and current status. The presence of infectious diseases often relates to social, economic, environmental, and other factors. Students who reside in states with several large metropolitan centers, for instance, may find higher numbers of AIDS and TB cases reported than students who reside in states with smaller cities, with more rural environments, or those that are less densely populated.

The following are everyday precautions that can reduce one's risk of contracting infectious diseases: frequent handwashing; attention to proper food preparation; sanitization of cookware, countertops, and toilets; eating nutritious meals; exercising regularly; managing stress; taking vitamin supplements, if necessary; and taking precautions when in contact with infected friends, relatives, and colleagues.

Students' risks and perceptions of risks of contracting infectious diseases outside the ambulatory care setting environment will vary. All students, however, should cite specific factors that may affect their susceptibility, including general physical health and emotional well-being; living and workplace environments (ventilation, sanitization, amount of contact with highly susceptible or presently infected people); presence of other illnesses; impaired immune system functioning (from cancer treatments, surgery, or trauma); lifestyle factors, such as nonuse/use of drugs and alcohol and sexual activity (number of partners and use of protective barriers); and degree of attention to hygiene and sanitization, such as handwashing and cleaning of cookware, counters, and other potentially contaminated surfaces and items.

ANSWERS TO WORKBOOK CASE STUDY QUESTIONS

Case 1

1. Michelle's dermatitis may be the result of an allergy to the latex material in the gloves she uses at work. She should have her condition evaluated by a physician, as this kind of allergy can be very serious, even life-threatening. Sensitivity may remain localized (dermatitis) or can cause a systemic reaction, such as anaphylaxis.

2. Medical assistants with latex allergies should switch to vinyl gloves at work. All people with latex sensitivity should wear a bracelet or other identification to alert health care professionals (who wear latex gloves during many procedures) about their condition, should they be treated for a medical emergency.

Case 2

1. On a daily basis, the inner chamber of the autoclave should be washed with a mild detergent and cloth, then rinsed and dried. The outer jacket should be wiped clean of dust and soil. The manufacturer's instructions and recommendations for cleansers should be followed.

2. The autoclave is drained, filled with cleaning solution, run through a 20-minute heated cycle, drained of solution, filled with distilled rinse water, run through another 20-minute heated cycle, drained of rinse solution, and filled with distilled water again. Then the inner shelves are removed and scrubbed and the inner chamber is wiped clean. During the cleaning process, the autoclave's rubber seal should be inspected for cracks or wear.

3. Proper cleaning and maintenance of the autoclave are essential to ensuring the sterility of instruments and equipment used in the ambulatory care setting, preventing the use of contaminated instruments in patient care.

Case 3

1. Joe should not administer the vaccination to the child without the consent of the mother. The DPT formulation carries a small risk of neurological damage, but many physicians advise that the risk of complication is far less than the risk of the child developing diphtheria, tetanus, or pertussis. In addition, a new formula, DTaP, greatly reduces the risk of neurological side effects. The ICD-9-CM code for the DTP vaccination is V06.1.
2. Although Joe should not dismiss Mary's concerns, he should encourage her to maintain Marissa's vaccination schedule, which allows for a 6-month window (from 12 to 18 months) for the DPT vaccine: "The new DTaP has almost no side effects. Why don't I get Dr. King? She'll explain the benefits and risks of vaccination to you. And we do have a window of time here, so you'll be able to think about the procedure and schedule a follow-up visit for the vaccination if you need more time to consider it after you've spoken to Dr. King."

Chapter

23

Taking a Medical History, the Patient's Chart, and Methods of Documentation

OVERVIEW

The medical assisting student is introduced to the importance of an accurate, complete, and up-to-date patient medical history to the quality of care provided by the physician and the health care team. Students explore the communication issues and challenges of taking histories from patients, emphasizing respect and attention to the patient's emotional needs while maintaining the level of information necessary to complete the history for the patient's permanent record.

PROFICIENCY EVALUATION OUTCOME ASSESSMENT

Students are evaluated for their understanding of performance objectives. All components of a patient medical history are understood and described. POMR and SOMR record-keeping methods, as well as the SOAP approach to charting, are described. Students are able to chart information accurately and also understand the correct procedures for correcting errors in charting. Therapeutic communication techniques for taking histories from patients are mastered. Ethical issues that may arise in the process of obtaining patient medical histories are explored.

Procedure 23-1   Taking a Medical History

SUPPLEMENTARY RESOURCES

Medical Assisting Videos: Appropriate content is available on Delmar's Medical Assisting Videos, 2nd ed., Tape 8, for the following topics:

Interview and Take Patient History
Take an In-depth Patient History
Introduction to Health Promotion, Disease Prevention, and Self-Responsibility

ANSWERS TO TEXT REVIEW QUESTIONS

1. a. set up the appointment for the patient and obtain the services of an interpreter to be present as well
2. c. treat the patient the same as all other patients
3. c. Have you noticed any changes in your condition since your last visit?
4. b. ask helpful questions to help the patient express specific problems or symptoms
5. a. are chronological, and usually over a long period of time

ANSWERS TO TEXT CRITICAL THINKING QUESTIONS

1. There are seven sections in the medical history:
   1. Personal data (or administrative information)
   2. Chief complaint
   3. Present illness
   4. Past medical history
   5. Family history
   6. Social history
   7. Review of systems
2. For the definition and importance of each section of the medical history, see the textbook.
3. The new patient may make a first appointment by telephone, by personal contact through a referral from another physician, or as an emergency patient.
4. The medical assistant helps take a patient's medical history by creating a positive atmosphere of confidence and concern for the patient's well-being. The medical assistant may need to make arrangements for an interpreter to enable full communication with the physician.
5. There are many aids available to the physician and the medical assistant for patients with special needs. Home health agencies have home health aids who can accompany older or physically challenged patients to office visits. Interpreters are available for non-English-speaking patients. Telecommunication devices for the deaf (TDDs/TTYs) are available for hearing-impaired patients, as are the services of qualified, certified American Sign Language (ASL) interpreters.
6. A medical assistant needs to be prepared to encounter patients who are in pain, grieving, silent, depressed, resentful, giddy, joyful, or angry, as well as patients who are friendly and fully cooperative. Patients' moods will change with their circumstances and the same patient may express different moods and emotions at different times. At all times, respect for patients' emotional needs must be shown in medical assistants' therapeutic communications.
7. There are three primary methods of charting, including:
   1. *Source-oriented medical records (SOMR).* All reports are filed chronologically according to specialty with the latest information on top because this information is the most important for patient current care and treatment.
   2. *Problem-oriented medical records (POMR).* Systematic way to record data pertinent to patient care. This record-keeping method consists of a numbered list of patient problems with plans and progress notes components of charting.
   3. *Computer-modified records.* These chart notes combine both SOMR and POMR charting methods in that the problems are stated but the record grows in a chronological order.
8. A discharge summary can be found under the hospital notes section. A follow-up visit for a consultation would be found in the consult section. A copy of the Worker's Compensation claim form is found in the correspondence section.
9. All allergies to medications should be noted on the cover of the chart in a significant place, as well as within the chart notes.
10. A correction should be made by making a line through the error, writing "error" over the correction, initialing and dating the correction, and inserting the correct notation.

ANSWERS TO WORKBOOK EXERCISES AND ACTIVITIES

Vocabulary Builder

1. C. The chart note means: On March 10, the patient's chief complaint was nausea, vomiting, and diarrhea lasting four days, with a temperature of over 100 degrees Fahrenheit for two days, and loss of appetite.
   The correction to 3 days is inserted properly as follows:

   ⟨error⟩ 3 days   3/10   Students Initials _____

   3/10/xx CC: NVD × ~~4~~ days. T > 100°F × 2 days. Loss of appetite.
2. G.
3. E.
4. L.
5. H.
6. F. The proper insurance coding for the laboratory tests is
CBC	85024
Urinalysis	81000
Abdominal ultrasound	76700

The diagnosis codes for the two suspected conditions are
Acute appendicitis   540.0
Ovarian cyst, twisted   620.2
The physician will not code a diagnosis for the patient until a diagnosis is confirmed. The medical assistant
will code symptoms until a diagnosis is confirmed by the physician.

7. D.
8. B.
9. K.
10. J.
11. A.
12. I.

Learning Review

1. Students' answers will vary. Some appropriate questions include
    What do you think caused the problem?
    When do you think it started?
    What does it do to your body?
    What do you expect from the course of this problem?
    What do you fear from this problem?
    What kind of treatment do you expect?
2. Nine characteristics of chief complaints are: location, radiation, quality, quantity, associated manifestations, aggravating factors, alleviating factors, setting, and timing.
3. A. The date of the examination and the taking of this chart note.
    B. A chief complaint of lower abdominal pain lasting one week with increasing malaise or fatigue and listlessness.
    C. Weight is 135 pounds. Height is 5 feet 4 inches. Temperature is 99.8°F, slightly elevated above normal. Respiration is 19 breaths per minute and is clear. Pulse is 78 beats per minute and is regular. Blood pressure reading is 134 (systolic) / 82 (diastolic).
    D. Patient describes an increasing urge to urinate with a burning sensation upon urination; pressure in abdomen; lack of energy.
    E. The patient has a past medical history that is positive for frequent urinary tract infections. The patient was diagnosed with Type II diabetes mellitus in 1987 and takes a prescribed dosage of 3 milligrams of Glynase by mouth every day in tablet form. The patient quit smoking 20 years ago and has lost 10 pounds in the last 2 years.
    F. The patient has no known allergies.
    G. There is no change in family history.
    H. The patient has less than two glasses of wine per week, does not smoke, and exercises regularly.
4. The student will choose from the list of systems included in textbook.

Multiple Choice Questions

1. d. family
2. b. chief complaint
3. a. medical problem

4. c. POMR
5. c. referrals for insurance companies

Investigation Activity

Use this investigation activity to encourage students to think about the relationship of family medical histories to the quality of care the physician and health care team can provide when they are given the proper, complete family history information. The genogram can be used as a method of patient education, helping patients think about their health and the preventive measures that may be appropriate for them to initiate and follow to maintain an optimum state of health, fitness, and well-being.

ANSWERS TO WORKBOOK CASE STUDY QUESTIONS

1. Liz will want to use active listening to make sure that the patient understands her questions and that she, Liz, correctly takes down the patient's information. Liz will use nonverbal cues to gauge the patient's comfort level as she provides information and gives clues about any discomfort or distress the patient may be experiencing. Liz will be sure to adjust her vocabulary to the patient's level of understanding. Liz will want to communicate a respect for the patient's age and her obvious strong attachment to familiar people and events evidenced in the patient's attachment to past events, her long-term relationship with her previous primary care physician, her request for a new physician of Italian descent, and her close relationship with her granddaughter.

2. Liz will want to look for signs of confused thinking that may be evidenced in the patient's unannounced segues between past and present events. The physician may want to explore the distinction between the patient's personal style of relating information and the possibility of mild dementia. The patient's awareness, when reminded of the correct time frame, is significant. Liz should carefully document her observations regarding the patient's mental state.

3. Nancy's granddaughter can provide clues to the mental and physical state of the patient. However, extensive or repeated interruptions could inhibit Liz's ability to make a good assessment of the patient's responses. Liz may politely ask Leslie to remain silent during the remainder of the patient history. Liz could speak to Leslie separately for further insights into or specific information about her grandmother's state of physical and mental health.

Chapter 24

Vital Signs and Measurements

OVERVIEW

Medical assisting students learn the theory and the practice of taking vital signs, which will be one of the most important responsibilities in their careers as medical assistants. They must understand the reasons why vital signs are important, know the clues to disease that these measurements can provide, follow standard precautions, and be comfortable with all the required equipment and procedures. They must also have the ability to explain vital sign procedures for temperature, pulse rate, respiration, and blood pressure readings to patients. Possessing a knowledge of normal vital sign expectations for patients across the life span will help medical assistants perform the procedures with efficiency and accuracy, recognizing both inaccurate readings and also abnormal readings and measurements that may signal patient illness. As always, the medical assistant must act to ensure patient safety and comfort.

PROFICIENCY EVALUATION OUTCOME ASSESSMENT

Students are evaluated for their knowledge of performance objectives and their ability to perform all of the vital signs measurements covered in this chapter, including each variation. Students gain an understanding of the body processes at work for each vital sign in both the healthy and diseased states. Students should be able to discuss the procedures they perform and justify the actions they take to complete each measurement, also learning to differentiate between inaccurate results and results that may signify illness. They should be able to explain each procedure to the patient and to answer patient questions about the equipment used, the safety precautions taken, and the amount of time each procedure should take.

Procedure 24–1   Measuring an Oral Temperature Using a Mercury Thermometer

Procedure 24–2   Measuring an Oral Temperature Using a Disposable Oral Strip Thermometer

Procedure 24–3   Measuring an Oral Temperature Using a Digital Thermometer

Procedure 24–4   Measuring an Aural Temperature Using a Tympanic Thermometer

Procedure 24–5   Measuring a Rectal Temperature Using a Mercury Thermometer
Students of opposite sexes may be uncomfortable practicing this procedure. Encourage same-sex pairs and provide privacy.

Procedure 24–6   Measuring a Rectal Temperature Using a Digital Thermometer
Students of opposite sexes may be uncomfortable practicing this procedure. Encourage same-sex pairs and provide privacy.

Procedure 24–7   Measuring an Axillary Temperature

Procedure 24–8   Measuring a Radial Pulse

Procedure 24–9   Measuring an Apical Pulse

SUPPLEMENTARY RESOURCES

Medical Assisting Videos: Appropriate content is available on Delmar's Medical Assisting Videos, 2nd ed., for the following topics:

Tape 6   Take Vital Signs
　　　　 Take and Record Oral Temperature Using a Glass Thermometer
　　　　 Take and Record Rectal Temperature
　　　　 Take and Record Oral Temperature Using an Electronic Thermometer
　　　　 Take and Record an Aural (Ear) Temperature
　　　　 Take and Record Axillary (Underarm) Temperature
　　　　 Take and Record a Radial Pulse
　　　　 Take and Record a Brachial Pulse (Infant)
　　　　 Use a Stethoscope to Take an Apical Pulse (Adult)
　　　　 Use a Stethoscope to Take an Apical Pulse (Infant)
　　　　 Take and Record Respiration
Tape 7   Take and Record Blood Pressure
　　　　 Measure Height and Weight Using an Upright Scale

ANSWERS TO TEXT REVIEW QUESTIONS

1. c. 98.6°F
2. c. radial
3. c. give an arbitrarily high result
4. b. cool soapy water
5. b. tachycardia

ANSWERS TO TEXTBOOK CRITICAL THINKING QUESTIONS

1. The medical assistant may gain patient cooperation by explaining the procedure, recognizing patient anxieties and responding accordingly, reassuring the patient, and positioning the patient comfortably.
2. The appropriate charting procedure for normal vital sign results is
    Date:
    Time:
    T. 98.6°F–P. 72–R. 18 　　　　　　　　B/P 120/80
    Temperature: T. 98.6°F (note route if other than oral)
    Pulse: P. 72
    Respirations: R. 18
    Blood pressure: B/P 120/80
3. The responsibilities of the medical assistant in measuring vital signs are to recognize and correct factors that may produce inaccurate results, obtain vital signs using appropriate methods to ensure accurate results; record results accurately, and alert the physician to abnormal findings.
4. The following describes the care and use of oral, tympanic, and digital thermometers.
    Oral mercury, by mouth: The thermometer is sanitized (washed with soap and cool water), rinsed, dried, and soaked in disinfectant for the appropriate length of time in a covered container, for example, soaked in alcohol (70 percent solution) for 30 minutes. Timing begins after the last thermometer is added to the disinfectant solution. Because they are fragile, care should be taken to prevent breaking thermometers. After the appropriate length of disinfection time, remove thermometers from the disinfectant, rinse, dry, check for cracks, nicks, and so on, and store in a dry container. Disinfectant solution is discarded after soaking time has elapsed.
    Oral disposable strip, by mouth: This type of oral thermometer is used only one time then discarded in a biohazard waste container. It does not produce a completely accurate reading of body temperature.
    Digital thermometer, by mouth: This is a battery-operated electronic thermometer. The battery charge must be maintained for proper operation by replacing the unit in its charging holder after use.
    Tympanic thermometer: This is a battery-operated aural thermometer. Eject and dispose of the probe cover after each use. Replace the three AAA batteries when the indicator light goes on.

5. The procedure for converting temperatures from one scale to the other is shown in calculating the following conversions:
   • To calculate °F to °C: take degrees Fahrenheit, subtract 32, multiply by 5/9
   • To calculate °C to °F: take degrees Celsius, multiply by 9/5 and add 32
     A. 98.6°F = 37.0°C
     B. 39.1°C = 102.3°F
6. The rationale for not using the thumb for taking the pulse rate of a patient is as follows. The thumb has a pulse of its own and may mistakenly be counted in place of the patient's pulse.
7. The reason for taking the respiratory rate of a patient without the patient's knowledge is that the patient may, unconsciously, alter breathing if aware of respirations being counted.
8. The importance of using the appropriate blood pressure cuff size when measuring a patient's blood pressure is that an improperly sized cuff can produce an inaccurate blood pressure reading. A cuff that is too small will give an artificially high blood pressure reading, whereas a cuff that is too large will give an artificially low reading.
9. The normal vital signs variations expected between an infant and an adult are these: a child's respiratory and circulatory rates are higher than an adult's, whereas the blood pressure of a child is normally lower.
10. Definitions are as follows:
    • Hypertension: blood pressure readings consistently above 140/90 mm Hg.
    • Tachycardia: abnormally fast heart rate, usually ↑100/min or usually ↑100 bpm.
    • Apnea: cessation of breathing.
    • Remittent fever: fever that fluctuates but does not return to the baseline temperature.

ANSWERS TO WORKBOOK EXERCISES AND ACTIVITIES

Vocabulary Builder

1. orthopnea	9. hyperventilation	18. hypoventilation
2. emphysema	10. apnea	19. eupnea
3. tachypnea	11. rhonchi	20. bradypnea
4. A. hypotension	12. systole	21. arrhythmia
B. diastole	13. hypertension	22. stertorous
5. rales	14. Cheyne-Stokes	23. tachycardia
6. frenulum	15. baseline	24. hyperpnea
7. stridor	16. dyspnea	25. pyrexia
8. bradycardia	17. wheezes	

Learning Review

1. A. Body heat is produced by the actions of voluntary and involuntary muscles. As the muscles move, they use energy that, in response, produces heat. Cellular metabolic activities—such as the process of breaking down food sugars to simpler components, catabolism—are another source of heat. The hypothalamus maintains the body's balance of heat production and loss.
   B. A. Conduction; B. Evaporation; C. Radiation; D. Convection; E. Elimination.
   C. In their lists of temperature-increasing factors, students may include bacterial infection; increased physical activity; food intake; exposure to heat; pregnancy; metabolism-increasing drugs; stress; time of day (afternoon and early evening); and age, in that an infant's temperature is one or two degrees higher than an adult's.
   D. In their lists of temperature-decreasing factors, students may include viral infection; decreased physical activity; fasting; emotional depression; exposure to cold; metabolism-decreasing drugs; time of day (during sleep and early morning); and age, in that an elderly person's normal temperature may be slightly lower than that of a young or middle-aged adult.
   E. Fever is also called pyrexia. A. Remittent; B. Relapsing; C. Intermittent; D. Continuous.
2. A. Normal blood pressure ranges are Infant: 50–52/25–30; Child, age 6: 95/62; Child, age 10: 100/65; Adolescent, age 16: 118/75; Adult: < 140/< 89.
   B. *Blood volume* is the amount of blood in the arteries. Increased volume increases blood pressure, whereas a decrease in volume will decrease blood pressure, as in the case of a hemorrhage.
   Peripheral resistance is the resistance to blood flow in the arterioles. The smaller the lumen of the arterioles, the more pressure is needed to push blood through. The larger the lumen, the less resistance and therefore less pressure is needed to push blood through. Lumen can become smaller from deposits of fatty cholesterol, resulting in an increase in blood pressure.
   Vessel elasticity refers to the ability of arteries to expand and contract to provide a steady flow of blood. As a person ages, elasticity of vessels is reduced. It can cause an increase in arterial wall resistance, resulting in an increase in blood pressure.

Condition of the heart muscle is extremely important to blood flow and pressure. A weak heart muscle results in an inefficient pumping action of the heart, leading to a decrease in blood pressure and blood flow. Four other factors include genetics, diet and weight, activity, and emotional state.

C. The sounds are called Korotkoff sounds. The act of listening is called auscultation.

   A. Phase IV. Blood is now passing through the vessels fairly easily. The sounds heard are muffling and fading of the tapping sounds.

   B. Phase II. More blood passes through the vessels. The sound is that of a soft swishing sound.

   C. Phase V. Blood is flowing freely at this time; all sounds disappear.

   D. Phase I. Blood is first allowed to enter the vessels as the cuff begins the deflation process. A sharp tapping sound is heard.

   E. Phase III. Blood continues to pass through the vessels. The sound is a rhythmic tapping sound.

3. A. The four types of hypertension are primary (essential), secondary, benign, and malignant. Hypertension is blood pressure that is consistently above normal.

   B. Student choices will vary, but they may include as possible causes of hypotension: hemorrhage, traumatic shock, emotional shock, central nervous system disorder, chronic wasting disease, and rapid change from supine to standing position (orthostatic hypotension). Hypotension is blood pressure that is consistently below normal in which the patient is unable to function.

4. Normal pulse rate ranges are: Birth: 130–160; Infant, < 1 year: 110–130; Child, age 1–7: 80–120; Child > 7: 80–90; Adult: 60–80 beats per minute.

5. *Bradycardia* is an adult pulse rate under 60. *Tachycardia* is an adult pulse rate over 100 beats per minute. *PVC* or premature contraction is a type of arrhythmia in which a pulsation is felt before it is expected. In *sinus arrhythmia*, the pulse rate increases on inspiration and decreases on expiration.

6.

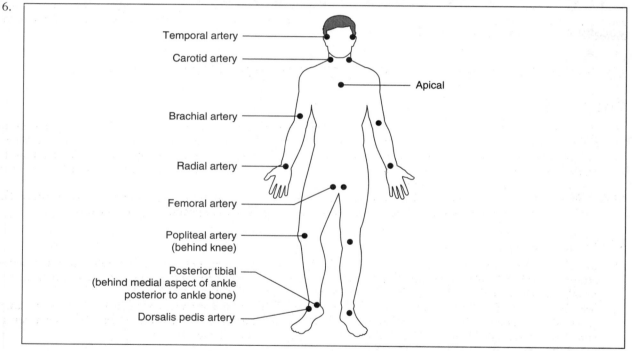

7. Normal ranges of respiratory rates are as follows: Infant: 30–60; Child, age 1–7: 18–30; Adult: 12–20 respirations per minute.

8. Five abnormal breath sounds include (1) rales: rattling sound heard on inspiration and expiration; (2) rhonchi: snoring sound produced in the throat; (3) wheezes: high-pitched musical sound heard on expiration; (4) stridor: crowing sound heard on inspiration; (5) stertorous respiration: snoring sound with labored breathing, produced in the trachea and bronchi.

9. A. Four characteristics of pulse include rate, rhythm, volume of pulse, and condition of the arterial wall. Rate is the number of pulsations or beats felt for 1 minute. Rhythm of pulse refers to the time between pulsations and regularity of the beat. Volume refers to the strength of the beat that is felt. Normal arteries feel soft and elastic, whereas abnormal arteries may feel hard, knotty, wiry, or a combination.

   B. The three characteristics of respiration include rate, rhythm, and depth. Rate is the number of respirations per minute. Rhythm refers to the pattern of breathing. Depth is the amount of air that is inspired or expired with each respiration.

C. The normal respiration rate is usually a 1:4 ratio relationship to the pulse rate.

D. Students answers will vary according to their own results for resting, active, and aerobic pulse and respiration rates.

Multiple Choice Questions

1. a. two-tenths of a degree
2. b. ear
3. d. apical
4. d. eupnea
5. c. life threatening

Investigation Activity

This investigation activity will give students a practical demonstration of the normal variations in body temperature they should expect to see as medical assistants. Performing this common routine on several different subjects gives them additional practice, not just in temperature taking but also in patient interaction. Ask students about the reactions their subjects had to the procedure. What kind of questions did they ask? How cooperative were they? How did the students answer questions and handle problems? On completion of the activity, students should recognize that the medical definition of *normal*—even in relation to something like body temperature, which everyone knows "should be" a standard 98.6°F—must always be flexible. Students should also be able to discuss reasons (such as time of day or age) why body temperature may deviate from the standard.

Part B of the activity examines variations in measurement caused by the different types of equipment used to take patient temperatures. Students should recall from their study of the text that, for example, rectal temperature is generally 1 degree higher than oral temperature. This exercise gives them a chance to see this phenomenon firsthand and to make observations of their own in regard to other methods. It also gives them additional practice with the equipment and with patient interaction. Discuss with students their observations, their experiences with the different types of equipment, and their experiences with a more in-depth patient contact.

ANSWERS TO WORKBOOK CASE STUDY QUESTIONS

Case 1

1. Wanda will take Wayne's temperature using the axillary method. Because of Wayne's possible ear infection in the right ear and history of infections in both ears, she cannot use a tympanic thermometer. Because the patient has recently drunk hot coffee, any oral method will give an inaccurate result. This patient, who is developmentally disabled, would most likely become agitated at the idea of a rectal procedure, even though the rectal temperature would produce the most accurate result.

2. "Sometimes the things we eat or drink can make a difference in the way we can take someone's temperature. The coffee might have made your mouth too warm, so I have to take your temperature in another way."

Case 2

1. In an emergency situation like this, Bruce will probably choose the strong and easy-to-find pulse site at the carotid artery to check the child's heart rate. A second choice might be the pulse site at the temporal artery, which can also be used to help control the bleeding from Henry's cut.

2. "Ms. Hansen, the first thing I have to do is find out how seriously injured your son might be. We need to know about his respiration and heartbeat before we can do anything else. Dr. Whitney is on his way. Why don't you go with Karen Ritter; she'll take care of you while the physician examines your son."

Case 3

A. 1. To obtain an accurate respiration rate—and to hear any possible unusual breath sounds—Audrey will have to observe Abigail's breathing pattern at a different time in the examination, and in a different way than she usually does. Audrey should simply observe the rise and fall of Abigail's chest wall for 1 minute at a later time, perhaps while checking the patient's weight.

2. Audrey should say nothing to Abigail about the alteration of her breathing pattern. Whether the change is conscious or unconscious, calling it to Abigail's attention will only make her less likely to breathe naturally.

B. 1. Audrey will measure Abigail's weight in a private environment, assisting Abigail throughout the procedure to ensure her safety and comfort. She will inform the patient of the results in a discreet and professional manner.

2. "Ms. Johnson, because of your diabetes and your flu symptoms today we really need to have a weight measurement; Dr. King will need the information. I promise to help you through the procedure; you'll be able to rest comfortably for a few minutes afterward while I go get Dr. King for your examination."

Chapter

25

The Physical Examination

OVERVIEW

Medical assistants perform a vital function when assisting the physician with patients' physical examinations. Medical assisting students discover the methods, components, and sequence of routine physical examinations. The basic examination positions are covered, as well as draping techniques. Students learn the importance of accurately assessing the potential requirements of the physician during a physical examination and preparing the patient and examination room to meet those requirements. Observance of aseptic technique and standard precautions is reinforced. Empathy and respect for the patient must also be shown by all health care professionals.

PROFICIENCY EVALUATION OUTCOME ASSESSMENT

Students are evaluated for their understanding of performance objectives. An understanding of all aspects of the routine physical examination, including methods of examination, components of the examination, and the correct sequence of events during examination is required. Students demonstrate the ability to position and drape patients for physical examination and possess a knowledge of equipment and supplies routinely used. Students are encouraged to explore the role of the medical assistant in patient and room preparation, with emphasis also placed on following aseptic techniques and standard precautions and on exhibiting respect for the patient's conditions and needs at all times.

SUPPLEMENTARY RESOURCES

Medical Assisting Videos: Appropriate content is available on Delmar's Medical Assisting Videos, 2nd edition, Tape 8, for the following topics:

Clean Examination Table and Countertop
Assist Physician with Examination and Treatments
Position and Drape the Patient
Role of the Medical Assistant During the Examination
Introduction to Health Promotion, Disease Prevention, and Self-Responsibility

ANSWERS TO TEXT REVIEW QUESTIONS

1. c. auscultation
2. a. horizontal recumbent
3. c. body movement
4. c. answer questions to the extent of knowledge; refer others to the physician
5. a. supine position

ANSWERS TO TEXT CRITICAL THINKING QUESTIONS

1. Answers will vary depending on the physician and type of practice; however, the following responsibilities are likely, but may not be all-inclusive:
    Patient preparation: including explanations of what the patient will need to do as well as procedures to be performed, assistance if necessary with disrobing, gowning, positioning, draping, and specimen collection.
    Room preparation: including assembling proper instruments and equipment, checking batteries and light sources, and ensuring patient privacy and comfort.
    Maintain medical asepsis and adhere to Standard Precautions.
2. Six methods used in the physical examination are inspection: to view, look at; palpation: to feel, touch; percussion: **tapping to elicit body sounds;** auscultation: listening to sounds, usually with the aid of a stethoscope; mensuration: **measuring, usually with the aid of a measuring device;** and manipulation: passive, forceful movement of a joint.
3. Two reasons why positioning and draping are done are
    1. Each position is designed to make examination of a particular area of the body easier and more efficient.
    2. Draping is done for modesty and to protect the patient against embarrassment; draping also maintains the patient's warmth.
    4. A. lithotomy: pelvic and rectal examinations
        B. Sims': rectal examination
        C. knee-chest: examination of rectum and sigmoid colon
        D. supine: examination of the anterior surface of the body, including the head, neck, chest (heart, lung, and breast), abdomen, and extremities
    5. The various components of a physical examination are
        General appearance: skin color, grooming, ease of conversation
        Gait: manner or style of walking, maintaining coordination and balance
        Stature: height and trunk to limb proportion
        Posture: normal and abnormal curvatures of the spine
        Body movements: voluntary and involuntary movements
        Speech: ability to use and understand language
        Breath odors: abnormal odors may indicate a disease process
        Nutrition: body weight and proportion
        Skin and appendages: skin color and elasticity; abnormal shape of nails may indicate a disease process or nutrition abnormality
6. The sequence for a physical examination is as follows.
    1. **Patient preparation:** obtaining vital signs; height and weight; visual and/or auditory acuity; specimen collection; electrocardiography; disrobing, gowning, draping, positioning.
    2. **Physical examination:** head, eyes, ears, mouth and throat, nose, neck, chest, breast, lungs, heart, abdomen, female or male genitalia, pelvic and rectal examinations, and reflexes.
7. Instruments and/or supplies needed for examining the following body areas:
    Head: light, ophthalmoscope, otoscope, tongue depressor, nasal speculum, emesis basin, tissues.
    Reflexes: percussion hammer.
    Chest: tape measure, stethoscope, drape, gown.
    Abdomen: stethoscope, tape measure, drape, gown.
8. The cleaning process for each instrument is as follows.
    A. **Nasal speculum:** Wash with soap and water, rinse, dry. Wipe with alcohol. May be boiled.
    B. **Tuning fork:** Wash with soap and water, rinse, dry. Wipe with alcohol.
    C. **Percussion hammer:** Wash with soap and water, rinse, dry. Wipe with alcohol.
    D. **Reusable otoscope speculum:** Wash with soap and water, rinse, dry. Wipe with alcohol or boil.
9. Three sources of information the physician uses to aid in making a diagnosis are
    Health history: includes past medical problems, current medications, allergies, and factors such as family and social history that may make an impact on patient health
    Physical exam: a head-to-toe exam of each body system
    Laboratory tests and other diagnostic tests: includes urine and blood testing, x-rays, ultrasound, ECG, and other tests used to help identify a patient's problems.

10. Two procedures or tests the medical assistant might perform as part of a basic physical examination include
    - temperature
    - pulse
    - blood pressure
    - height and weight
    - Snellen chart
    - audiometry
    - electrocardiogram
    - urinalysis
    - venipuncture and blood testing

ANSWERS TO WORKBOOK EXERCISES AND ACTIVITIES

Vocabulary Builder

1. scleroderma
2. pyorrhea
3. ataxia
4. jaundice
5. cyanosis
6. pallor
7. vitiligo
8. bruits
9. symmetry
10. tinnitus
11. vertigo and labyrinthitis

Learning Review

1. A. Observation or Inspection
   B. Auscultation
   C. Manipulation
   D. Percussion
   E. Mensuration
   F. Palpation

2. A. Dorsal recumbent position
   B. Supine or horizontal recumbent position
   C. Lithotomy position
   D. Sims' position
   E. Prone position
   F. Fowler's or Semi-Fowler's position
   G. Trendelenburg position
   H. Knee-Chest position

3. A. ME; vital signs
   B. PI; speech
   C. BP; neck
   D. PI; nutrition-extremities
   E. ME; eyes
   F. PI; rectum
   G. PI; chest
   H. ME; mouth and throat
   I. BP; male genitalia
   J. BP; breast
   K. LP; chest
   L. PI; posture
   M. PI; speech
   N. LP; prior to examination
   O. BP; reflexes
   P. BP; ears
   Q. PI; breath odor

Multiple Choice Questions

1. d. observation
2. b. horizontal recumbent
3. a. blood pressure drops
4. d. Sims'
5. a. mensuration

Investigation Activity

Use this activity to raise students' awareness of the need to accurately triage patient conditions in order to correctly prepare the patient and examination room for the physician's examination. Students are also challenged by the "human" factor—the possible complicating effect that patients' attitudes, demeanors, and physical and/or personality characteristics may have on the process of successful patient preparation for examination. The activity will encourage students to sharpen both their triage and communications skills, while reinforcing their understanding of patient and examination room preparation.

ANSWERS TO WORKBOOK CASE STUDY QUESTIONS

1. Bruce will provide a short gown or drape for the boy and assist him in covering up. The boy may be experiencing discomfort and embarrassment while sitting on the examination table in only his underwear. Bruce will reassure the boy with a soothing tone and comforting body language. He will make a game out of pre-examination procedures, such as the recording of vital signs, to distract the child and calm him down.
2. Bruce will reassure the child as well as the mother, acknowledging the pain and discomfort caused by the child's condition. It is only reasonable that the boy would be fearful and upset. If he senses that it will calm the child further, Bruce may want to engage the mother in assisting him while he performs pre-examination procedures by asking her to hold the child or to stand close at hand. He may ask whether the child has brought a favorite toy, which may serve as a further calming distraction.

Chapter

26

Obstetrics and Gynecology

OVERVIEW

Medical assisting students must possess knowledge of the female reproductive system and the common disorders and diseases that can affect it. Students learn the importance of accurately assessing the potential requirements of the physician during the examination of the female patient and preparing the patient and examination room to meet those needs. The examination of the female patient during her nonpregnant and pregnant states along with tests and procedures that are a part of the female examination are covered.

PROFICIENCY EVALUATION OUTCOME ASSESSMENT

Students are evaluated for their understanding of performance objectives. Students are able to describe the female reproductive system and identify common disorders and disease that affect it both during the nonpregnancy and pregnancy states. An understanding of the initial prenatal visit and examination and all subsequent visits the pregnant patient will make is necessary. Students demonstrate the ability to position and drape the patient during the examination and possess a knowledge of the equipment and supplies used during the prenatal visits as well as during gynecological visits.

Procedure 26–1   Assisting with Routine Prenatal Visits
Procedure 26–2   Instructing Patient in Breast Self-Examination
Procedure 26–3   Assisting with Gynecologic or Pelvic Examination and a Paparicoloaou (Pap) Test

SUPPLEMENTARY RESOURCES

Medical Assisting Videos: Appropriate content is available on Delmar's Medical Assisting Videos, 2nd ed., for the following topics:

Tape 1   Communication Skills
Tape 8   Taking a Patient History
                Positioning and Draping the Patient
                Role of the Medical Assistant During the Examination
                Breast Self-Examination

TIP   *Nagele's Rule:* A method for calculating the estimated (or expected) date of confinement (EDC) or of delivery (EDD): count back three months from the first day of the last menstrual period, and add one year and seven days. An unavoidable error of plus or minus two weeks may occur.

ANSWERS TO TEXT REVIEW QUESTIONS

1. d. poor nutritional habits
2. c. May 27, 2001
3. a. alphafetal protein analysis (AFP)

4. c. oxytoxin
5. d. number of weeks of gestation
6. c. a strong, foul odor to vaginal discharge
7. c. wet mount
8. e. ultrasonography
9. c. condylomata
10. b. detect dysplastic cells of cervix following a positive Pap smear

ANSWERS TO TEXT CRITICAL THINKING QUESTIONS

1a. Some likely preliminary tests and procedures are abdominal and vaginal examination, complete blood count, Rh factor, blood type, hepatitis B and C, HIV, venereal research laboratory test, and ultrasonography.

1b. The physician will make a diagnosis based on the laboratory tests and procedures as outlined in 1a. The most likely diagnosis will be pregnancy of 6 months' gestation with spotting, possibly a threatened abortion.

2. The physician will perform a pelvic examination and a pregnancy test to confirm the diagnosis of ectopic pregnancy. Appendicitis has similar symptoms, but with amenorrhea, pregnancy is suspected and confirmed.

3. Certain human papilloma viruses can cause lesions on the cervix that can become cancerous. The patient should be examined more frequently to determine cervical involvement with HPV.

4. There should not be bright red bleeding following intercourse. The physician will ask the medical assistant to set up for a gynecological examination. The bleeding can be caused by intercourse-related injury or from a vaginal or cervical lesion. A Pap smear will be done, because many cervical cancers can have symptoms of bright red bleeding.

5. The physician may prescribe oral contraceptives for this patient because she suspects that the patient may have endometriosis. The hormones in the contraceptives help to lessen the endometrial buildup; therefore, the patient usually experiences less pain prior to and during menses. If there is little or no improvement, a laparoscopy may be performed to identify the extent of the endometriosis. Additional treatment with different hormones may be indicated.

ANSWERS TO WORKBOOK EXERCISES AND ACTIVITIES

Vocabulary Builder

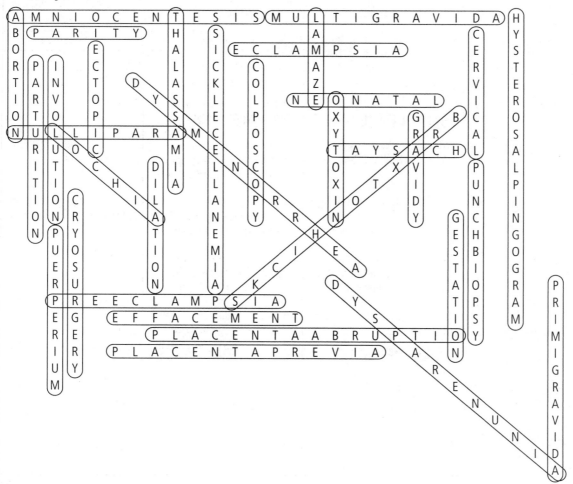

Learning Review

A. Identification
   1. Ovary: female sex cells, also known as female gonads. Are responsible for producing mature ova (eggs) and releasing them at monthly intervals (ovulation). Also responsible for producing hormones that are necessary for the normal growth and development of the female, and for maintaining pregnancy, should it occur.
   2. Cervix: neck of the uterus.
   3. Anus: opening to the rectum.
   4. Fallopian tubes: also known as the uterine tubes or the oviducts. Serve as a passageway for the ova (eggs) as they exit the ovary en route to the uterus.
   5. Uterus: pear-shaped, hollow, muscular organ that houses the fertilized, implanted ovum as it develops throughout the pregnancy. Also the source of monthly menstrual flow if pregnancy does not occur.
   6. Urinary bladder: hollow, muscular sac in the pelvic cavity that serves as a temporary reservoir for urine. Lies between the symphysis pubis and uterus and vagina.
   7. Symphysis pubis: pubic bones midline on the front of the body.
   8. Urethra: tubelike opening to the bladder.
   9. Vagina: muscular tube that connects the uterus with the vulva.

B. Matching:
   Match each female condition or disease to its description.

D	1.	PID	A. Malignant cells found in the ovaries.
C	2.	Menopause	B. Painful menstruation.
E	3.	Endometriosis	C. Period of time that marks permanent cessation of menstrual activity.
A	4.	Ovarian cancer	D. Pelvic inflammatory disease, involving some or all of the reproductive organs, usually transmitted sexually.
F	5.	Ovarian cysts	E. Painful condition characterized by endometrial cells adhering to tissues and organs outside of the uterus.
B	6.	Dysmennorhea	F. Cysts located on the ovaries.

C. The chart below lists complications of pregnancy. Fill in the description, symptoms, and treatments that correspond to the complication.

Complication	Description	Symptoms	Treatment
Abortion/Interruption of pregnancy			
1. Spontaneous	1. Unknown etiology. Expulsion of products of conception	1. Bleeding from vagina with expulsion of products of conception	1. Bedrest, D&C
2. Complete	2. Unknown etiology	2. Expulsion of all products of conception, fetus, and placenta	2. Bedrest, D&C
3. Missed	3. Fetus dies in the uterus and must be removed	3. Lack of movement of fetus; no heartbeat heard	3. D&C
4. Incomplete	4. Only parts of the fetus and placenta are expelled, with tissue remaining in the uterus	4. Expulsion of parts of fetus and placenta	4. D&C
5. Threatened	5. Bleeding from the uterus, no contractions or dilation of the cervix. Pregnancy continues	5. Bleeding from uterus, heartbeat may be present	5. Bedrest
6. Induced	6. Evacuation of the fetus and placenta from the uterus at the mother's request or due to health problems	6. None	6. D&C

continued

Continued

Eclampsia	Also called toxemia; can result in convulsions and is potentially life-threatening. Unknown cause	Hypertension, generalized edema, proteinuria	Monitor blood pressure, weight, routine urinalysis, bedrest, medications
Pre-eclampsia	Less severe than eclampsia; same symptoms but without convulsions	Hypertension, generalized edema, proteinuria	Monitor blood pressure, weight, routine urinalysis, bedrest, medications
Gestational diabetes	Appears in the second or third trimester, and disappears after delivery. Can lead to fetal and neonatal illness and death	High blood glucose levels	Prompt detection of glucose levels, medication
Hyperemesis gravidarum	Excessive vomiting during pregnancy. Unknown cause	Uncontrollable nausea and vomiting, inability to eat and exhaustion from inability to sleep, dehydration, and possible starvation	Intravenous fluids to replace those lost through vomiting, mild sedation to aid rest and sleep
Placenta previa	Placenta implants low in the uterus and partially or completely covers the cervical os. Cause is unknown, leading to maternal blood loss and fetal anoxia and death	Painless bleeding during third trimester or bleeding during labor	Depends on gestational age of fetus and percent of placenta that covers os. Cesarean section may be necessary
Placenta abruptio	Placenta prematurely and abruptly separates from the uterine lining. May result in fetal distress and death and maternal shock	Sudden release of amniotic fluid, pain, contractions	Delivery as soon as possible, either vaginally or by Cesarean section

D&C = Dilation and curretage.

D.

Obstetrical history	Number of pregnancies	Number of live births	Number of abortions
Gravida 1 Para 1 Abortion 1	1	1	1
Gravida 6 Para 4 Abortion 0	6	4	0
Gravida 3 Para 1 Abortion 2	3	1	2

Multiple Choice Questions

1. c. obstetrics
2. d. all of the above
3. c. eclampsia

4. a. monthly
5. d. pelvic inflammatory disease

ANSWERS TO WORKBOOK CASE STUDY QUESTIONS

The role of the medical assistant during a Pap smear and pelvic examination is to
1. Assemble the supplies needed.
2. Explain to the patient the procedures to be performed.
3. Position the patient in the lithotomy position and drape appropriately for privacy.
4. Assist the physician with obtaining specimens.
5. Label specimens correctly.
6. Send specimens to a reference lab, if indicated.

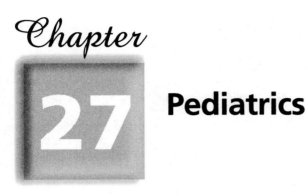

Chapter 27

Pediatrics

OVERVIEW

The medical assisting student is introduced to the branch of medicine that cares for new-borns, infants, children, and adolescents. Students learn the needs of this population, including the stages of growth and development and the diseases that affect them.

PROFICIENCY EVALUATION OUTCOME ASSESSMENT

Students are evaluated for their understanding of performance objectives. Students recognize the importance of possessing knowledge of the care and treatment of pediatric patients. Students learn procedures specific to this population such as measuring height, weight, head, chest circumference, and vital signs. Students are able to recognize the developmental stages and diseases of infants and children. Students are able to identify immunizations accurately and have a basic knowledge of the childhood diseases they prevent.

Procedure 27-1   Measuring the Infant: Weight, Height, Head, and Chest Circumference
Procedure 27-2   Taking and Infant's Rectal Temperature with a Mercury or Digital Thermometer
Procedure 27-3   Taking an Apical Pulse on an Infant
Procedure 27-4   Measuring Infant's Respiration Rate
Procedure 27-5   Obtaining a Urine Specimen from an Infant or Young Child

SUPPLEMENTARY RESOURCES

Medical Assisting Videos: Appropriate content is available on Delmar's Medical Assisting Videos, 2nd ed., for the following topics:

Tape 6: Vital Signs: Brachial Pulse on Infant
Apical Pulse on Infant Using a Stethoscope
Tape 7: Blood Pressure, Measurements, and Screening Procedures
Weigh and Measure an Infant
Growth Chart as a Screening Procedure
Big E Vision Chart for Children

ANSWERS TO REVIEW QUESTIONS

1. c. 2 months
2. b. tympanostomy
3. c. beta-hemolytic streptococcus group A
4. d. 6 years
5. c. 5th intercostal space on the left side

ANSWERS TO CRITICAL THINKING QUESTIONS

1. Talk to the physician immediately and report your findings and suspicions of abuse before the physician sees the child. This information is confidential and must be reported to the authorities. State laws vary, but both the medical assistant and physician may be required to file reports. The physician is responsible for speaking to the caregivers and informing them of his suspicions and that report(s) will be filed with the appropriate social service agencies and the police.

2. Head circumference measurement is important because an abnormal measurement can alert the physician to a problem. Rapid growth may indicate **hydrocephalus**, excessive fluid around the brain that can damage the brain. A slowly growing head can indicate **microencephaly**, an abnormally small brain resulting in mental retardation.

3. Growth charts aid in the diagnosis of growth abnormalities, nutritional disorders, and disease.

4. Place the child on his or her side with knees flexed or in prone position on the examination table or on the parent's lap.

5. It is clear plastic with adhesive tabs for application to the **perineum** of the child. The area must be washed and dried before applying the bag to reduce microorganism level and to obtain a good quality specimen. The bag must be secured to the perineum with the adhesive tabs. For a specimen from a female, place the bag over the labia; for males, place the bag over the penis and scrotum.

6. The chart used to check the visual acuity of young children is known as the kindergarten chart. It contains pictures on the chart in descending size and the lines on the chart are labeled in the same manner as the Snellen chart. The child is asked to identify a picture, one at a time, as the medical assistant points to it.

7. Aural temperatures should be taken on children over the age of 2 and on a child who has neither impacted cerumen in the ear nor is experiencing otitis media.

8. Restraint of infant movement may be necessary when taking a rectal temperature. Insert the thermometer gently past the anal sphincter to about ½ inch. Both of these actions help to ensure the infant's safety and comfort.

9. Chest measurements are taken on an infant when there is a suspicion of overdevelopment or underdevelopment of the heart and/or lungs or calcification of rib cartilage.

10. The printed lines across growth charts indicate the normal ranges of growth of infants and children in the United States. When growth is plotted on the growth charts, the charts become part of the infant's permanent record.

ANSWERS TO WORKBOOK EXERCISES AND ACTIVITIES

Vocabulary Builder

Exudate: accumulated fluid in a cavity; an oozing of pus.
Myringotomy: incision into the tympanic membrane. Part of the treatment for otitis media.
Suppurative: producing or associated with the generation of pus.
Tympanostomy: placement of a tube through the tympanic membrane of the ear to allow ongoing drainage.
Otitis Media: inflammation of the middle ear.
Tonsillitis: inflammation of the tonsils.
Pediculosis: infestation of lice.

Learning Review/Case Study

1. Gloves, mercury thermometer, sheath, paper towels, pediatric stethoscope, watch with second hand, sphygmomanometer, alcohol wipes, otoscope, sterile culture collection tube and gloves, biohazard waste container.

2. A. *Temperature:* For a 3-year-old child, the best method for taking the temperature is the axillary method. Note that the axillary method is the least accurate method for measuring temperature. Axillary temperature is at least 1 degree lower than an oral temperature because the axilla is an open body cavity. The thermometer must be kept in place for 5 minutes before reading. The child is exhibiting pyrexia.

   Pulse: A stethoscope is used to take the apical pulse, the preferred location for taking a child's pulse rate. The apical pulse is heard at the apex of the heart, located at the fifth intercostal space left side, mid-clavicular line. The heart rate is at the high end of the normal range for a child of this age. Heart rate increases in response to fever, excitement, and anxiety. Sinus arrhythmia is a normal cycle of irregular rhythm commonly seen in children, characterized by a faster heart rate on inspiration and a slower heart rate on expiration.

   Respiration: The rate of respiration is at the high end of the normal range for a 3-year-old child. Rhonchi, rattling sounds heard during inspiration and expiration, are noted. Rhonchi are exhibited, then the lung passageways contain secretions. The normal respiration rate is usually a 1:4 ratio with the pulse rate.

   Blood *pressure:* A pediatric cuff and stethoscope are used. The cuff for a child should cover two thirds of the upper arm. For children whose blood pressure can still be read to zero, the beginning of Korotkoff Phase IV and zero are both recorded. The blood pressure measurement is in the normal range for a 3-year-old child.

B. The medical assistant should distract the child by trying to make a game of the vital sign procedures that will enlist the child's attention and cooperation. The medical assistant may also involve the parent in the process of the examination by having the parent hold or comfort the child while vital signs are taken. A favorite toy brought from home, or a toy from the office's reception area toybox, also can help occupy the child and can be offered as long as it does not interfere with the procedure being performed.

3. The medical assistant's role is to attend to the emotional needs of the patient and his mother during the examination and to assist the physician as necessary. The medical assistant will hand instruments to the physician during the examination and will assist in the proper collection, handling, and processing of the laboratory specimen. The physician will collect the specimen due to the age of the child and the risk of causing further injury to the ear during the collection process.

4. A. To make a clinical diagnosis, the physician requires subjective and objective information such as the vital sign measurements, patient history (verbalized by both the patient and his mother), and the results of a physical examination. A clinical diagnosis does not include the results of laboratory testing; laboratory testing will be done to confirm the physician's clinical diagnosis.

B. Otitis media is an inflammation of the middle ear, occurring as a result of an upper respiratory tract infection. Children are likely at higher risk because their eustachian tubes are shorter than an adult's. Effective treatment involves identifying the microorganism causing the upper respiratory infection. Otitis media is commonly treated with antibiotics and analgesics. Local heat and nasal decongestants also are used. Patient education includes teaching the parent(s) to recognize the warning signs of otitis media and to use vaporizers and decongestants as preventive measures against the inflammatory condition when their child suffers an upper respiratory tract infection.

Multiple Choice Questions

1. d. hearing
2. a. 12.5 to 14.5 inches
3. c. in the armpit

4. b. 20 to 40
5. a. an inflammation of the middle ear

Investigation Activity: information obtained from the Centers for Disease Control and Prevention Web site: www.cdc.gov

Diphtheria

Description	A respiratory disease caused by bacteria
Symptoms	Gradual onset of a sore throat and low-grade fever
Complications	Airway obstruction, coma, and death if not treated
Transmission	Spread by coughing and sneezing
Vaccine	Diphtheria toxoid (contained in DTP, DTaP, DT or Td vaccines) can prevent this disease.

Haemophilus influenzae type b (Hib)

Description	A severe bacterial infection, occurring primarily in infants
Symptoms	Skin and throat infections, meningitis, pneumonia, sepsis, and arthritis (Can be serious in children under age 1, but there is little risk of getting the disease after age 5)
Complications	Hib meningitis (death in 1 out of 20 children, and permanent brain damage in 10 to 30 percent of the survivors)
Transmission	Spread by coughing and sneezing
Vaccine	Hib vaccine can prevent this disease.

Hepatitis A

Description	A disease of the liver caused by hepatitis A virus
Symptoms	Potentially none (likelihood of symptoms increases with the person's age). If present: yellow skin or eyes, tiredness, stomachache, loss of appetite, or nausea
Complications	Because young children might not have symptoms, the disease is often not recognized until the child's caregiver becomes ill with hepatitis A.
Transmission	*Most often:* spread by the fecal-oral route (an object contaminated with the stool of a person with hepatitis A is put into another person's mouth) *Less often:* spread by swallowing food or water that contains the virus
Vaccine	Hepatitis A vaccine will prevent this disease.

Hepatitis B

Description	A disease of the liver caused by hepatitis B virus
Symptoms	Potentially none when first infected (likelihood of early symptoms increases with the person's age) If present: yellow skin or eyes, tiredness, stomachache, loss of appetite, nausea, or joint pain

Complications	The younger the person, the greater the likelihood of staying infected and having lifelong liver problems, such as scarring of the liver and liver cancer
Transmission	Spread through contact with the blood of an infected person or by having sex with an infected person
Vaccine	Hepatitis B vaccine will prevent this disease.

Measles

Description	A respiratory disease caused by a virus
Symptoms	Measles virus causes rash, high fever, cough, runny nose, and red, watery eyes, lasting about a week.
Complications	Diarrhea, ear infections, pneumonia, encephalitis, seizures, and death
Transmission	Spread by coughing and sneezing (highly contagious)
Vaccine	Measles vaccine (contained in MMR, MR, and measles vaccines) can prevent this disease.

Mumps

Description	A disease of the lymph nodes caused by a virus
Symptoms	Fever, headache, muscle ache, and swelling of the lymph nodes close to the jaw
Complications	Meningitis, inflammation of the testicles or ovaries, inflammation of the pancreas and deafness (usually permanent)
Transmission	Spread by coughing and sneezing
Vaccine	Mumps vaccine (contained in MMR) can prevent this disease.

Pertussis (whooping cough)

Description	A respiratory disease caused by bacteria
Symptoms	Severe spasms of coughing that can interfere with eating, drinking, and breathing
Complications	Pneumonia, encephalitis (owing to lack of oxygen), and death, especially in infants
Transmission	Spread by coughing and sneezing (highly contagious)
Vaccine	Pertussis vaccine (contained in DTP and DTaP) can prevent this disease.

Polio

Description	A disease of the lymphatic and nervous systems
Symptoms	Fever, sore throat, nausea, headaches, stomachaches, and stiffness in the neck, back, and legs
Complications	Paralysis that can lead to permanent disability and death
Transmission	Contact with an infected person
Vaccine	Polio vaccine (IPV) can prevent this disease.

Rubella (German measles)

Description	A respiratory disease caused by a virus
Symptoms	Rash and fever for two to three days (mild disease in children and young adults)
Complications	Birth defects if acquired by a pregnant woman such as deafness, cataracts, heart defects, mental retardation, and liver and spleen damage (at least a 20 percent chance of damage to the fetus if a woman is infected early in pregnancy)
Transmission	Spread by coughing and sneezing
Vaccine	Rubella vaccine (contained in MMR vaccine) can prevent this disease.

Tetanus (lockjaw)

Description	A disease of the nervous system caused by bacteria
Symptoms	*Early symptoms:* lockjaw, stiffness in the neck and abdomen, and difficulty swallowing *Later symptoms:* fever, elevated blood pressure, and severe muscle spasms
Complications	Death in one third of the cases, especially people over age 50
Transmission	Enters the body through a break in the skin
Vaccine	Tetanus toxoid (contained in DTP, DT, DTaP and Td vaccines) can prevent this disease.

Varicella (chickenpox)

Description	A virus of the herpes family
Symptoms	A skin rash of blister-like lesions, usually on the face, scalp, or trunk
Complications	Bacterial infection of the skin, swelling of the brain, and pneumonia (usually more severe in children 13 or older and adults)
Transmission	Spread by coughing and sneezing (highly contagious)
Vaccine	Varicella vaccine can prevent this disease.

Chapter 28

Male Reproductive System

OVERVIEW

Medical assisting students must possess knowledge of the male reproductive system and the common disorders and diseases that can affect it. The student must be aware of treatments and procedures that they will encounter in the office when assisting the physician with the male patient, and must become comfortable with the terminology used.

PROFICIENCY EVALUATION OUTCOME ASSESSMENT

Students are evaluated for their understanding of the performance objectives. Students are able to describe the male reproductive system and identify common disorders and diseases that affect the system. A knowledge of the diagnostic tests and procedures that may be performed in the office is necessary for the student to possess. Students recognize the importance of health promotion and prevention of disease.

Procedure 28-1   Instructing Patient in Testicular Self-Examination

SUPPLEMENTARY RESOURCES

Medical Assisting Videos: Appropriate content is available on Delmar's Medical Assisting Videos, 2nd ed., for the following topics:

Tape 8   Taking a Patient History
Testicular Self-Examination

ANSWERS TO TEXT REVIEW QUESTIONS

1. a. prostate-specific antigen
2. c. monthly self-examination
3. b. aging and hormonal changes
4. a. painful urination
5. c. biopsy of the prostate

ANSWERS TO TEXT CRITICAL THINKING QUESTIONS

1. Slowly roll the testicle between the thumb and finger, applying slight pressure. Try to find hard, painless lumps.

   Examine the epididymis, the comma-shaped cord behind each testicle. It may be tender to the touch. It also is the location of most noncancerous problems.

   Continue by examining the vas (sperm-carrying tube that runs up from the epididymis). Feels firm and smooth. Repeat examination on the other side.

2. The purpose of severing the vas deferens in a vasectomy is to disconnect the flow of sperm from going up the testicle, the epididymis to the vas deferens, and to the urethra for ejaculation in semen. It prevents ejaculation of sperm, rendering the male infertile.

3. Symptoms of BPH are
   a. Cystitis from urine pooling in the bladder and providing a medium for bacteria to grow because the enlarged prostate constricts the urethra, impending urine flow.
   b. Diminished flow of urine.
   c. Difficulty to start urinating.
   d. Inability to empty the bladder.
   All of these symptoms are caused by the enlarged prostate constricting the urethra and diminishing urine flow.

4. The blood test prostate-specific antigen will help diagnose prostate cancer. Tumor cells release the antigen into the circulation and they can be measured in a blood sample.

5. Benign prostatic hypertrophy is more common in men over 50 years of age because it is a disease of aging.

6. The age group afflicted by testicular cancer is 20 to 35 years. Monthly testicular self-examination helps with early detection.

7. Semen analysis can be done to count the number of sperm per ejaculation in order to determine the male's ability to procreate. It is also used post vasectomy to be certain there are no sperm in the semen.

8. Males can contract any of the following STDs:

   gonorrhea   condylomata
   syphilis   AIDS
   chlamydia   hepatitis B
   herpes type II

9. A patient with nocturia gets up several times during the night to urinate. The physician will suspect an enlarged prostate gland. The gland can be palpated when the physician does a digital rectal examination, which can determine if the gland is enlarged and blocking urine flow, making the patient feel the urge to urinate more frequently, including during the night.

10. Benign hypertrophy of the prostate (BHP) is treated with medication that can relax prostate muscles, hormones that can block prostate growth, or bladder relaxants. A transurethral resection of prostate is the surgery performed if the patient does not respond to medication.

ANSWERS TO WORKBOOK EXERCISES AND ACTIVITIES

Vocabulary Builder

1. E.
2. D.
3. A.
4. B.

5. F.
6. G.
7. C.

Learning Review

1. Epididymis: epididymitis
2. Testicle: anorchism
                        orchitis
                        cryptorchidism
3. Urinary bladder: cystitis
                        carcinoma of the bladder
4. Prostate gland: benign prostatic hypertrophy
                        carcinoma of the prostate
5. Urethra: urethritis
6. Glans penis: balanitis

Multiple Choice Questions

1. d. all of the above
2. c. prostate cancer
3. b. PSA blood test

4. a. hyperplasia
5. c. annually

Investigation Activity

The chart below lists diseases of the male reproductive system. Fill in the cause, symptoms, and treatments that correspond to the disease.

Disease	Cause	Symptoms	Treatment
Benign prostatic hypertrophy	Enlargement of the prostate gland	Obstruction of urine flow: difficulty in starting urination, a weak stream of urine, the inability to empty the bladder completely, dribbling at the end of voiding	Medication, surgery
Cancer of the prostate	Malignant growth within the prostate gland	Frequency of urination, inability to urinate, dribbling during urination, pain or burning upon urination	Chemotherapy, hormone therapy, radiation therapy, surgery
Epididymitis	Inflammation of the epididymis, can result from a chlamydial infection	Pain, fever, tenderness, and difficulty walking	Antibiotics, analgesics
Prostatitis	Inflammation of the prostate	Low back pain, fullness or pain in the perineal area, urinary frequency, and discharge from the urethra	Medication for infection, pain, fever
Genital herpes	STD viral infection of the genitalia caused by herpes simplex	Multiple shallow ulcerations of the penis and scrotal sac, flulike symptoms of fever, headache, malaise, painful urination	Medication to reduce swelling and pain
Gonorrhea	STD bacterial infection of the mucous membrane of the genital tract	Greenish-yellow drainage of pus from the urethra, painful urination, frequent urination	Antibiotics
Syphilis	STD caused by spirochete, Treponema pallidum; chancre appears on the penis	Three stages: primary with lesion on the penis; secondary with nonitching rash on the hands and feet, flulike symptoms, bone and joint pain; tertiary with lesions invading body organs and symptoms	Penicillin
Testicular cancer	Malignant growth of the testicle	Painless lump in the testicle	Chemotherapy, radiation therapy, surgery

ANSWERS TO WORBOOK CASE STUDY QUESTION

Often, patient information brochures and instructions are available in the office for the medical assistant to review and give to the patient. With the older patient, especially when confronted with a life-threatening disease, empathy and compassion must be part of the care and treatment. Asking the patient to repeat what the physician has explained will help the medical assistant understand and evaluate the patient's level of knowledge. Informing the physician of the patient's fear and lack of understanding is important.

Chapter 29

Gerontology

OVERVIEW

Medical assistants assist with the care of the geriatric patient on a regular basis. With the population aging, students are expected to identify the changes that the elderly undergo with their body, their mind, and the social stigma attached to the older adult in society. Communication skills are stressed to the student, who will be instrumental in assisting the geriatric patient in the ambulatory setting.

PROFICIENCY EVALUATION OUTCOME ASSESSMENT

Medical assisting students are introduced to the concepts surrounding the geriatric patient. The importance for students to identify and understand the social, psychological, and physiological changes that confront the elderly patient is stressed. Students will be able to define key glossary terms, describe how to improve communication with the aged, and describe the increasing problem of elderly abuse. They will be able to assist those with sight difficulties to maneuver safely in the ambulatory setting.

SUPPLEMENTARY RESOURCES

Medical Assisting Videos: Appropriate content is available on Delmar's Medical Assisting Videos, 2nd ed., for the following topics:

Tape 1   Communication Skills
Tape 8   Taking a Patient History
Tape 9   Introduction to Body Mechanics
          Transfer Wheelchair to Examination Table and Back
          Instructing Patients with Special Needs

ANSWERS TO TEXT REVIEW QUESTIONS

1. a. arteriosclerotic heart disease
2. d. glaucoma
3. a. cartilage erodes in the joints
4. c. pneumonia
5. c. amount of urine left in bladder after voiding

ANSWERS TO TEXT CRITICAL THINKING QUESTIONS

1. Adding different herbs and seasonings can make the food more appealing.
2. To keep mentally and physically stimulated, seniors can learn a foreign language, play a musical instrument, garden, volunteer, and engage in regular exercise.
3. Regular exercise, calcium supplements, hormone replacement therapy, and medication all help to keep bones from becoming brittle.

4. Color intensity is diminished when a person suffers from macular degeneration.
5. Four reasons for incontinence are urinary tract infection, diabetes, prostatitis, and certain medications.
6. The most common myth about seniors is that "to be old is to be sick."
7. Students will have their own personal answers.
8. Speak slowly, clearly, and face the individual in order to enhance communication.
9. First make the person aware of your presence.
10. Some of the reasons older Americans are living longer are because of good nutrition, exercise, a positive attitude, technology and financial resources.

ANSWERS TO WORKBOOK EXERCISES AND ACTIVITIES

Vocabulary Builder

1. C.
2. E.
3. G.
4. J.
5. I.
6. H.
7. D.
8. F.
9. B.
10. A.

Learning Review

A. Identification of System Problems
1. Dry, red, irritated eyes, sensitivity to light, inability to see clearly, inability to tell colors apart, inability to see small print, loss of hearing.
2. Diminished taste, diminished smell.
3. Thinning of skin, wrinkles, age spots, smaller sweat glands, loss of hair color, thinning of hair, drying of skin.
4. Memory loss, delay in memory functions, confusion, inability to do tasks, balance problems, temperature regulation problems, diminished pain sensation, insomnia.
5. Loss of muscle strength, loss of mobility, stiffening of joints, loss of height, brittle bones, prolonged healing time.
6. Diminished breathing capacity, shortness of breath, loss of lung elasticity.
7. Blood vessels lose elasticity, narrow, and build up with plaque; high blood pressure, congestive heart failure, myocardial infarction.
8. Stomach secretions and mobility decrease, peristalsis slows, metabolism slows, dental problems.
9. Decrease urine output, loss of kidney function, loss of bladder elasticity, inability to urinate completely, hypertrophy of prostate gland.
10. Estrogen production decreases, decrease in vaginal secretions, diminished testosterone levels, benign prostatic hypertrophy.

B. List ten ways to improve communication with the geriatric patient.
1. Talk to the person in a nondistracting place.
2. Begin conversations with orienting information, introducing yourself and calling the patient by name.
3. Use short words and short, simple sentences.
4. Speak slowly and clearly, lower the pitch of your voice, speak in a warm and pleasant manner.
5. Never talk down to a patient or be condescending.
6. Give clear, simple instructions; allow time for information to be absorbed and understood. Ask for the patient to repeat instructions and information given.
7. Ask the person to do one task at a time.
8. Listen actively.
9. Use humor when appropriate.
10. Protect confidentiality by talking in private.

Multiple Choice Questions

1. d. the average lifespan is increasing
2. b. presbycusis
3. a. taste buds decrease in size
4. c. increased pain sensation
5. c. arteriosclerosis

Investigation Activity

A. List of techniques used to help the elderly maneuver. Role-playing techniques can be performed when one student takes the role of the medical assistant and another of the patient as they explore the difficulties encountered by the geriatric patient.
1. Making contact.

2. Grip just above the elbow.
3. Stand next to and one-half step behind the person.
4. Set a comfortable pace.
5. Explain to the person when approaching a narrow passageway. Have the person put an arm in back, and you should assist by holding the arm above the elbow.
6. Give information when approaching doors and doorways, with the guide going through the doorway first, assisting the person through.
7. Revolving doors should be avoided, but if you are not able to, wait until traffic through the revolving door has stopped. Stop the door, and guide the person through the door. The person, after getting through, should wait for the guide to join him or her.
8. Inform the person about stairways, letting the person know if they go up or down. Have the person stand with the handrail at the side, and have the person hold your arm above the elbow. Slowly take one step at a time until you reach the top or bottom.
9. When guiding someone to a seat, walk up to the chair, and place your hand on the back of the chair. Have the follower trail your arm down to the back, tell him or her the way the chair is facing, and assist him or her in sitting down.

B. The student may describe feelings of confusion, apprehension, or pressure when assisting the person who cannot see.
C. The student may express feelings of apprehension and helplessness when blindfolded.

ANSWERS TO WORKBOOK CASE STUDY QUESTIONS

A suggestion that you can give Mr. Jones is to use a pill dispenser that he can put his pills in by the time of day and day of the week. This can be purchased at drug stores and pharmacies. Using an alarm clock to ring when he must take his next medication may be helpful in reminding him to take his medications.

Explain to the granddaughter that normal physiological changes in the older person include a diminish of taste and smell, leading to food being less appealing as it does not taste as good as it once did. Loss of smell also contributes to the decrease in the desire for food. Eating may also be thought of as a social activity, where pleasure is obtained during the eating process by interacting with others. Since Mr. Jones lives alone, and therefore eats alone, the pleasure he once got when interacting with others during meals is gone, contributing to the loss in the interest in food.

Chapter

30

Examinations and Procedures of Body Systems

OVERVIEW

Medical assisting students' thorough knowledge and understanding of the various specialty examinations and clinical procedures routinely performed as a part of patient care are essential to their successful preparation for employment in specialists' offices or ambulatory care settings where a variety of patient problems are treated. This chapter introduces students to specialty and body systems examinations and appropriate clinical procedures used during each. Students are challenged to broaden their knowledge and skills, assisting the physician or specialist to provide the highest-quality patient care.

PROFICIENCY EVALUATION OUTCOME ASSESSMENT

Students are evaluated for their understanding of performance objectives. They should demonstrate the ability to assist the physician during a specialty examination. This includes specialty and body system examinations and appropriate clinical procedures in urology; endoscopy; sensory system; the respiratory system; the musculoskeletal, neurological, and circulatory systems; blood and lymph; and integumentary system. The student is able to discuss the role of the medical assistant during the physician's examination of the patient; describe the equipment and supplies necessary for clinical procedures, including use, care, cleaning, and storage; identify laboratory test and analysis procedures the physician may order for a patient specimen; and discuss the pharmacological properties and safe administration of drugs prescribed by the physician for the patient. All quality control guidelines and safety guidelines should be followed, including standard precautions for infection control. The importance of developing strong therapeutic communication skills to facilitate patient cooperation, education, and attendance to the patient's emotional needs is emphasized.

Procedure 30-1	Performing a Urine Drug Screening
Procedure 30-2	Performing a Urinary Catheterization on a Female Patient
Procedure 30-3	Urinary Catheterization of a Male Patient
Procedure 30-4	Assisting with Proctosigmoidoscopy
Procedure 30-5	Fecal Occult Blood Test
Procedure 30-6	Performing Visual Acuity Testing Using a Snellen Chart
Procedure 30-7	Measuring Near Visual Acuity
Procedure 30-8	Performing Color Vision Test Using the Ishihara Plates
Procedure 30-9	Performing Eye Instillation
Procedure 30-10	Performing Eye Patch Dressing Application
Procedure 30-11	Performing Eye Irrigation
Procedure 30-12	Assisting with Audiometry
Procedure 30-13	Performing Ear Irrigation
Procedure 30-14	Performing Ear Instillation
Procedure 30-15	Assisting with Nasal Examination
Procedure 30-16	Performing Nasal Irrigation
Procedure 30-17	Performing Nasal Instillation
Procedure 30-18	Obtaining a Sputum Specimen

Procedure 30-19 Administer Oxygen by Nasal Cannula for Minor Respiratory Distress
Procedure 30-20 Instructing Patient in Use of Metered Dose Nebulizer
Procedure 30-21 Spirometry Testing
Procedure 30-22 Assisting with Plaster-of-Paris Cast Application
Procedure 30-23 Assisting with Cast Removal
Procedure 30-24 Assisting the Physician During a Lumbar Puncture
Procedure 30-25 Assisting the Physician with a Neurological Screening Examination

SUPPLEMENTARY RESOURCES

Medical Assisting Videos: Appropriate content is available on Delmar's Medical Assisting Videos, 2nd ed., for the following topics:

Tape 6   Take Vital Signs
         Take and Record Rectal Temperature
         Take and Record a Brachial Pulse (infant)
         Use a Stethoscope to Take an Apical Pulse (infant)
Tape 7   Take and Record Blood Pressure
         Weigh and Measure an Infant
         Growth Chart as a Screening Procedure
         Vision Screen
         Using an Audiometer to Perform a Hearing Screen
Tape 8   Take an In-depth Patient History
         Clean Examination Table and Countertops
         Assist Physician with Examination and Treatments
         Position and Drape the Patient
         Role of the Medical Assistant During the Examination
         Introduction to Health Promotion, Disease Prevention, and Self-Responsibility
         Testicular Self-Examination
         Breast Self-Examination
Tape 11 Prepare and Administer Medication as Directed by Physician
         Administer Eye Medications
         Administer Ear Medications
         Administer Sublingual Medications
         Administer Rectal Suppositories
         Topical Applications
         Transdermal Patch Applications

ANSWERS TO TEXT REVIEW QUESTIONS

1. d. warts
2. d. fibromyalgia
3. b. impacted
4. c. Parkinson's
5. c. furuncle

ANSWERS TO TEXT CRITICAL THINKING QUESTIONS

1. A urinary catheterization is a sterile procedure that is performed by inserting a catheter through the urethra into the bladder to withdraw urine. The urinary meatus and labia are cleansed with sterile cotton balls, using sterile forceps and a sterile antiseptic solution, while wearing sterile gloves. Dispose of the forceps with the sterile gloved hand used to cleanse. The lubricated catheter is inserted into the urinary meatus approximately 5 to 6 inches. Allow urine to flow into a sterile specimen container for a urinalysis.
2. Rules of evidence are followed during a drug screen to ascertain that the urine specimen offered by the patient is in fact the patient's own urine.
3. Dietary restrictions for fecal occult blood include no red meat, processed meats, liver, turnips, broccoli, cauliflower, and melon. Avoid aspirin and vitamin C. Consume a high-fiber diet. Other directions to the patient include not doing the test during menses or if bleeding from hemorrhoids.
    Store the slides out of direct sunlight. The supplies given to the patient include three guaiac slides, three wooden spatulas, and an envelope addressed to the physician.

The guaiac slides are obtained by opening the window flag on the front side of the slide. Use one end of the applicator to smear a thin amount of stool from the toilet onto box "A." Repeat, using the other end of the applicator, taking a specimen from a different section of the same stool and applying a thin smear to box "B." Close the corner and date. Repeat the process for the next two bowel movements on subsequent days.

To develop the slides, the medical assistant puts on gloves, opens the window flap on the back of the slide, and applies two drops of developer to the box and directly over each smear. Interpret results within 30 to 60 seconds. A positive reaction for the presence of hidden blood will show a blue halo around the outside edges of the smear of feces. The quality control procedures must be performed by processing the negative and positive monitor strips on each slide. Place one drop of developer between the positive and negative areas (where noted). The guaiac paper should test positive on the positive side and negative on the other side. This confirms that the test system is functional.

4. a. Preparation for a barium enema: clear liquids one day before the X ray; 8 oz. of water every hour until bedtime; laxative after dinner the night before the exam; light evening meal; nothing by mouth except for water after dinner; cleansing enemas until clear returns are achieved.

    b. Preparation for an upper GI (barium swallow): light evening meal the night before the test; nothing by mouth after midnight.

    c. Preparation of a cholecystogram: A fat-free dinner the evening before; dye tablets taken one at a time, each with 8 oz. of water; laxative and cleansing enemas may be prescribed; nothing by mouth after dinner, and dye tablets.

    d. Preparation of intravenous pyelogram: light evening meal the night before the exam; laxative the night before; nothing by mouth after 9 p.m.; cleansing enemas in the morning.

5. Visual acuity test for an adult includes the following steps: Perform the test while the patient is wearing eyeglasses or contact lenses; stand at the 20 ft. mark and cover the left eye with an occluder, keeping the left eye open; stand next to the Snellen chart and point to line 3 (to line 2 or line 1 if the patient cannot read line 3). Record the results of the line of smallest letters that the patient can read with two or less errors. Vision is recorded in the right eye, left eye, and both eyes, checking each eye separately. Wipe the occluders with alcohol. Visual acuity for a 9-year-old child follows the same steps as those for checking visual acuity for an adult. Visual acuity testing for a 4-year-old toddler is performed by using the kindergarten chart. It consists of pictures of objects that a young child can recognize, and the objects are shown in descending size. The line of pictures are labeled as they are on the adult Snellen chart.

6. The audiometer is a device used to test hearing acuity and assess hearing loss. Frequency of sound waves tests the patient's ability to hear. The patient listens for one frequency at a time. When the patient hears a new frequency, the tester is signaled. The test is conducted in a soundproof room or a room free of outside noise. The patient is seated and headphones are placed over the ears. Each ear is tested separately. The audiometer is started at a low frequency. The patient indicates by signaling (raising the hand) that the sound is heard. The results are plotted on a graph (audiogram). The frequencies gradually increase to higher frequencies until the test is completed. The other ear is tested in the same manner. The physician interprets the results.

7. When performing an eye irrigation, the flow of the irrigating solution must move from inner canthus to outer canthus to prevent the solution from reaching the other eye and causing it to become contaminated from the solution that has been used on the affected eye. Flowing from inner to outer canthus requires the patient's head to be tipped in the direction of the affected eye.

8. Bronchitis is an inflammation of the bronchi caused by either a bacterium or virus, and it produces a dry, painful cough that becomes productive. The sputum is yellow-green in color. Emphysema is the enlargement or stretching of alveoli in the lungs resulting in loss of elasticity and the capacity to completely exhale. Some carbon dioxide remains trapped in the alveoli. Dyspnea, chronic cough, weight loss, and barrel chest are some of the signs and symptoms. Emphysema is an irreversible, debilitating lung disease. Asthma is usually caused by an allergen and is characterized by spasms of the smooth muscles of the bronchi. Dyspnea and wheezing are common symptoms.

9. The medical assistant wears personal protective equipment while helping the patient obtain a sputum specimen. The patient must cough deeply and expectorate directly into a sterile specimen container. The top of the container is secured and a laboratory request form is completed and secured to the specimen container. The specimen is sent to the laboratory within 30 minutes in a plastic bag.

10. The medical assistant's role in spirometry is to explain the procedure and allow the patient to become familiar with the equipment. The patient is either seated or may remain standing, but should be comfortable. The patient must take deep breaths to fill the lungs to his or her maximum capacity. The patient exhales for as long as possible and until told to stop. The test results are given to the physician for interpretation.

11. The various kinds of cast materials used in the clinic or office are plaster-of-paris; synthetic, such as plastic; and the air cast. Cast care guidelines for the patient include: Allow the cast to dry by exposing it to the air and keeping it uncovered, even at night; elevate the extremity with the cast to aid in reducing swelling and pain; observe fingers and toes for changes in color, changes in temperature, decreased sensation, and tingling; do not place objects into the cast to scratch irritated skin; do not get the cast wet. Cover with waterproof covering when bathing; clean cast with a damp cloth; if decorating a cast, use water-based paints or marking pens.

12. The components of a neurological examination include checking for the following: mental status, cranial nerve function, cerebral function, motor function, and deep tendon reflexes.

13. The five areas that are reviewed as part of a mental status exam are: (1) Level of consciousness; (2) Memory; (3) Cognition; (4) Mood; and (5) Ideation content.

14. When assisting with a lumbar puncture, the medical assistant's role is to prepare the room; set up the equipment; have the patient void; cleanse the site with antiseptic soap and water; position the patient in a lateral recumbent position with the back at the edge of the table and have the patient draw up the knees to the chest, grasp onto the knees and flex the chin onto the chest; and assist the physician to aspirate anesthetic. Help the patient maintain his or her position. Remind the patient not to hold the breath or talk and to take deep breaths to help with relaxation. The medical assistant prepares the specimen of cerebral spinal fluid for transportation to the laboratory. Cleansing of equipment, supplies, and treatment area also are part of the medical assistant's job.

ANSWERS TO WORKBOOK EXERCISES AND CASE STUDY

Vocabulary Builder

1. J.
2. I.
3. H.
4. G.
5. F.
6. E.
7. D.
8. C.
9. B.
10. A.
11. T.
12. S.
13. R.
14. Q.
15. P.
16. O.
17. N.
18. M.
19. L.
20. K.

Multiple Choice Questions

1. b. hematogenous
2. c. uremia
3. c. colon
4. a. occult blood in the stool
5. c. cholecystogram

Learning Review/Case Study

1. Gloves, mercury thermometer, sheath, paper towels, pediatric stethoscope, watch with second hand, sphygmomanometer, alcohol wipes, otoscope, sterile culture collection tube and gloves, biohazard waste container.

2. A. *Temperature:* For a 3-year-old child, the best method for taking the temperature is the axillary method. Note that the axillary method is the least accurate method for measuring temperature. Axillary temperature is at least 1 degree lower than an oral temperature because the axilla is an open body cavity. The thermometer must be kept in place for 5 minutes before reading. The child is exhibiting pyrexia.

    Pulse: A stethoscope is used to take the apical pulse, the preferred location for taking a child's pulse rate. The apical pulse is heard at the apex of the heart, located at the fifth intercostal space left side, mid-clavicular line. The heart rate is at the high end of the normal range for a child of this age. Heart rate increases in response to fever, excitement, and anxiety. Sinus arrhythmia is a normal cycle of irregular rhythm commonly seen in children, characterized by a faster heart rate on inspiration and a slower heart rate on expiration.

    Respiration: The rate of respiration is at the high end of the normal range for a 3-year-old child. Rhonchi, rattling sounds heard during inspiration and expiration, are noted. Rhonchi are exhibited, then the lung passageways contain secretions. The normal respiration rate is usually a 1:4 ratio with the pulse rate.

    Blood pressure: A pediatric cuff and stethoscope are used. The cuff for a child should cover two-thirds of the upper arm. For children whose blood pressure can still be read to zero, the beginning of Korotkoff Phase IV and zero are both recorded. The blood pressure measurement is in the normal range for a 3-year-old child.

    B. The medical assistant should distract the child by trying to make a game of the vital sign procedures that will enlist the child's attention and cooperation. The medical assistant may also involve the parent in the process of the examination by having the parent hold or comfort the child while vital signs are taken. A favorite toy brought from home, or a toy from the office's reception area toybox, also can help occupy the child and can be offered as long as it does not interfere with the procedure being performed.

3. The medical assistant's role is to attend to the emotional needs of the patient and his mother during the examination and to assist the physician as necessary. The medical assistant will hand instruments to the physician during the examination and will assist in the proper collection, handling, and processing of the laboratory specimen. The physician will collect the specimen due to the age of the child and the risk of causing further injury to the ear during the collection process.

4. A. To make a clinical diagnosis, the physician requires subjective and objective information such as the vital sign measurements, patient history (verbalized by both the patient and his mother), and the results of a physical examination. A clinical diagnosis does not include the results of laboratory testing; laboratory testing will be done to confirm the physician's clinical diagnosis.

    B. Otitis media is an inflammation of the middle ear, occurring as a result of an upper respiratory tract infection. Children are likely at higher risk because their eustachian tubes are shorter than an adult's. Effective treatment involves identifying the microorganism causing the upper respiratory infection. Otitis media is commonly treated with antibiotics and analgesics. Local heat and nasal decongestants also are used. Patient education includes teaching the parent(s) to recognize the warning signs of otitis media and to use vaporizers and decongestants as preventive measures against the inflammatory condition when their child suffers an upper respiratory tract infection.

Chapter

Assisting with Minor Surgery

OVERVIEW

To assist with minor surgery in the ambulatory care setting, medical assistants need to be able to understand and apply sterile technique. To assist the physician effectively, medical assistants need to be aware of the steps involved in commonly performed minor surgical procedures and must recognize the function of equipment and supplies necessary for each. Therapeutic communication skills are also essential in allaying patients' apprehension and promoting patients' understanding of procedures performed as well as any post-operative care.

PROFICIENCY EVALUATION OUTCOME ASSESSMENT

Students are evaluated for their understanding of performance objectives. The ability to effectively assist the physician during minor surgical procedures commonly performed in the ambulatory care setting is demonstrated. Students distinguish between medical aseptic and surgical aseptic techniques and possess the ability to identify situations where each is appropriate. A knowledge of suture materials, surgical instruments, and other supplies, such as dressings and bandages, is demonstrated. An awareness of standard precautions necessary for specific procedures is exhibited. Students are able to establish a sterile field and place instruments and supplies correctly within the sterile field; sterile guidelines are understood and applied. Therapeutic communication skills in patient preparation, comforting the patient during procedures, and providing postoperative care and instructions are emphasized.

SUPPLEMENTARY RESOURCES

Medical Assisting Videos: Appropriate content is available on Delmar's Medical Assisting Videos, 2nd ed., for the following topics:

Tape 5   Set a Sterile Field
Open a Sterile Pack
Open a Peel Pack
Use Disposable Trays of Instruments
Perform Surgical Aseptic Procedures
Tape 6   Take Vital Signs
Tape 8   Assist Physician with Examination and Treatments
Position and Drape the Patient
Role of the Medical Assistant During the Examination

ANSWERS TO TEXT REVIEW QUESTIONS

1.   c.   to prevent microorganisms from entering the body during an invasive procedure
2.   c.   provide the physician a separate container for contaminated instruments
3.   c.   4-0
4.   a.   gut
5.   b.   to reduce blood flow in the operative site through vasoconstriction
6.   d.   incise and drain the cyst

ANSWERS TO TEXT CRITICAL THINKING QUESTIONS

1.   If the instrument pack is to be used immediately, it is acceptable to consider the inner contents sterile. If the instrument pack is to be stored for later use, the contents must be rewrapped and re-sterilized. Wrapped items that will pierce body tissue, such as surgical instruments, must be wrapped in two layers to maintain sterility during storage. If the outer layer of the wrap is compromised with a tear, the intact single inner wrap will still protect the contents, but only for a short time, and is not considered sufficient protection for storage purposes.

2.   One of the options is to place the unopened suture package onto the side counter. Once the physician has applied sterile gloves, the nonsterile outer wrap of the suture package may be peeled back with ungloved hands and held out for the physician to remove the sterile suture package. This option is advantageous if the medical assistant is to be present during the surgery. The disadvantage of this option is that the medical assistant would need to be present during the surgery at some point between the time the physician applies the sterile gloves and the suturing.

Another option is to peel back the nonsterile outer wrap of the suture package and "flip" the sterile suture package onto the sterile surgical field on top of the other items. The advantage of this option is that the surgery tray is complete and would not necessitate an assistant being present during the surgery. A disadvantage of this option is that the suture package might not be in the most logical and organized location on the tray.

A third option is to request another medical assistant to peel back the outer wrap and offer the sterile inner suture package to you. You could then place the suture package onto the sterile surgery tray with your sterile gloves and proceed with the tray set-up. This method is advantageous only if another medical assistant is available. This method has the disadvantage of requiring another person to assist, which may be disruptive to the office flow. Any of these three options is certainly acceptable and the choice would be made with consideration regarding the advantages and disadvantages within each particular office and situation.

3.   Students may need additional references to determine their answer to this question. The determination to suture a wound takes into consideration its location, depth complexity, and size, as well as whether or not the wound is gaping. If a wound is gaping, it will usually heal quicker and with less scarring if the edges are approximated with sutures. Even if the wound is not gaping, but is located on a portion of the body that bends, such as a knee or an elbow, suturing is desirable to minimize scarring. If a wound is deep and/or larger than a centimeter, suturing will probably aid healing and lessen complications. If a wound is several hours old, it is usually not suitable for suturing due to the healing process that takes place in the first few hours. Sometimes a physician may choose to trim the healed edges to expose fresh tissue, then proceed with suturing. If a determination is made not to suture a wound because of advanced healing, adhesive sterile strips may be used to pull the edges of the wound closer for the completion of the healing process. Sometimes a wound is infected and a decision will be made to leave a wound open to allow drainage. Occasionally a "wick" is placed into the wound to facilitate the drainage. Even though puncture wounds are often deep, they are usually not wide enough for suturing and are often left open for drainage.

4.   If a patient is weak or impaired after surgery and hurts himself or herself or others while driving home, the physician may be held liable. If no one is available to drive the patient home, the patient should stay in the clinic until it is determined that he or she is no longer impaired.

5. Written instructions are always given to the patient and caregiver and are explained to each until they are clearly understood. The clinic or office phone number and an "after hours" number should also be written for patients so they can call if they experience any complications or need further instructions. Assure patients that comfort and safety are very important and encourage them to call with concerns and questions if need be. A follow-up call later in the day or the next day should be standard practice.
6. The area has become contaminated and must be set up again with new equipment and supplies.
7. Explain the situation to Dr. Woo. Examine the torn gloves; apply a new pair of sterile gloves.
8. Wear PPE, including mask, goggles, gown, and gloves. Discard soiled items in a biohazard container according to OSHA guidelines.

ANSWERS TO WORKBOOK EXERCISES AND ACTIVITIES

Vocabulary Builder

A. 1. I.
2. D.
3. H.
4. J.
5. G.
6. C.
7. A.
8. B.
9. L.
10. M.
11. F.
12. K.
13. E.

B. 1. F.
2. J.
3. A.
4. N.
5. M.
6. O.
7. C.
8. G.
9. H.
10. K.
11. I.
12. L.
13. B.
14. E.
15. D.

Multiple Choice Questions

1. a. 1 inch
2. d. 18 inches
3. b. chromion
4. d. cauterization
5. c. ratchet

Learning Review/Case Study

1. A. Sterile.
   B. Contaminated. Do not turn your back on a sterile field. If you cannot see the field, you cannot be aware of what touched it. If work must be interrupted, apply a sterile field cover and move the tray to a place where it will not be disturbed.
   C. Contaminated. Reaching over a sterile field with contaminated waste will contaminate the field. The biohazard container should be placed away from the sterile area and in a position that does not necessitate reaching over or near the sterile field.
   D. Sterile.
   E. Contaminated. Anything below the waist is considered out of the sterile range and, therefore, contaminated. All articles should be held above the waist; gloved hands should be held in front of and away from the body, above waist height.
2. A. SAH; B. MAH; C. MAH; D. SAH; E. MAH; F. SAH; G. MAH; H. SAH.
3. A. Choices C, D, and F are correct instruments for the suturing procedure.
      The identification and use of instruments illustrated in the exercise is as follows.
      A. Walther urethral sound. This probe is used to determine the size and shape of the urethra or to detect the presence of an unseen foreign body.
      B. Foerster sponge forceps. These are used to hold gauze sponges.
      C. Iris scissors (curved). Delicately bladed operating scissors, used to cut tissues.
      D. Rochester Ochsner forceps (curved). Hemostatic forceps, or hemostats, are used to grasp and clamp blood vessels.
      E. Lister bandage scissors, large. These are used to remove bandages without causing injury to the patient.
      F. Adson tissue forceps. Thumb forceps with teeth, which are used to grasp tissue.
      G. Jones towel clamp. Used to attach surgical field drapes to each other.

B. The medical assistant will also need syringe and needle for anesthetic, suture material and needle, needle holder, and gauze sponges for the surgical tray. The medical assistant will need anesthetic as ordered by the physician; dressings, bandages, and tape; splint/brace (optional); and sterile gloves for the side table.

C. Suturing is recommended if a laceration or incision is gaping, bleeding uncontrollably, or is located on the face, neck, or a bend of a body part or extends deep into underlying tissue. Suturing facilitates healing by approximating the edges; it decreases scarring, helps decrease the likelihood of infection, and promotes healing. Before suturing, the laceration must be carefully cleaned of any dirt and debris that could cause infection and impede the healing process.

4. A. The medical assistant will require sponge forceps (B) and bandage scissors (E).

B. The medical assistant will also require gauze sponges, a biohazard waste container, tape, suture removal kit, sterile latex gloves, and Betadine solution or wash.

C. To removes sutures, grasp the suture knot with thumb forceps. Place the curved tip of the suture removal scissors just next to the skin under the suture. Clip. Gently pull the suture knot up and toward the incision with thumb forceps to remove.

D. Audrey will check the patient's vital signs. She will explain wound care, providing written instructions as well. The patient must be checked for any unusual or adverse reactions to the procedure. Instructions must be given to the patient, both verbally and in writing, to ensure that information is understood by the patient and can be easily and accurately followed by the patient at home.

Chapter

Diagnostic Imaging

OVERVIEW

Medical assisting students are introduced to the terminology and concepts surrounding radiology and diagnostic imaging. Students become aware of the three types of radiology and their uses in the ambulatory setting. Radiation safety is a key issue the student must be aware of for their own safety and for the safety of the patient.

PROFICIENCY EVALUATION OUTCOME ASSESSMENT

Students are evaluated for their understanding of performance objectives. Students will be able to define the key terms related to radiology and diagnostic imaging. Students will be able to describe the various positions used during X-ray procedures and the safety precautions necessary for personnel and patients. Students will describe fluoroscopy and the various procedures that require patient preparation. An understanding of ultrasound, CT scans, and MRIs will be demonstrated by the students. In this chapter, students explain the differences among radiology, radiation therapy, and nuclear medicine.

SUPPLEMENTARY RESOURCES

Medical Assisting Videos: Appropriate content is available on Delmar's Medical Assisting Videos, 2nd ed., for the following topics:

Tape 1 Professionalism and Communication Skills
Display Professionalism
Communication Skills
Tape 9 Body Mechanics, Therapeutic and Rehabilitative Procedures
Ultrasound Procedures

ANSWERS TO TEXT REVIEW QUESTIONS

1. b. mammogram
2. b. tablets
3. c. bile ducts
4. c. posteroanterior
5. c. magnetic resonance imaging

ANSWERS TO TEXT CRITICAL THINKING QUESTIONS

1. Because X-ray beams can be harmful, lead-lined aprons and gloves are used by personnel taking X rays and an apron is worn by patients to protect their reproductive organs. Lead-lined walls in the X-ray department absorb X rays that tend to scatter about the room.
2. Thermography is a heat-sensing technique used to detect tumors.

3. X rays can diagnose many diseases and conditions such as fractured bones, poorly functioning organs, tumors, calculi, etc. Because X-rays can penetrate most materials, they are useful for making images to aid in diagnosing a patient condition.

4. X rays are used to treat certain diseases such as malignancies. Because X rays can penetrate tissues and cells, the aim is to interfere with cell growth and to disrupt DNA. The object is to destroy as many malignant cells as possible without harming healthy surrounding cells.

5. Four types of contrast media are barium sulfate, given by mouth or enema. It is radiopaque and useful for identifying abnormalities in the gastrointestinal tract. Iodine salts, given either by mouth or injection, is also radiopaque and useful for identifying problems in the urinary tract or gallbladder. Air and carbon dioxide are used to identify problems in the spinal cord and joints.

6. Exposure to radiation while pregnant can have serious effects on the developing embryo or fetus. It can cause severe damage or even death to the embryo or fetus.

7. Once X rays are taken and processed, they belong to the facility that was responsible for taking them.

8. Radiation therapy helps to destroy malignant neoplasms by disrupting cell DNA and interfering with cell growth.

9. When patients are having an intravenous pyelogram, it is important to ask if they have allergies, especially to fish, because it contains iodine. Many people who are allergic to fish will be allergic to the iodine salts used as a contrast medium for an intravenous pyelogram.

10. State laws vary, but many states forbid nonlicensed persons from taking and processing X rays. Because medical assistants are not licensed to take and process X rays, they are forbidden by law in certain states to do so.

ANSWERS TO WORKBOOK EXERCISES AND ACTIVITIES

Vocabulary Builder

1. B.
2. F.
3. I.
4. H.
5. G.

6. D.
7. J.
8. A.
9. C.
10. E.

Learning Review

A. Description of positions used during X rays and direction of X rays.

Position	Description	Direction of X rays
Anteroposterior view (AP)	Anterior surface of the body faces the X-ray tube	X rays are directed from the front toward the back of the body
Posteroanterior view (PA)	Posterior surface of the body faces the X-ray tube	X rays are directed from back to front
Lateral view	Side to side	X rays pass through the body from one side to the opposite side
Right lateral view (RL)	Right side of the body is next to the film	X rays are directed through the body from the left to the right side
Left lateral view (LL)	Left side of body is next to the film	X rays are directed through the body from the right to the left side
Oblique view	Body is positioned at an angle	X rays are directed through the body at an angle
Supine view	Body is lying face up, on the back	X rays are directed through the body from front to back while the patient is lying down
Prone view	Body is lying face down, on the abdomen	X rays are directed through the body from back to front while the patient is lying down

B. Radiology tests, purpose and procedures

Test	Purpose	Patient Preparation
Angiography	To visualize the inside of blood vessel walls, to diagnose heart attacks, stroke, and aneurysms	NPO 6-8 hours before the exam
Barium swallow (upper GI series)	To study the esophagus, stomach, duodenum, and small intestines for diseases such as ulcers, tumors, hiatal hernia, esophageal varices	Day before X ray 1. Light evening meal 2. NPO after midnight Day of test 1. NPO Postprocedure 1. Increase fluid intake 2. take laxative as prescribed
Barium enema (lower GI series)	To study the colon for diseases such as polyps, tumors, lesions	Clear liquid one day before the test. 8 oz. of water every hour until bedtime Day before X ray 1. Late afternoon: drink a bottle of magnesium citrate 2. Early evening: take Dulcolax tablet(s) as prescribed 3. Light evening meal. NPO except water after dinner Morning procedure 1. NPO 2. Cleaning enema Postprocedure 1. Increase fluid intake and dietary fiber Report to physician if no bowel movement within 24 hours of the test
Cholangiography	To view the bile ducts for possible calculi or lesions	May have cleaning enema 1 hour before the exam. Meal preceding the exam is withheld
Cholecystography	To study the gallbladder for disease such as stones, duct obstruction, inflammation	1. Evening before test: fat-free dinner 2. Patient takes dye tablets with 8 oz. water as prescribed 3. Cathartic or cleansing enema may be prescribed 4. NPO after dinner and tablets
Cystography	To view the urinary bladder for lesions, calculi	1. Light meal the night before the exam 2. Laxative the evening before the exam 3. NPO after midnight
Hysterosalpingography	To view the uterus and fallopian tubes for blockage and lesions and to check for pelvic masses	1. Laxative the evening before the exam 2. Cleansing enema the day of the exam 3. Meal before the exam is withheld
Intravenous pyelography (IVP)	To visualize the kidneys, ureters, and bladder to detect kidney stones, lesions, strictures of the urinary tract	1. Eat a light evening meal and NPO after midnight 2. Laxative and enema are used to clean out intestines
Mammography	To detect abnormalities in the breast especially breast cancer	Shower before the test. Do not wear lotion, deodorant, or powders to test. Clothing is removed from waist up
Retrograde pyelography	To view the kidneys and urinary tract for abnormalities	Drink 4-5 glasses of water before the examination, then NPO

Multiple Choice Questions

1. b. the tube
2. d. all of the above
3. b. radiopaque

4. a. barium enema
5. d. is a noninvasive procedure

Investigation Activity

The Internet has many different sites that can assist the student in gathering information about their state laws concerning radiology. Some of the Web sites are

> http://www.asrt.org/
> http://www.medsch.wisc.edu/chslib/hw/allied/radiotec.htm
> http://www.fda.gov/cdrh
> http://www.DelmarAlliedHealth.com/members/weblinks/radtechweb.html

ANSWERS TO WORKBOOK CASE STUDY QUESTION

As a new employee, you need to talk with the office manager about your concerns of safety with radiation. Explain that you are uncomfortable with the procedures and ways the office handles X rays, and you are willing to educate everyone on radiation safety. You need to suggest that the office develop radiation safety policies that include the use of dosimeters to measure exposure to radiation, and the use of lead aprons over patients' reproductive organs, especially those of child-bearing ages. If the office does not appear interested in improving safety, consider leaving for a different position.

Chapter

33

Rehabilitation and Therapeutic Modalities

OVERVIEW

Rehabilitation medicine is a field of medical discipline that uses physical and mechanical agents to aid in the diagnosis, treatment, and prevention of diseases or bodily injuries. Medical assisting students learn how to safely transfer patients from a wheelchair to an examination table and from an examination table to a wheelchair, how to assist a patient to safely stand and walk, and how to help a falling patient. Each assistive device is described, along with the correct methods for instructing patients in their use. Therapeutic exercises are described; medical assisting students learn how to perform various types of range of motion exercises on patients. The use of therapeutic modalities such as cold, heat, light, and electricity are discussed, and the situations where each modality is used are delineated. Medical assisting students recognize the importance of supporting and encouraging patients with physical disabilities, to better help them complete their rehabilitation programs.

PROFICIENCY EVALUATION OUTCOME ASSESSMENT

Students are evaluated for their understanding of performance objectives. They gain an understanding of the importance of rehabilitative medicine, learn to employ correct body mechanics, and demonstrate the ability to safely transfer patients. The techniques and safety precautions to be used when helping a patient safely stand and walk are outlined. Students gain a working knowledge of the types of assistive devices, learn how to help a patient ambulate using each device, and master safe methods for pushing a wheelchair. Therapeutic exercises used in patient rehabilitation are explored. Proper methods of performing range of motion exercises are mastered. Students recognize the various types of hot and cold modalities, the safety precautions of each, and how the body reacts to each.

SUPPLEMENTARY RESOURCES

Medical Assisting Videos: Appropriate content is available on Delmar's Medical Assisting Videos, 2nd ed., Tape 9, for the following topics:

> Introduction to Body Mechanics
> > Body Mechanics
> > Transfer Wheelchair to Examination Table and Back
> > Ultrasound Procedures
> > Rehabilitative Care
> > Passive Range of Motion Exercises
> > Instructing Patients with Special Needs

ANSWERS TO TEXT REVIEW QUESTIONS

1. b. activities of daily living (ADL)
2. c. paralysis of one side of the body
3. b. walkers, canes, and crutches
4. d. abduction
5. b. moving the arm so the palm is up

ANSWERS TO TEXTBOOK CRITICAL THINKING QUESTIONS

1. Rehabilitation medicine uses physical and mechanical agents to diagnose, treat, and prevent diseases or bodily injuries. It aids in restoring any body functions that have been affected by disease or injury; and for those who have permanent loss of ability, it seeks to find practical substitutions for that loss while assisting patients to make the most of their remaining abilities.
2. Move your foot in the direction the patient is falling and steady him or her back on his feet. Ask if the patient wants to end or continue ambulating. Check for fatigue, and call for assistance if necessary.
3. The procedure for measuring a patient for axillary crutches is as follows. Have the patient stand tall and position the crutch tips about 6 inches in front and to the outside of each foot. Adjust the height of the crutches so they are two to three fingers, or 2 inches, below the patient's armpit. Adjust the handgrips so the patient's elbows are bent at a 20° to 30° angle.
4. Patients who need a forearm crutch are those who will be using crutches permanently or for long periods of time.
5. In crutch-walking gaits, a point is the number of feet or crutch tips that are on the ground at the same time.
6. The five different types of crutch gaits are as follows.
   1. *Two-Point Gaits.* A. Non–weight-bearing gait; both crutch tips are out in front. The patient pushes off, takes the weight off his or her body and transfers it to his or her hands, then brings the strong leg forward past the crutches and places it down. B. Two-point alternating gait: Opposite foot and crutch are advanced at the same time.
   2. *Three-Point Gait.* Advance both the crutches and the weak leg at the same time. Transfer the body weight forward to the crutches, and advance the stronger leg slightly in front of the crutches.
   3. *Four-Point Alternating Gait.* Move one crutch forward, then the opposite foot. Move the other crutch forward, then the opposite foot.
   4. *Swing-to Gait.* With crutches at the side, move both forward. Transfer the weight forward and swing both feet together up to the crutches.
   5. *Swing-through Gait.* With crutches at the side, move both crutches forward. Transfer the weight and swing both feet through the crutches, stopping slightly in front of the crutches.
7. The six safety rules for transporting a patient in a wheelchair are as follows. (1) Make sure the brakes are locked if transferring a patient into or out of a wheelchair or if you must leave the patient for any time. (2) Make sure the patient's feet are always placed on the footrests when in use. (3) Guide the wheelchair from behind. (4) Always back into and out of elevators. (5) Stay to the right in corridors. (6) Back down slanted ramps.
8. Joint range of motion refers to the amount of movement present in a joint. It is measured with an instrument called a goniometer and is always expressed in degrees.
9. Heat causes vasodilation, or dilation of the blood vessels. It increases circulation to an area and speeds up the repair process. Heat is used to relax muscle spasms, relieve pain in a strained muscle or sprained joint, relieve localized congestion and swelling, increase drainage from an infected area, and increase tissue metabolism and repair.
   Cold causes vasoconstriction, or constriction of the blood vessels. It slows or stops the flow of blood to an area, thereby slowing down the inflammatory process. Cold is used to reduce or prevent swelling of inflamed tissues, reduce bleeding, numb pain by acting as a topical anesthetic, and reduce drainage to an area.

10. Ultrasound converts high-frequency sound waves into heat in the deeper tissues. It is used for treating chronic pain or acute injuries like sprains or strains. It relaxes muscle spasms, increases the elasticity of tissues such as tendons and ligaments, and stimulates circulation.

ANSWERS TO WORKBOOK EXERCISES AND ACTIVITIES

Vocabulary Builder

A. 1. G.
2. H.
3. P.
4. L.
5. A.
6. M.
7. S.
8. C.
9. K.
10. B.
11. J.
12. D.
13. R.
14. N.
15. F.
16. E.
17. Q.
18. T.
19. O.
20. I.

B. 1. K. Supination
2. E. Eversion
3. A. Extension
4. F. Adduction
5. I. Inversion
6. L. Rotation
7. G. Hyperextension
8. M. Abduction
9. B. Circumduction
10. J. Pronation
11. C. Plantar Flexion
12. D. Dorsiflexion
13. H. Abduction

Learning Review

1. A. CANES
Standard. Identifying feature may be one of the following: single leg, curved handle, rubber tip. The standard cane is good for patients with only one good arm, lateral instability, or balance conditions.
Quad. Identifying feature may be one of the following: single cane resting on a platform with four wheels, rubber tips on legs. The quad cane is good for patients with more serious conditions.
Walkcane or hemiwalker. Identifying feature may be one of the following: has four legs that come all the way up to a handlebar, rubber tips on all legs. These canes are best for hemiplegic patients who require extra support on one side.
B. WALKERS
Standard. Identifying feature may be one of the following: adjustable, rubber tips. Standard walkers are excellent for geriatric patients.
Rolling. Identifying feature: legs have wheels. Rolling walkers are good for patients who need a walker for balance but not support.
C. CRUTCHES
Axillary. Identifying feature may be one of the following: wooden or steel, worn under axillae. Axillary crutches are good for younger persons with lower extremity or hip fractures that will heal in a short time and are not recommended for older persons.
Forearm, Lofstrand, or Canadian. Identifying feature may be one of the following: shorter than axillary crutches, has metal cuff worn around upper arm. These crutches are good for long-term crutch use.
Platform. Identifying feature may be one of the following: platform affixed to a crutch, patient bears weight on forearm. Platform crutches are best for patients with severe arthritis or poor use of hands.
2. A. Assisted exercises.
B. Active exercises.
C. Passive exercises.
D. Active resistance exercises.
3. A. Six precautionary measures when performing ROM exercises on a patient are as follows: (1) Always move the patient's limbs gently, within pain tolerance and the flexibility of the limb. (2) Use slow, careful movements that allow the muscles time to adjust to the movement. (3) Always support the limb above and below the joint. (4) Perform passive ROM with the patient in the supine position. (5) ROM should never cause pain to the patient. Discontinue if pain occurs and consult the physician or rehabilitation therapist. (6) Repeat each motion several times.
B. (1) Hip and knee flexion. (2) Shoulder abduction. (3) Wrist inversion and eversion. (4) Ankle dorsiflexion.
4. Correct answers include any six of the following precautions when using hot and cold modalities: infants and patients who cannot report a burning sensation should be watched carefully; check patients frequently and never leave patients alone; never have a patient lie on a heating pad; always wrap appliances with cloth before applying them to skin; soak or immerse patients in water only between 104°F and 113°F (40°C and 45°C); do not use heat on pregnant or menstruating women as it can cause uterine contractions; never apply heat to the abdomen if appendicitis is suspected; never use heat within the first 48 hours of an acute inflammatory process; never apply heat to newly burned skin; carefully monitor persons with impaired circulation or cardiovascular, renal, sensorineural, or respiratory conditions or osteoporosis; be aware that lack of sensation to a therapy may mean impaired circulation to an area and that the patient may be unable to report a burning sensation; have patients remove all jewelry and other metal objects and administer the treatment on nonmetal tables and chairs.

5. A. DCT: Ice packs can be performed at home without assistance.
   B. MHT: This modality, ordered by a physician, is carried out in the physical therapy department by a professional therapist. The use of hot wax and oil can be dangerous to attempt for an untrained individual.
   C. MCT: Cold compresses can be performed at home without assistance.
   D. DHT: Hot water bottle can be used at home by the patient or with the assistance of a caregiver. Supervision is recommended for small children and elderly patients, especially those suffering dementia.
   E. MHT: Hot compresses can be administered at home by the patient or a caregiver.
   F. MHT: Immersion in a whirlpool bath can be administered at home, if the home is equipped with a whirlpool tub, or in a health care setting.
   G. DHT: Heating pads can be administered in the home by the patient or caregiver. Special care should be used with heating pads to prevent burns. Small children and elderly persons should be supervised.
   H. MHT: Hot soaks of one extremity can easily be administered in the home.
   I. MHT: Hot packs generally are administered in the clinical setting to treat large areas such as the back or shoulders.
   J. MHT: Total body immersion in a Hubbard tank occurs in a clinical setting and provides room for limited body exercise without the effects of gravity.
6. A. Water temperature between 105°F and 115°F (41°C and 46°C); administered for no more than 30 minutes.
   B. Several layers of seven parts paraffin to one part mineral oil mixture heated to melting (about 127°F); administered for no longer than 30 minutes.
   C. The temperature can be as cold as the patient can tolerate. The colder the temperature, the shorter the exposure. Administered for 30 to 60 minutes.
   D. Water heated to no more than 125°F (32°C). Temperature should be checked and bottle refilled periodically to maintain correct level of warmth; administered for 20 to 30 minutes, rewarming as necessary.
   E. A clean washcloth is soaked in hot water. Temperature should be high enough to warm but not hot enough to burn the skin, 110°F to 115°F, which is not quite as hot as a water faucet will run. The cloth should be rewarmed periodically, as necessary.
   F. Plain or medicated water is heated to no more than 115°F (44°C); administered for no more than 15 minutes. If patient's skin develops redness, remove from limb immediately.
7. Ultrasound waves travel best in tissue high in water, such as muscles, but they cannot penetrate and move through tissue such as bone that has a low water content. Ultrasound treatment should be used carefully near bones as the waves are capable of concentrating in one area and causing damage. Treatment lasts from 5 to 15 minutes, depending on the patient's condition and the physician's or therapist's instructions. Ultrasound may be performed only by a medical assistant or other health care professional specifically trained in its use.

Multiple Choice Questions

1. c. legs and arms
2. c. crutches
3. d. 30 degrees
4. a. axillary
5. b. four legged

Investigation Activity

By performing this investigation activity with a friend or family member—an unskilled, "real" person—the medical assisting student realizes the importance of proper training in body mechanics and transfer techniques to successfully perform everyday tasks. Students experience firsthand the benefits of properly educating patients and caregivers so daily living activities are performed as efficiently as possible in the home setting, with a maximum of dignity and respect for the patient. Students also learn to deal with the range of emotions displayed by both the patient and caregiver and how these emotions and the levels of support and encouragement provided by each person can affect the quality of care given and received.

Students are encouraged to bring their friends' or family members' assessments of the activity to class. A discussion of various laypersons' points of view can be used as a springboard for exploring issues important to caregivers and for highlighting specific areas medical assistants can focus on for patient and caregiver education.

ANSWERS TO WORKBOOK CASE STUDY QUESTIONS

Case 1

1. The medical assistant should use the proper technique for lifting heavy objects. Instead of bending from the waist, Ellen should bend from the hips and knees, squat down, and push up with the leg muscles. She should position herself as close to the boxes as possible, to allow the center of gravity to be maintained over the base of support. Although Ellen is tired, she should carry only one box at a time, as she will need to lift each box to shoulder height to place it on the appropriate shelf.

2. Ellen should take a few moments to rest and remind herself that it is better to move the cartons properly and avoid injury than to rush, use bad technique, and risk injury.
3. The situation can be easily avoided by following proper lifting techniques.

Case 2

1. As Mary throws her arms around Wanda's neck, Wanda should maintain a firm grasp on the gait belt worn around the patient's waist and plant herself firmly on her center of gravity in the attempt to keep her balance and steady the patient. Once Wanda has confirmed that she and her patient are steady, and the patient is calm, the transfer can be continued. Wanda will instruct the patient to remove her arms from around Wanda's neck and will ask the patient's son to stand clear. If the patient drags Wanda off balance by pulling on Wanda's neck and the medical assistant senses that the patient may fall, the medical assistant should follow proper procedures for preventing or cushioning the patient's fall to prevent injury.
2. "Mary, don't be afraid. I need you to take your hands away from my neck, okay? I've got enough strength to lift you into the wheelchair. John, please stand clear. I need an unobstructed pathway to get your mom into the wheelchair. Mary, let's steady ourselves for a moment and catch our breath. All right, now? Good. We'll count to three and continue on into the wheelchair. Remember, we're moving to the right."
3. Wanda has correctly explained the procedure to the patient and her son. She could not have anticipated the patient's panicked response. However, because Wanda must perform the transfer on the patient's weaker side, she might have benefited from obtaining the help of a colleague. A two-person transfer is likely the best choice in this situation.

Case 3

1. Bruce will explain to the patient why she must wear the belt to ensure her protection while learning to maneuver with an assistive device. He will take into consideration the patient's fatigued state and will not hurry Dottie or push her beyond her current level of endurance.
2. "Dottie, I'm especially concerned that you are tired now, and we need to make sure you are safe so we must use the gait belt. When you've mastered the technique and are well rested at home, you'll do just fine on your own with the walker. Let's rest a moment before we start."
3. The medical assistant cannot control the patient's level of energy or mood; however, he can act to protect the patient's safety by following correct procedures and monitoring the patient's balance and level of fatigue.

Chapter

34 Nutrition in Health and Disease

OVERVIEW

Medical assisting students learn the elements of the digestive system and the role each plays in digestion. The seven basic nutrient types and how each contributes to a healthy diet are discussed. The elements that make up fats, proteins, and carbohydrates are discussed. The differences between water-soluble and fat-soluble vitamins are explored as well as in what foods each are found. The importance of nutrition labels is emphasized; students learn to analyze food labels from the perspective of good nutrition and health. This knowledge of the nutritive value of processed and other foods leads students to an awareness of the profound effect of nutrition on health. Students will be better able to educate patients on the importance of complying with the physician's treatment plan concerning nutrition and diet issues. Various therapeutic diets are discussed as well as the role each can play in controlling a disease state. The need for an individual to modify diet throughout the life span is explored. Medical assisting students learn to become nutrition advocates, encouraging patients to adopt healthy eating habits in their lifestyles.

PROFICIENCY EVALUATION OUTCOME ASSESSMENT

Students are evaluated for their understanding of performance objectives. The functions of the digestive system and the parts of the body that make up the digestive system are explored. The seven basic nutrient types, along with the role each plays in a healthy diet, are discussed. Students recognize the composition of the three energy nutrients and their proper balance for the body's optimum health. Students understand how to interpret nutrition labels on food packaging. They understand that nutritional needs change at various points in the life cycle and know how to modify diets in response to a particular disease state or to accommodate a change in the life cycle. Students become aware of the cultural diversity in patients' diets and the potential impact this culture dietary influence can have on patients' overall health. Students discover the role of the medical assistant as a patient educator and vital source of patient support.

SUPPLEMENTARY RESOURCES

Medical Assisting Videos: Appropriate content is available on Delmar's Medical Assisting Videos, 2nd ed., Tape 8, for the following topics:

Take an In-Depth Patient History
Introduction to Health Promotion, Disease Prevention, and Self-Responsibility

ANSWERS TO TEXT REVIEW QUESTIONS

1. c. absorption
2. c. energy nutrient
3. b. metabolism
4. a. have 3 to 5 servings of vegetables a day
5. a. tocopherol

ANSWERS TO TEXTBOOK CRITICAL THINKING QUESTIONS

1. Student answers will vary depending on their individual dietary intakes. The balance of energy nutrients can be calculated, as shown in textbook Figure 34-6. With the new labeling of food products, percentages of mineral and vitamin requirements can be found on the label or calculated from a good medical dictionary. The average person should get 15 to 20 grams of fiber per day.

2. For each of the following vitamins and minerals, these symptoms might appear if there were a deficiency.

   Vitamin A   A deficiency in vitamin A leads to vision problems especially in relation to night vision, because of the role in rhodopsin. It will also lead to cracking skin.

   Vitamin K   Because of the role of vitamin K in clotting, a deficiency of this vitamin will lead to easy bleeding and bruising.

   Vitamin C   A deficiency in vitamin C will also lead to easy bleeding because the integrity of the capillary wall is decreased. There will also be bleeding gums, sores that will not heal, and iron absorption will decrease. This deficiency is called scurvy.

   Thiamin   This deficiency is called beriberi. Symptoms are paralysis and edema.

   Riboflavin   With this deficiency there is decreased protein production and energy production.

   Cobalamin   A deficiency in this vitamin leads to pernicious anemia, where there is a decreased synthesis of heme protein.

   Calcium   With prolonged calcium deficiency there is a decreased bone mass, as calcium that is needed for other bodily functions is taken from the bones. This deficiency is called osteoporosis.

3. For each of the procedures below, these are problems that might exist if diet modifications do not take place.

   Colostomy   A colostomy removes part of the colon and creates an opening on the outside of the body from the remaining part. With this, the function of the colon is lost. Without diet modification, the person will become dehydrated as adequate reabsorption of fluids does not occur.

   Gastroileostomy   This is a surgical connection between the stomach and ileum, bypassing the duodenum and jejunum. It is in these two parts that a great portion of digestive enzymes are secreted. Without modifications, the food will not be well digested.

   Gastrectomy   This is the removal of the stomach. The individual will not be able to eat as much at a single meal, thus would have to eat more frequently to prevent starvation.

4. A breakfast high in complex carbohydrates is an important goal because complex carbohydrates will be slowly digested and glucose will be released into the bloodstream over time. Simple sugars would give a quick burst of glucose; but then glucose would be taken up by the cells, and levels would quickly decrease again.

5. The new pyramid shape is an accurate portrayal of the ideal diet because by putting the carbohydrates at the foundation of the pyramid, the new shape puts the greatest emphasis on carbohydrates, which should make up 50 to 60 percent of the diet. Likewise, it puts the least emphasis on fats, which should make up less than 30 percent of the diet.

6. A therapeutic response to a teenage girl who refuses to gain weight during her pregnancy includes the following information. The increased need for nutrients will ensure healthy development of the fetus, placenta, and other structures associated with pregnancy. It is also important for the health of the mother that nutrients are plentiful. Weight gain is normal during pregnancy; the time to worry about weight is after the birth of the child, unless the mother decides to breastfeed.

7. Here are some things to consider when assessing the diet of an elderly person. Physiologically, consider the activity level of the person. A decrease in activity would require a decrease in caloric intake. Illness and decreased absorption capability in the gastrointestinal tract would require an increase in nutrient levels. Aging causes a decrease in taste ability, salivary secretions, and gastrointestinal motility. In addition, problems with teeth can lead to discomfort upon eating. Psychologically, depression and loneliness might occur as the person becomes more isolated. All of these may cause a decreased desire to eat.

8. Typical things a person can do to decrease the risk of heart disease include exercise regularly, decrease fat intake, adjust cholesterol intake (increase HDL and decrease LDL), stop smoking, decrease salt intake, maintain a healthy weight, and stop using drugs.

9. Diet can be used to control diabetes by controlling the levels of glucose in the blood. By eating foods that release glucose slowly, drastic fluctuations in blood glucose levels can be avoided and thus better managed by the body. Even after insulin therapy has started, the patient can help control blood glucose levels in the body in this way.

10. Below is information from a label for peanut butter. Calculate the percentage of calories due to fat, protein, and carbohydrate.

   Serving size . . . . 2 tbs.
   Calories 204
   Protein . . . . 9 grams
   Carbohydrates . . . . 6 grams
   Fat . . . . 16 grams

Fat:

$$16 \text{ grams of fat} \times \frac{9 \text{ calories}}{\text{gram}} = 144 \text{ calories due to fat}$$

$$\frac{144 \text{ calories due to fat}}{204 \text{ total calories}} = 71\% \text{ of calories due to fat}$$

Protein:

$$9 \text{ grams of protein} \times \frac{4 \text{ calories}}{\text{gram}} = 36 \text{ calories due to protein}$$

$$\frac{36 \text{ calories due to protein}}{204 \text{ total calories}} = 18\% \text{ of calories due to protein}$$

Carbohydrate:

$$6 \text{ grams of carbohydrate} \times \frac{4 \text{ calories}}{\text{gram}} = 24 \text{ calories due to carbohydrate}$$

$$\frac{24 \text{ calories due to carbohydrate}}{204 \text{ total calories}} = 12\% \text{ calories due to carbohydrate}$$

ANSWERS TO WORKBOOK EXERCISES AND ACTIVITIES

Vocabulary Builder

A. The two functions of vitamins in the body are to facilitate cellular metabolism by acting as a coenzyme with a catalyst and to act as a component of tissue structure.

B. A. Niacin works with both thiamin and riboflavin in the production of energy and is important throughout the body.
   B. Thiamin helps in the conversion of glucose to energy.
   C. Tocopherol is an antioxidant, which reduces the likelihood of oxidation of substances.
   D. Cholecalciferol is involved in the metabolism of calcium in the body. It helps with calcium absorption and also with formation and maintenance of bone tissue.
   E. Folic acid is involved in the formation of DNA and the formation of red blood cells.
   F. Carotene is converted into retinol in the body. Retinol, vitamin A, is responsible in part for vision, especially night vision. Vitamin A also gives strength to epithelial tissue and is required for healthy skin and mucous membranes.
   G. Cobalamin is important to the functioning of red blood cells. It is responsible for the synthesis of the heme portion of hemoglobin.
   H. Ascorbic acid is a constituent of connective tissue and acts to hold cells together.
   I. Riboflavin is involved in energy production and is important in the production of proteins; it is necessary for normal growth.
   J. Pyridoxine has an important role in protein metabolism, especially the synthesis of proteins. It is also important in the metabolism and fats and carbohydrates.

C. 1. Preservatives.
   2. Nutrition.
   3. Fat-soluble.
   4. Amino acids.
   5. Diuretics.
   6. Coenzyme.
   7. Absorption.
   8. Extracellular.
   9. Metabolism.
   10. Electrolytes.
   11. Digestion.
   12. Nutrients.
   13. Homeostasis.
   14. Catalyst.
   15. Processed foods.
   16. Saturated fats.
   17. Oxidation.
   18. Elimination.
   19. Calories.
   20. Major minerals.
   21. Water soluble.
   22. Antioxidant.
   23. Trace minerals.
   24. Ingestion.
   25. Basal metabolic rate (BMR).
   26. Cellulose.
   27. Glycogen.

Learning Review

1. Students will identify the organs of the digestive system on the diagram to correspond to the order and numbering listed.

   (1) The liver produces bile. Common disorders include liver disease from alcohol abuse, hepatitis, cirrhosis, liver cancer, hemochromatosis (too much iron), and Wilson's disease (too much copper).

   (2) The salivary glands begin chemical digestion as ptyalin begins to change starch to maltose. Common disorders include the mumps virus, dry mouth, the formation of calculi (stones), and sarcoidosis.

   (3) The gallbladder stores bile and releases it into the small intestine to emulsify fats. Common disorders include gallstones and cholecystitis.

   (4) In the stomach, hydrochloric acid prepares the gastric area for enzyme action. Pepsin breaks down proteins. Lipase acts on emulsified fats. Common disorders include peptic ulcers, gastritis, and pernicious anemia.

   (5) The large intestine absorbs water and some other nutrients and collects food residue for excretion. Common disorders include diverticular disease, irritable bowel syndrome, peptic ulcer of the duodenum, bowel cancer, and ulcerative colitis.

   (6) In the esophagus, peristalsis and gravity move food along. Common disorders are esophagitis, esophageal stricture, and esophageal diverticulum.

   (7) The small intestine produces enzymes and prepares foods for absorption: lactase converts lactose, maltase converts maltose, sucrase converts sucrose to simple sugars. Peptidases reduce proteins to amino acids. Common disorders include ulceration of the small intestine in typhoid, Crohn's disease, and helminths (worms).

   (8) In the mouth, the teeth and tongue begin mechanical digestion by breaking food apart. Common disorders could include mouth ulcers or sores and toothache.

   (9) The pancreas releases enzymes into the small intestine. Amylase breaks down starch. Steapsin breaks down fats. Pancreatic proteases break down proteins. Disorders of the pancreas include pancreatic cancer, pancreatitis, and diabetes mellitus.

2. A. (1) No energy.
      (2) Energy.
      (3) No energy.
      (4) No energy.
      (5) Energy.
      (6) Energy.
      (7) No energy.

   B. The three chemical elements are carbon, oxygen, and hydrogen.
   C. The most important dietary complex carbohydrate is starch.
   D. The only true essential fatty acid in the human diet is linoleic acid.
   E. Protein also includes nitrogen.
   F. When carbohydrates and fats are in short supply, the body diverts its use of protein for structural purpose to use it as an energy source; this diversion can create dangerous deficiencies.
   G. PEM stands for protein-energy malnutrition and occurs along with deficiencies in total calories.
   H. Two diseases associated with PEM are marasmus and kwashiorkor.

3. A. Two ways in which minerals differ from vitamins are: Vitamins are complex molecules, whereas minerals are single elements; and vitamins are required by the body in minute quantities, whereas some minerals are required in larger amounts.

   B. (1) Sulfur, sodium.
      (2) Sodium, calcium, phosphorus.
      (3) Sodium, phosphorus.
      (4) Calcium.
      (5) Potassium.
      (6) Calcium, magnesium.

4. 1. MM, H.
   2. WSV, F.
   3. TM, C.
   4. FSV, I.
   5. MM, A.
   6. WSV, G.
   7. TM, J.
   8. WSV, E.
   9. FSV, B.
   10. FSV, D.

5. A. The six types of fiber that are carbohydrates are cellulose, gums, mucilages, algal polysaccharides, pectins, and hemicellulose.

   B. Lignin, an important fiber, is not a carbohydrate. Americans should consume 15 to 20 grams of fiber each day. Brown rice contains more fiber than white rice because the husk is not removed.

6. A. When the body takes in more calories than it will use, the energy is stored as fat. When the body uses more energy than the amount of calories it takes in, the body depletes the fat stores. If the fat stores are not sufficient, the body will break down its protein structures. The ideal percentages of energy nutrients to be consumed daily are: 50 to 60 percent of total calories from carbohydrates, 20 to 30 percent of total calories from fat, and 10 to 20 percent of calories from protein.

   B. Number of calories from fat: 18
      Number of calories from carbohydrates: 80
      Number of calories from protein: 16
      Percent of calories from fat: 16%
      Percent of calories from carbohydrates: 73%
      Percent of calories from protein: 14.5%

C. The peanut butter is a good source of protein, but the soy milk provides almost as much protein without the excessive amount of fat the peanut butter contains. The soy milk is also a rich source of carbohydrates, not provided by the peanut butter. Soy milk is well within the dietary guidelines, while peanut butter provides only the requirement for protein—and is way over the amount recommended for fat and well under the amount recommended for carbohydrates.

7. A. Calcium and phosphorus are two minerals that must be increased during pregnancy.
   B. The student may give any three of the following reasons why a woman needs to increase her intake of calories and nutrients when pregnant: to aid in the growth of the fetus, to aid in the growth of the placenta, because of the increase in adipose tissue in the mother, because of the increased volume of blood, and to aid in the growth of breast tissue.
   C. Iron usually needs to be added as a supplement to a baby's diet.

8. A. The percentage of daily values are based on one serving and a 2,000-calorie diet. The listing for total carbohydrates is broken down into dietary fiber and sugars. Dietary fiber is more beneficial because sugar has no nutritive value and converts easily to fat. Individuals should consume less than 2,400 milligrams of sodium per day. A high-fiber diet is important to aid in the proper functioning of the gastrointestinal tract by adding bulk to fecal matter as it is passed through the intestines. Lack of dietary fiber leads to gastrointestinal disorders such as colorectal cancer and diverticulitis.
   B. The muesli is more nutritious, providing more nutrients and in greater quantities than the pretzels. Students must double values for the pretzels to arrive at a comparison of the two products: two pretzel servings = 1 muesli serving. The muesli does contain more sugar, but far less sodium than the pretzels (two servings contain 720 milligrams versus the 30 milligrams in the muesli) and more dietary fiber (5 grams per serving for muesli and 2 grams for pretzels). Neither product contains cholesterol. Two servings of pretzels have roughly the same percentage of total calories from fat as the muesli: about 14 percent.

9. The U.S. southern diet contains a great deal of carbohydrates and fat and limited amounts of protein. Iron, calcium, and vitamins A and C may sometimes be deficient. The Jewish diet can be deficient in fresh vegetables and milk. The Jewish diet includes meat and other sources of protein; generally, the food is rich. The Jewish diet also involves respecting strict dietary laws. These laws had their origins in practical matters of hygiene and proper food sterilization as well as matters of religious significance. The Japanese diet is based on fish; rice, soy, and curd; fruits; and vegetables. The Japanese diet is a low-fat diet, high in protein and nutrient-rich. Currently, however, the influence of Western culture is affecting the Japanese diet and increasing the levels of fat consumed. The Japanese diet is the healthiest. The Jewish and U. S. southern diets can include too much fat and both contain potential areas for deficiency.

Multiple Choice Questions

1. b. their ability to convert into energy
2. c. a and d
3. a. fats

4. b. amino acids
5. d. BMR

Investigation Activity

Use this exercise to encourage students to examine their own, and their family's, eating habits and preferences. By going into the kitchen and actually analyzing what is there, students can relate firsthand to patients who are suddenly asked to observe dietary restrictions for health reasons and do not know where or how to start. The exercise encourages students to consider the impact of foods they may have taken for granted as being healthy or nutritious.

In class, students should compile a list of the products they have chosen and compare the nutritive values of each. Determine the variety of products students consume: how diverse is the list?

By studying the impact of food packaging on a consumer's decision to purchase a product, students become aware of the subconscious signals sent to us by manufacturers regarding the products they sell. Students consider whether the messages match the true nutritional value of the products and gain an insight into the challenges patients face when shopping for groceries, with advertising as the primary guiding influence, instead of a sound knowledge of nutritional principles. For example, just because a product says it is low-fat or fat-free does not mean you can eat twice as much and not gain weight!

ANSWERS TO WORKBOOK CASE STUDY QUESTIONS

1. Cancer patients require increased calories and nutrients because the cancerous growth has the ability to divert nutrients from the body to itself, causing the body to break down its own tissues for energy. More energy and nutrients will also boost the immune system in its attempt to destroy cancerous cells. When receiving radiation or chemotherapy, cancer patients have an even greater need for increased nutrients, as therapy is directed at killing any rapidly dividing cell, whether it is a cancer cell or a healthy body cell such as a cell in the lining of the gastrointestinal tract or a hair follicle. Increased nutrients help repair and replace lost cells. Protein levels should be increased.

2. Food should be made as appealing as possible. If the patient has difficulty swallowing, food can be liquefied in a food processor. Food is generally better tolerated if chilled; temperature extremes should be avoided. Several smaller meals may be easier than three large ones.

3. Macrobiotics is derived from Zen Buddhism. Adherents progress from the lower number diet to the higher, gradually giving up foods in the following order: desserts, salads, fruits, animal foods, soups, and ultimately vegetables, until only cereals—usually brown rice—are consumed. Beverages are kept to a minimum and only organic foods are consumed. These diets can be dangerous, becoming increasingly inadequate as followers give up foods. Medical cures from the diet cannot be attained; adherents should not delay appropriate medical treatment in favor of adherence to the diet. One good element of the diet is the importance of eating organic foods; however, the diet has little merit to cancer patients otherwise.

4. The medical assistant is providing a valuable community service while also reinforcing the moral and good nutrition habits of Lourdes, the patient who invites the medical assistant to speak to the support group. The responsible behavior and professional appearance of the medical assistant reflects positively on the medical practice and increases the likelihood of attracting new patients.

Chapter

35

Basic Pharmacology

OVERVIEW

It is essential that medical assisting students have a working knowledge of basic pharmacology, including uses, sources, forms, and delivery routes of drugs. In addition, they should recognize the governmental laws and regulations that oversee the distribution and administration of medications and demonstrate a knowledge of drug classifications and actions that will allow them to caution patients in the use of drugs. Students understand how to access medical resources and reference books for information relating to pharmaceutical products, including drug classification, routes, form of storage, and side effects, as well as contraindications. Medical assisting students also display the skills to recognize the signs of drug abuse and misuse and understand their roles and responsibilities in cases of suspected misuse and abuse in patients and in the workplace. Students should be reminded that only a licensed physician may prescribe drugs or recommend over-the-counter (OTC) medications to patients.

PROFICIENCY EVALUATION OUTCOME ASSESSMENT

Students are evaluated for their understanding of performance objectives. They must show a working knowledge of governmental regulations regarding controlled substances and other medications and become aware of the legal responsibilities of medical assistants and the need to document and report accurately and in compliance with the law. A thorough understanding of basic pharmacological concepts and the role of the medical assistant in dispensing or administering medications to patients as directed by the physician are emphasized. The need for proper risk management with regard to drug-related issues is stressed. Students become aware of the need to develop sharp observational skills to detect any drug side effects, adverse reactions, or potential drug misuse or abuse when assisting in the care of patients and to report such findings to the physician.

SUPPLEMENTARY RESOURCES

Medical Assisting Videos: Appropriate content is available on Delmar's Medical Assisting Videos, 2nd ed., for the following topics:

> Tape 2   Dispose of Controlled Substances in Compliance with Government
> Regulations
> Perform within Ethical Boundaries
> Tape 11 Prepare and Administer Medication as Directed by Physician
> Tape 12 Prepare and Administer Parenteral Medications

ANSWERS TO TEXT REVIEW QUESTIONS

1. d. epinephrine
2. d. brand
3. b. insulin
4. a. nembutal
5. d. dispose of it down the sink and document

ANSWERS TO TEXTBOOK CRITICAL THINKING QUESTIONS

1. Drug sources are (1) animals, (2) minerals, (3) plants, (4) synthetics, and (5) biotechnology (genetics).
2. The FDA protects the public by ensuring purity, strength, and composition of food, drugs, and cosmetics. It prohibits the movement in interstate commerce of adulterated and misbranded food, drugs, devices, and cosmetics.
3. The *U.S. Pharmacopeia,* or *National Formulary*, is recognized by the federal government as the official list of standardized drugs.
4. Factors that affect drug action are
   (1) Absorption: drug passes into body fluids and tissues.
   (2) Distribution: drug transported from blood to intended site of action.
   (3) Biotransformation: chemical changes that the drug undergoes in the body.
   (4) Elimination: process of substance being excreted from the body (e.g., kidneys, respiratory tract, and gastrointestinal tract).
5. While preparing an injection of Demerol® (meperidine), you accidentally drop and break the ampule, spilling its contents. Have a coworker witness that the ampule containing the narcotic broke and the contents spilled on the floor. Both medical assistant and coworker should sign the narcotic sheet and document the incident.
6. Students will choose emergency drugs from textbook Table 35-2.
7. A medical assistant may dispense stock medication under a physician's supervision.
8. Information regarding medical assistants administering medication can be obtained from the state attorney general, the physician's attorney, and associations such as the AAMA and the local or state medical society. Information about the storage and handling of narcotics can be obtained from the DEA.
9. Drug references include the *PDR, USP/NF*, and *New Drugs Publication*. There are seven main sections of the *PDR*: (1) manufacturer's index, (2) product name index, (3) product category index, (4) generic and chemical name index, (5) product identification, (6) product information section, and (7) diagnostic product information. Also included are discontinued products, poison control 800 numbers, and a guide to managing a drug overdose.
10. The medical assistant's potential substance abuse should be reported immediately to the office manager or physician-employer.

ANSWERS TO WORKBOOK EXERCISES AND ACTIVITIES

Vocabulary Builder

A. 1. G.   4. F.   6. D.
    2. C.   5. B.   7. A.
    3. E.

B. Key terms are inserted in the paragraph in the following order: curative, preventive or prophylactic, therapeutic, replacement, diagnostic, generic, chemical, trade or brand, plant, animal, synthetic, mineral, genetic engineering, gene splicing.

Learning Review

1. A. Federal Food, Drug, and Cosmetic Act.
2. C. must be counted, verified by two individuals, and recorded on an audit sheet.
3. C. two years.
4. A. the antibiotic penicillin.
5. A. the analgesic ibuprofen.
6. C. local action.
7. A. elimination.
8. C. returned to the pharmacy.
9. C. both A and B.
10. C. oral and parenteral.

11. Schedule I specifies drugs that have a high potential for abuse and are not accepted for medical use within the United States: LSD, heroin.

    Schedule II includes drugs with a high abuse potential but that do have an accepted medical use within the United States: amphetamines and cocaine.

    Schedule III drugs have a low-to-moderate potential for physical dependence, yet have a high potential for psychological dependency: barbiturates and various drug combinations containing codeine and paregoric.

    Schedule IV includes drugs, which when misused or abused, can lead to limited physical or psychological dependency: chloral hydrate and diazepam.

    Schedule V drugs have the lowest potential for abuse of controlled substances: Lomotil and Donnagel.

12. A. OTC. The patient is using an OTC drug instead of seeking appropriate medical care. Because the safe minimum dose is not effective for her, she takes too much ibuprofen to relieve the pain of her arthritis and risks any bad effects associated with misuse of that drug.

    B. PM. The patient should not take any medication prescribed for another person. All warning labels on medication containers should be heeded. Unused medication should be discarded properly, and no medication should be used without checking the expiration date.

    C. OTC. Many OTC medications have several active ingredients, which may prove to be undesirable or unnecessary to properly treat the condition.

    D. PM. The physician should be consulted before stopping any prescribed medication. Suddenly stopping the antihypertensive drug could cause Abigail's blood pressure to rise dangerously. Also, medications should be taken exactly as prescribed.

    E. PM. The patient should continue to take the medication for the duration of the prescribed number of days, weeks, and so on.

13. A. Liquids and ointments must be rinsed down the drain.

    B. Powdered drugs must be mixed with water and disposed of by rinsing down the drain.

    C. Pills and capsules must be flushed down the toilet.

    D. Vials and ampules must be opened and their contents poured down the drain.

    E. Outdated and expired controlled substances must be returned to the pharmacy (as required by law). If a controlled substance is dropped or spilled and is unfit to give to a patient, a witness should verify the action and proper documentation should take place.

    F. If a medication is removed from its container it should not be used or replaced in the container. This medication should be disposed of according to proper guidelines.

14. A. (1) The characteristics of the drug must be considered. Insulin is destroyed by digestive enzymes; therefore, the route of administration must be parenteral. (2) The action of the medication on the body, local or systemic, must be considered. Intravenous medication reaches the systemic circulation rapidly via the bloodstream and quickly becomes effective, thus it is the best choice for systemic chemotherapeutic agents. (3) The physical and emotional state of the patient must be considered. Here, because of the patient's inability to swallow easily and the presence of dementia, the patient may not be able to understand or tolerate the administration of nitroglycerin by a sublingual or an oral route. This patient is better served by a transdermal route.

    B. Seven additional routes of drug administration are topical, sublingual, buccal, rectal, vaginal, inhalation, and instillation.

    C. Three new systems of drug delivery are: (1) transdermal, where medication is received by means of a medicated adhesive patch applied to intact skin near the treatment site; (2) eye-curing lens system, where the drug is contained between two ultrathin plastic membranes and is placed inside the lower eyelid; and (3) implantable devices, which are positioned just beneath the skin near blood vessels that lead directly to the area to be medicated. The transdermal method is good for patients who cannot accept medications by mouth or for its convenience. The eye-curing lens allows for controlled release of medication over an extended period of time, causes little or no discomfort, and is convenient. Implantable devices allow for a continuous supply of medication and have the advantage of delivering higher doses with fewer side effects than can be realized through the systemic route.

15. A. Four examples are drugs used to treat or prevent disease, drugs that have a principal action on the body, drugs that act on specific body systems or organs, and drug preparation.

    B. (1) Hemostatic: Humafac,® Amitar,® vitamin K.

    (2) Antiemetic: Tigan,® dramamine, phenergan, Reglan,® Marinol®

    (3) Antacid: Amphojel,® Gelusil,® Mylanta®, milk of magnesia.

    (4) Vasodilator: isosorbide dinitrate (Isordil®), nitroglycerin.

    (5) Antipyretic: aspirin, acetaminophen (Tylenol®).

    (6) Laxative: Metamucil® powder, Dulcolax®.

    (7) Contraceptive: Envid-E® 21; Ortho-Novum® 10/11-21, 10/11-28; Triphasil®-21.

    (8) Antineoplastic: busulfan (Myleran®), cyclophosphamide (Cytoxan®).

    (9) Antidiarrheal: Pepto-Bismol®, Kaopectate®, diphenoxylate HCL (Lomotil®).

    (10) Sedative: amobarbital (Amytal®), butabarbital sodium (Buticaps®), phenobarbital.

16. A. Chronulac Syrup's® generic name is lactulose. The sugar it contains is galactose. The drug's source is plant.
    B. Humulin's® generic name is insulin. The animal source it is derived from is porcine. The drug's source is genetically engineered (chemically altered porcine insulin).
    C. Pepcid's® generic name is famotidine. The drug's active ingredient is the enzyme pepsin. The drug's source is animal.
    D. Ortho-Tri-Cyclen® may interact with drugs used in the treatment of epilepsy, such as barbiturates (e.g., phenobarbital), and anticonvulsants (e.g., carbamazepine; Tegretol® is one brand of this). The drug's source is synthetic, or chemical.

Multiple Choice Questions

1. b. interferon
2. d. 17 years
3. a. cortisone
4. c. DEA
5. a. two years

Investigation Activity

Use this activity to increase student awareness of the nature of drugs commonly contained in the home medicine cabinet. In a class discussion, students compare the variety of drugs they have at home and what these drugs are commonly used for. Compile a class list of the most common illnesses or conditions for which over-the-counter drugs are purchased for use in the home. What drugs are considered home staples and what drugs are purchased for an occasional, specific purpose?

Students are also encouraged to consider the contraindications and potential interactions of common drugs. How aware are the students of the potential danger of taking OTC medications incorrectly or of taking OTC medications concurrently? How aware are students' family members of taking OTC drugs incorrectly? By addressing these issues, students recognize that most patients are not aware of the potential interactions between the medications they take and often do not heed warnings. Or patients will assume that OTC medications are not harmful and can be taken with other OTC medications or with prescribed medications without potentially harmful effects.

A discussion of how drugs are stored in the home will encourage students to become effective patient educators and recognize that the same care should be taken in the use and storage of medications in the home as in the ambulatory care setting.

Above all, students should not assume that patients have a knowledge of the effects of the drugs they are taking, that patients will ask questions about medications, or that patients will understand the importance of revealing what medications they take on a regular basis—including vitamins and supplements—to health care professionals who are prescribing or administering medications to them. Medical assistants must fully inform patients about the medications they are taking and must stay alert to the signs of harmful effects or the misuse or abuse of legal or illegal drugs.

ANSWERS TO WORKBOOK CASE STUDY QUESTIONS

1. Anna's first action is to report the missing drugs to the office manager. She should also report Audrey's erratic behavior, but may do so without placing direct blame on Audrey or accusing her of stealing the controlled substance without firm evidence that Audrey has done so. Anna should not confront Audrey. The office manager will investigate both the missing bottle of phenobarbital and Audrey's erratic behavior. If the two events are linked, the office manager will take appropriate action.

2. There is a tremendous rise in the number of abuse cases involving legal and illegal drugs, and this increase is reflected in the workplace. All health care professionals, including medical assistants, have a responsibility to provide their patients with the highest-quality care and competent treatment. To maintain this quality of care, intentional misuse or abuse of drugs is not tolerated. Medical assistants may encounter patients and/or fellow health care professionals who are misusing or abusing drugs, and they have a responsibility to report such individuals to the proper authorities. Health care professionals also have the responsibility of becoming role models for good health practices and behaviors for their patients.

Chapter

36

Calculation of Medication Dosage and Medication Administration

OVERVIEW

Medical assisting students learn the importance of dosage calculation and medication administration in the ambulatory care setting. Students discover that a knowledge of pharmacology, dosage measurement systems and calculation formulas, and methods of medication administration are all needed to safely administer medications to patients. The importance of following all laws and regulations governing the administration of medications is stressed, as is the need to follow OSHA guidelines and standard precautions for infection control.

PROFICIENCY EVALUATION OUTCOME ASSESSMENT

Students are evaluated for their understanding of performance objectives. Students possess the ability to read and understand medication labels, describe the parts of a medicine order and prescription, and understand prescription abbreviations. A knowledge of dosage factors and the ability to calculate adult and pediatric dosages in metric, apothecary, household, and unit systems is required. Procedures for preparing and administering medications as directed by a physician are correctly performed. Inhalation medication and its administration is described. Students demonstrate a knowledge of quality control and safety guidelines, with special emphasis on the safe handling and disposal of sharps. Ethical and legal aspects of medication administration are explored.

The importance of therapeutic communication and attention to the patient's emotional needs is stressed.

Procedure 36-1	Administration of Oral Medications
Procedure 36-2	Administration of Subcutaneous, Intramuscular, and/or Intradermal Injections
Procedure 36-3	Withdrawing (Aspirating) Medication from a Vial
Procedure 36-4	Withdrawing (Aspirating) Medication from an Ampule
Procedure 36-5	Administering a Subcutaneous Injection
Procedure 36-6	Administering an Intramuscular Injection
Procedure 36-7	Administering an Intradermal Injection
Procedure 36-8	Reconstituting a Powder Medication for Administration
Procedure 36-9	Z-Track Intramuscular Injection Technique

SUPPLEMENTARY RESOURCES

Medical Assisting Videos: Appropriate content is available on Delmar's Medical Assisting Videos, 2nd ed., for the following topics:

Tape 2   Practice Risk Management Measure to Prevent Professional Liability
Dispose of Controlled Substances in Compliance with Government
Regulations
Perform within Ethical Boundaries

ANSWERS TO TEXT REVIEW QUESTIONS

1. b. prescription
2. b. NPO
3. a. Type I
4. a. when calculating children's dosages
5. c. subcutaneous injection

ANSWERS TO TEXT CRITICAL THINKING QUESTIONS

1. To determine the state law regarding a medical assistant administering medication, place a telephone call or write to the state attorney general's office, contact the State Medical Society, or the executive director of the AAMA.

2. The medication order is given by the physician. It is for a specific patient and denotes the drug to be given, the dosage, the form of the drug, the time for or frequency of administration, and the route by which the drug is to be given. Its purpose is to give the complete information in the patient's medical record and to allow the medical assistant to extract the information before administering a medication. The medical assistant takes all of the information from the medication order and writes the information on a medicine ticket or card before administering the prescribed or ordered medication. The physician can write a prescription and this too is a medication order, giving the pharmacist information for compounding and dispensing the medication. The physician also includes information about administering the medication. The purpose of a prescription is to control the sale and use of drugs that can be safely and effectively used only under the supervision of a licensed physician.

3. The nine parts of a prescription are:
   1. The physician's name, address, telephone number, and registration number.
   2. The patient's name, address, and the date the prescription is written.
   3. The *superscription*, including the symbol Rx, signifying recipe (L). It is the beginning of the prescription.
   4. The *inscription* states the names and quantities of ingredients to be included in the medication.
   5. The *subscription* gives directions to the pharmacist for filling the prescription.
   6. The *signature* (sig) gives direction to the patient.
   7. Physician signature blanks, when signed, indicate whether a generic substitute is allowed or if the medication is to be dispensed as written.
   8. *Repetatur* 0 1 2 3 prn. The physician indicates whether or not the prescription can be refilled.
   9. The label gives directions to the pharmacist to label the medication appropriately.

4. Factors that affect medication dosage are:
   • Weight, sex and age of the patient. The usual adult dose is suitable for the 20-60 age group.
   • Infants, young children, adolescents, and the aged require individualized dosages.
   • If medication is required during pregnancy and/or lactation, the dosage is lower because of the concern for possible congenital anomalies occurring in the developing embryo, because medication crosses the placenta and is circulated through the embryo's cells and tissues. Medication can be found in breast milk, therefore the infant can be affected by absorbing the medication while breastfeeding.
   • Physical and emotional changes in the condition of the patient may require either a higher or lower dosage depending on the nature of the condition.
   • The presence of another disease process, the causative microorganisms, and the severity of the infection may require adjustments in dosages either greater or less than the average adult dose depending upon the disease or disease processes present.
   • The patient's past medical history, which includes allergies and idiosyncrasies, are important considerations when dosage is determined by the physician. Usually patients with sensitivities or allergic reactions to medications require smaller dosages of medication.

- The safest method, route, time, and amount to obtain the desired result must be considered factors that influence dosage. An intravenous injection bypasses the gastrointestinal tract, therefore, a lower dose of medication may give the maximum result.

5. The fundamental units of the metric system are
   Meter (m)   length
   Liter (L)   volume
   Gram (Gm, g)   mass and/or weight

6. To calculate children's dosages, use either the body surface area (BSA) or calculate according to kilogram of body weight.

7. The "Six Rights" are
   1. Right dose. Patient has the right to expect to be given the correct dose.
   2. Right drug. The patient must be given the correct medication.
   3. Right route. The correct route ensures accurate and maximum therapeutic effect of the medication.
   4. Right time. The medication must be given at the appropriate time to be therapeutically effective.
   5. Right patient. Identification of the patient before drug administration prevents errors.
   6. Right documentation. Correct documentation of medication administered, when and how administered, and patient's reaction. Initial and date entry.

8. The accident must be reported immediately to the supervisor in charge of the student. The supervisor will notify the physician that the accident has occurred so appropriate measures can be taken to correct the error. An antidote may be prescribed to counteract the medication if it was too large a dose, or if the dose was intended for another patient; or more medication or a different kind of medication may be prescribed instead. Check patient's vital signs, skin color, and orientation. Report to the physician. Careful documentation in the patient's record must be done.

9. If accidentally stuck by a used needle, immediately and thoroughly wash the area with soap and water, wipe site with antiseptic, report incident to the immediate supervisor, seek medical attention, make out an OSHA 200 form, and document the incident (keeping copies for yourself).

10. Allergenic extracts are injections of minute quantities of allergen(s) into the patient's subcutaneous tissues. The purpose is to desensitize an allergic individual. The desensitizing regimen is prescribed by the physician, and is given subcutaneously with a tuberculin syringe while the physician is present in the facility. A patient should be observed for 15 to 30 minutes following the injection, because severe allergic reactions can occur and immediate first aid treatment may be necessary.

11. Oxygen may be prescribed for patients with cardiac or certain pulmonary diseases. It is administered from a canister or cylinder through a tubing attached to a mask or cannula that is placed over the patient's nose and mouth (mask), or prongs are placed into the patient's nostrils (cannula). Oxygen supports combustion and fire is a danger that must be avoided. Friction, static electricity, or a lighted cigarette or cigar can cause ignition.

ANSWERS TO TEXT CALCULATION PROBLEMS

1. To calculate these dosages for a child, follow these formulas.

   $$\frac{\text{BSA of child (m}^2)}{1.7 \text{ (m}^2)} \times \text{adult dose} = \text{child's dose}$$

   A. Step 1 $\dfrac{0.57 \text{ (BSA)}}{1.7} \times 400 \text{ mg (adult dose)} = \text{child's dose}$

   Step 2 $0.57 \div 1.7 = 0.34$

   Step 3 $0.34 \times 400 \text{ mg} =$

   $$
   \begin{array}{r}
   400 \\
   \times\ 0.34 \\
   \hline
   1600 \\
   1200 \\
   \hline
   136.00
   \end{array}
   $$

   136 mg = child's dose

   B. Step 1 $\dfrac{0.56 \text{ (BSA)}}{1.7} \times 250 \text{ mg (adult dose)} = \text{child's dose}$

   Step 2 $0.56 \div 1.7 = 0.33$

   Step 3 $0.33 \times 250 \text{ mg} =$

   $$
   \begin{array}{r}
   250 \\
   \times\ 0.33 \\
   \hline
   750 \\
   750 \\
   \hline
   82.50
   \end{array}
   $$

   82.5 mg = child's dose

2. To calculate the children's dosages according to kilogram of body weight, follow this formula.
   Step 1: Convert pounds to kilograms by dividing pounds by 2.2 (1 kg = 2.2 lb)
   Step 2: Multiply the dose ordered by kilogram of body weight.
   Step 3: If dose ordered is in divided doses, divide the number of times into the answer obtained in Step 2.

   A. Step 1   Convert 72 pounds to kilograms

$$
2.2 \overline{\smash{\big)}\, 720.0} = 33 \text{ kg} \quad \substack{32.7}
$$

$$
\begin{array}{r}
32.7 \\
2.2 \overline{\smash{\big)}\, 720.0} = 33 \text{ kg} \\
\underline{66} \\
60 \\
\underline{44} \\
160 \\
\underline{154} \\
6
\end{array}
$$

   Step 2   Multiply dose ordered by kilogram of body weight
   dose ordered = 20 mg/kg/day
   20 × 33 =

$$
\begin{array}{r}
33 \\
\times\ 20 \\
\hline
660
\end{array} = \text{total dose per 24 hours}
$$

   Step 3   To be given in divided doses q8h, divide total daily dose by 3 (3 doses if giving q8h)

$$
\begin{array}{r}
220 \\
3 \overline{\smash{\big)}\, 660} = \textbf{220 mg \ q8h} \\
\underline{6} \\
6 \\
\underline{6} \\
0
\end{array}
$$

   B. Step 1   Convert 78 pounds to kg

$$
\begin{array}{r}
35.4 \\
2.2 \overline{\smash{\big)}\, 780.0} \\
\underline{66} \\
120 \\
\underline{110} \\
100 \\
\underline{88} \\
12
\end{array}
$$

   Step 2   Multiply 40 mg/kg/day × 35

$$
\begin{array}{r}
35 \\
\times\ 40 \\
\hline
1400
\end{array} = \text{total dose for 24 hours}
$$

   Step 3   Divide into four equal doses

$$
1400 \div 4 =
\begin{array}{r}
350 \\
4 \overline{\smash{\big)}\, 1400} = \textbf{350 mg each dose} \\
\underline{12} \\
20 \\
\underline{20} \\
00
\end{array}
$$

   C. Step 1   Convert 86 pounds to kg

$$
\begin{array}{r}
39 \\
2.2 \overline{\smash{\big)}\, 860.0} = 39 \text{ kg} \\
\underline{66} \\
200 \\
\underline{198} \\
2
\end{array}
$$

Step 2   Multiply dose ordered by kg of body weight
2 mg × 39 = 78 mg = correct dose

Step 3   Divide into three doses (q8h)

$$3\overline{)78} = \mathbf{26\ mg\quad q8h}$$

26
6
18

3.

4. To calculate this adult dose, follow this formula.
Desire (D) divided by what is on hand (H) times the Quantity (Q) divided by 1

$$\frac{D}{H} \times \frac{Q}{1} = dose$$

$$\frac{125\ (D)}{250\ (H)} \times \frac{1(Q)}{1} = dose \qquad \frac{125}{250} = \frac{1}{2} \qquad \frac{1}{2} \times \frac{1}{1} = \frac{1}{2}$$

Give ½ of 250 mg tab.

5. $$\frac{D}{H} \times \frac{Q}{1} = dose$$

$$\frac{250\ (D)}{300\ (H)} \times \frac{5\ mL}{1} = dose \qquad \frac{250}{250} = \frac{5}{6} \qquad \frac{5}{2} \times \frac{5\ mL}{1} = \frac{1}{2}$$

$$6\overline{)25.00} \text{ or } 4.2$$

4.16
24
10
6
40
36
4

Give 4.2 ml

ANSWERS TO WORKBOOK EXERCISES AND ACTIVITIES

Vocabulary Builder

1. Absence of breathing.
2. Body surface area. A highly accurate method for calculating medication dosages for infants and children up to twelve years of age.
3. A lack of oxygen in the blood.
4. The convex or concave upper surface of a column of liquid in a container. Crescent shaped.
5. A graph that shows the relationship among numerical values. An estimate of BSA of a patient can be determined by its use.
6. Injection of a liquid substance into the body via a route other than the alimentary canal.
7. A substance in the form of fine particles that separates from a solution if allowed to stand for a period of time.
8. To pull or draw tight a surface, such as the skin.
9. A premeasured amount of medication, individually packaged on a per-dose basis.
10. A slight elevation of skin that can be produced as a result of an intradermal injection.

Learning Review

1. Dr. King has prescribed 100 mg (1.67 gr) of Dilantin to be taken by mouth three times a day. The pharmacist is directed to dispense 90 tablets, a 30-day supply.

   Dr. Lewis has prescribed 5 cc, or 1 teaspoon, of Amoxicillin by mouth three times a day. The pharmacist is directed to dispense 150 cc (30 teaspoons) for a total of 30 doses to be administered over a period of 10 days.

2. A. Gm   weight, gram, metric
       gr   weight, grain, apothecary
       qt   volume, quart, household
       tbsp   volume, tablespoon, household
       mL   volume, millileter, metric
       fldr   volume, fluidram, apothecary
       gt   volume, drop, household
       mg   weight, microgram, metric

   B. (1) 4 tsp = 20 mL   (4) 30 mg = .5 gr
       (2) 3.5 in = 8.75 cm   (5) 8 mL = 120 gtt
       (3) 1,200 mg = 1.2 Gm

   C. Proportions express the comparative relationships between parts, shares, or portions with regard to size, number, or amount. In mathematics, proportions express the relationship between two ratios. In calculating dosages of medication, proportions are important to make conversions within or between systems of measurement, when converting amounts for adult and pediatric dosages, or when calculating unit dosages. A working knowledge of mathematics ensures that the correct dosage is administered to the patient.

3. A. (1) Type: hypodermic; size: 5 cc; calibration: 0.2 cc.
       (2) Type: insulin; size/calibration: U–100 (1cc).
       (3) Type: tuberculin; size: 1 cc; calibration: 0.1 cc and 0.01 cc.

   B. 1. IM, 90 degrees   2. ID, 10–15 degrees   3. SC, 90 degrees   4. SC, 45 degrees

Multiple Choice Questions

1. b. seven years
2. d. signature
3. a. kilo
4. c. units
5. c. lumen

Investigation Activity

Use this activity to help students connect the elements of safe medication administration: (1) knowledge of pharmacology, (2) ability to calculate dosages, and (3) competency in methods of medication administration. Students become aware that one drug may have several prescribed uses to treat different patient conditions; the drug may be administered in various forms (liquid, solid, semi-solid) through the appropriate routes (oral, parenteral, transdermal, buccal, sublingual, etc.) for each form. Health care professionals have a responsibility to know how a drug is properly administered for each condition it is used to treat, and the effects the drug(s) may and/or will have on the patient when administered to patients in specific dosages for specific treatment purposes.

Students gain a respect for the accuracy necessary when working with drugs and administering drugs to patients. Patients depend on the accuracy and competence of health care professionals in preparing and administering dosages of medications they receive in the ambulatory care setting. Medical assistants who demonstrate a knowledge of all elements of safe medication administration will be better able to assist the physician in patient treatment. They also will become better patient educators and therapeutic communicators, helping patients understand and comply with the medication administration component of the physician's treatment plan.

ANSWERS TO WORKBOOK CASE STUDY QUESTIONS

1. Liz has not given Louise the dosage the physician intended to be administered in the ambulatory care setting for immediate treatment of her migraine headache. Liz's error most likely has not endangered the patient. However, the patient's headache pain will be alleviated more quickly through immediate administration of the Imitrex® medication.

2. If the patient has not yet left the facility, Liz can locate her for immediate administration of the drug. If the patient has left the premises, the physician is notified and a telephone call should be made to follow up and make sure that Louise promptly filled the prescription and began taking the medication. All rules of confidentiality apply when attempting to reach a patient by telephone to discuss treatment issues. Liz should recognize her error; report the error immediately to the physician; stay calm; assess the patient's condition, when possible; follow the physician's order for correcting the error; and document the error in the patient's record or the facility's record form.

37 Electrocardiography

OVERVIEW

Medical assisting students are introduced to the electrical conduction system of the heart and learn the proper procedures for administering electrocardiograms (ECGs), which present graphic representations of the heart's electrical activity. Electrocardiograms are important diagnostic tools that help physicians accurately diagnose cardiac conditions.

PERFORMANCE EVALUATION OUTCOME ASSESSMENT

Students are evaluated for their knowledge of performance objectives. A knowledge of the circulation of blood through the heart and of the electrical conduction system of the heart is demonstrated. Students possess the ability to recognize the cardiac cycle on an ECG tracing and can describe various types of ECGs and their capabilities. Common artifacts and their sources are identified. Students recall several cardiac diagnostic tests and their purposes. Placement of Holter monitor electrodes is identified. The procedures for mounting ECG tracings in the patient's permanent record are mastered. The role of the medical assistant as a patient educator is emphasized.

Procedure 37-1	Perform Twelve-Lead Electrocardiogram, Single Channel
Procedure 37-2	Perform Twelve-Lead Electrocardiogram, Three Channel
Procedure 37-3	Perform Holter Monitor Application

SUPPLEMENTARY RESOURCES

Medical Assisting Videos: Appropriate content is available on Delmar's Medical Assisting Videos, 2nd ed., for the following topics:

Tape 15 Run an Electrocardiogram and Record the Results
   Mounting and ECG Tracing
   ECG Artifacts and Interference
   Holter Monitor

ANSWERS TO TEXT REVIEW QUESTIONS

1. a. somatic tremor
2. d. Parkinson's disease
3. d. 0.8 second
4. a. QRS complex
5. a. precordial

ANSWERS TO TEXT CRITICAL THINKING QUESTIONS

1. Some behaviors Mrs. Johnson can adopt to have a healthier heart are avoiding tobacco, taking medications as prescribed, eating a low-fat, low-cholesterol, low-sodium diet, exercising regularly (with a physician's permission), getting adequate rest, keeping weight under control and at an acceptable level, and practicing stress reduction behaviors.

2. To ensure an adequate ECG tracing from a patient with Parkinson's disease, try to have the patient slide both hands under the buttocks while the ECG is being recorded. This can help reduce somatic tremor.

3. If the equipment malfunctions during an ECG, the medical assistant should attempt to determine the cause. A probable cause may be a broken patient cable. A service person or maintenance person from the manufacturer may need to be consulted to determine the cause of the malfunction.

4. Four cardiac abnormalities that can be detected on an ECG include myocardial ischemia, damage caused by a myocardial infarction, arrhythmias, and electrolyte imbalance.

5. ECG graph paper is divided into 1 mm squares and 5 mm squares. Each large square consists of 25 small squares, and is 5 mm high and 5 mm wide.

   One small square = 0.04 sec. in time.

   One large square = $0.004 \times 5 = 0.2$ sec.

   Divide 60 seconds (1 min.) by 0.2 sec.: $60 \div 0.2 = 300$.

   If there are 2½ large boxes between each cardiac cycle, the heart rate is calculated as: $300 \div 2.5$ or 120 beats per minute.

6. The twelve leads of an ECG are placed as follows:

Lead I	V_1	Lead aVR	V_4
Lead II	V_2	Lead aVL	V_5
Lead III	V_3	Lead aVF	V_6

   Lead I – Right arm to left arm ⎤
   Lead II – Right arm to left leg ⎥ Limb leads or standard
   Lead III – Left arm to left leg ⎦ bipolar leads

   aVR – Right arm + (left arm and left leg) ⎤
   aVL – Left arm + (right arm + left leg) ⎥ Augmented leads
   aVF – Left leg + (right arm + left arm) ⎦

   V_1 – fourth intercostal space at right margin of sternum
   V_2 – fourth intercostal space at left margin of sternum
   V_3 – midway between V2 and V4
   V_4 – fifth intercostal space at junction of left midclavicular line.
   V_5 – horizontal to V4 at left anterior axillary line
   V_6 – horizontal to V4 at left midaxillary line

7. Coughing and movement result in somatic tremor, which is an artifact that interferes with a good-quality ECG.

8. Standardization is a quality assurance check to determine if the machine is set and working properly. Standardization measurements are internationally accepted and are used as a means of accurate calibration according to universal measurements. One millivolt of cardiac activity will deflect the stylus exactly 10 mm high. This is equivalent to 10 small squares on the ECG paper.

9. An interference is caused by electrical interferences and appears as a series of small regular peaks. Electricity present in equipment or wires in the area can leak a small amount of electricity into the room where the ECG is being recorded. To eliminate AC interference, properly ground the machine, unplug other electrical equipment in the room, move the ECG table away from walls, straighten lead wires and follow patient's body contours with them, and clean reusable electrodes and tips of lead wires. Wandering baseline occurs when the stylus suddenly moves or wanders from the center of the ECG paper, resulting in the complexes wandering across the paper in a bottom-to-top or top-to-bottom movement away from the center of the paper. To eliminate wandering baseline, there should be equal tension on all four limb leads, metal tips should be firmly attached to the electrodes and the patient cable should not be pulling or dangling so as to cause pulling on the electrodes, electrodes should be clear, and use the appropriate amount of electrolyte and remove lotions, oils, and creams from the patient's skin where the electrodes will be attached. Interrupted baseline is manifested by a break between complexes. A broken patient cable or lead wire may be responsible.

10. Three purposes for using a Holter monitor include diagnosing cardiac arrhythmias, assessing the function of an artificial pacemaker, and checking the effectiveness of antiarrhythmic drugs. Instructions for the patient include

    1. Keep a diary of daily activities, symptoms, and emotions, and note the time of occurrence.
    2. Do not shower, bathe, or swim because the recording can be damaged.
    3. Do not handle the electrodes.
    4. Do not remove the recorder from its case.
    5. Do not use an electric blanket.
    6. Depress the event button only briefly and when experiencing a significant symptom.

ANSWERS TO WORKBOOK EXERCISES AND ACTIVITIES

Vocabulary Builder

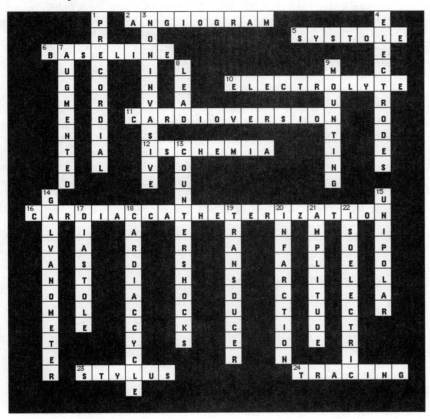

Learning Review

1. Five reasons electrocardiograms are performed include
   (1) To detect myocardial ischemia.
   (2) To detect and evaluate cardiac arrhythmia.
   (3) To estimate damage to the myocardium caused by a myocardial infarction.
   (4) To assess effects of cardiac medication on the heart.
   (5) To determine if electrolyte imbalance is present.
2. See textbook.
   A. bipolar
      • Lead I records electrical activity between the right arm and left arm.
      • Lead II records electrical activity between the right arm and left leg.
      • Lead III records electrical activity between the left arm and left leg.
   B. unipolar
      • Lead aVR records electrical activity from the midpoint between the left arm and the left leg to the right arm.
      • Lead aVL records electrical activity from the midpoint between the right arm and the left leg to the left arm.
      • Lead aVF records electrical activity from the midpoint between the right arm and the left arm to the left leg.
   C. precordial, unipolar
      • Chest or precordial leads record the heart's electrical impulse from a central point within the heart to one of six predesignated positions on the chest wall where an electrode is attached.
3.   D 1. Alternating current   A 3. Interrupted baseline
     B 2. Somatic tremor   C 4. Wandering baseline

Multiple Choice Questions

1. d. relaxes
2. b. Welch sensor
3. a. unipolar

4. b. 10 mm high
5. a. lotions, creams, or oils on the patient's skin

Investigation Activity

Use this activity to increase students' awareness of the many preventive measures patients can employ to reduce their risk of heart disease. Studies have shown that lifestyle choices and diet have a significant impact on heart health. As effective patient educators, medical assistants can encourage patients to choose heart-healthy habits. By researching medical organizations, medical studies, insurance programs and coverage, and community resources, medical assistants discover the wide range of support and data available to health care professionals and health care consumers on health topics, such as cardiovascular health and fitness. With this knowledge at their disposal, medical assistants increase their own understanding and are better able to direct patients to appropriate resources and information.

ANSWERS TO WORKBOOK CASE STUDY QUESTIONS

1. The exercise tolerance test is a treadmill stress test. The test is done to diagnose heart disorders, to diagnose the probable cause of the patient's chest pain, and to assess the patient's cardiac ability following cardiac surgery. The test is a noninvasive ECG tracing taken under controlled conditions while the patient is closely monitored by the physician. Frequent blood pressure readings are done. The patient wears comfortable clothing and flat shoes, such as sneakers with rubber soles, and exercises on a treadmill at prescribed rates of speed. Electrodes are applied to the chest only.
2. The test is discontinued if the patient experiences pain, shortness of breath, excess fatigue, or any other unusual symptom, because the symptoms could indicate cardiac disease.
3. At the conclusion of the test, the patient is told to rest. Monitoring continues until the vital signs and heart rate return to normal. The patient is instructed to rest, refrain from a hot bath or shower, avoid stimulants such as caffeine, and avoid extreme temperature changes for several hours.
4. The cardiovascular stress test is a procedure; the proper code is 93015.

Chapter

38

Safety and Regulatory Guidelines in the Medical Laboratory

OVERVIEW

Medical assisting students are introduced to the federal guidelines and regulations instituted to protect patients and health care professionals in the medical setting. The CDC's universal, standard, and transmission-based precautions are outlined and discussed both in this chapter and Chapter 22. Compliance with CLIA '88 standards for laboratory testing and the OSHA Bloodborne Pathogen Standard and the impact of these guidelines and regulations on the medical assistant's performance of duties in the ambulatory care setting are emphasized. Students learn about the types of blood and body fluids and discover pathways for possible infection from pathogens. The special risks of HIV and HBV transmission are highlighted. Students discover the importance of the strict use of and compliance with standard precautions, CLIA '88, and OSHA. Infectious diseases and accidents in the ambulatory care setting occur through lack of education and carelessness. Medical assisting students recognize the necessity of exhibiting professional behavior that will protect themselves and their patients from the spread of infectious diseases and maintain high safety standards in the ambulatory care setting.

PROFICIENCY EVALUATION OUTCOME ASSESSMENT

Students are evaluated for their understanding of performance objectives. Students must recognize the necessity of strict compliance with standard precautions, CLIA '88, and OSHA guidelines and regulations. Students should be able to identify and give strategies for implementing universal, standard, and transmission-based precautions and identify sources of potentially infectious materials from the human body, such as blood and OPIM. Students should cite the categories of testing under CLIA '88 and understand the process of obtaining facility certification to perform laboratory tests. Students outline the details of a chemical hygiene plan and understand the function and purpose of the MSDS manual, including coding of substances for chemical hazards. Students understand the purpose of the OSHA Bloodborne Pathogen Standard and can develop an exposure control plan. Students define and identify PPE. Students understand proper disposal of contaminated waste materials. In this chapter, the student gains insight into the scope and application of measures designed to protect both patients and health care professionals and the responsibility to obey all state and federal laws.

SUPPLEMENTARY RESOURCES

Medical Assisting Videos: Appropriate content is available on Delmar's Medical Assisting Videos, 2nd ed., for the following topics:

Tape 5   Infection Control and Standard Precautions
            Performing Medical Aseptic Procedure of Handwashing
Tape 10   Office Emergencies, Respiratory Emergencies, and First Aid
            Workplace Hazards and Material Safety Data Sheets
Tape 13   Venipuncture, Hematology, and Immunology
            Basic Information for Specimen Taking and Laboratory Work
Tape 14   Collect and Process Specimens
            Quality Control in Collecting and Processing Specimens

ANSWERS TO TEXT REVIEW QUESTIONS

1. b. CDC
2. c. laboratory tests performed on specimens taken from the human body
3. b. the Chemical Hygiene Plan
4. d. OSHA
5. c. orientation, periodic drills, and consistent enforcement of policy
6. d. the methods used in testing
7. c. HCFA (Health Care Financing Administration)
8. d. a medical assistant
9. c. Ergonomic Hazards
10. c. Health
11. d. Fire
12. a. Reactivity or Instability
13. b. Use PPE

ANSWERS TO TEXT CRITICAL THINKING QUESTIONS

1. The purpose of CLIA '88 is to protect patients by regulating all laboratory tests performed on specimens taken from the human body, i.e., blood and body secretions and excretions. The law was amended in 1988 because of patients' deaths that resulted from Pap tests that were misread.
2. Four categories of testing are waived, moderate complexity, high complexity, and physician-performed microscopy. Waived tests are simple and require a minimum of judgment and interpretation. Moderate- and high-complexity tests are categorized according to the degree of operator intervention needed, the necessary knowledge and experience the operator possesses, and the degree of troubleshooting needed to perform the tests. Physician-performed microscopy tests are in the waived category.
3. The fifteen major components of CLIA are
   (1) All laboratories are required to register with CLIA even if just one test is performed, regardless of which of the categories the test is found and regardless of whether there is Medicare and Medicaid reimbursement.
   (2) The regulations apply to all laboratories. Previously unregulated laboratories could enroll until January 1, 1994.
   (3) The regulations are specific to the *complexity* of the test. Standards become more stringent as the complexity of the test increases.
   (4) A laboratory must obtain a certificate to perform tests. An initial filing for a certificate is made on form 116 with HCFA of the Department of HHS. One of the following five certificates can be obtained (there can be a state exemption, as previously mentioned): (a) Certificate of Waiver (for laboratories that perform only waived tests), (b) Registration Certificate (for laboratories that perform tests of moderate- and high-complexity; issued for a period of 2 years until HCFA can determine that these laboratories are in compliance with all requirements), (c) Certificate (for laboratories that perform moderate- and high-complexity tests after HCFA has determined that the laboratories are in compliance with all requirements), (d) Certificate of Accreditation (for laboratories that have been accredited by an accrediting body recognized by HCFA), and (e) Physician Performed Microscopy Certificate (added in January 1993; includes wet mounts, e.g., preparation of vaginal, cervical, or skin specimens; all potassium hydroxide preparations; pinworm examinations; fern tests; postcoital exams of vaginal and cervical mucus, and urine sediment examinations). If physicians personally perform these tests on their patients, the laboratory can apply for the certificate of physician performed microscopy. Under this certificate, the laboratory is allowed to perform waived tests; however, no other tests can be performed. All five certification categories must be renewed every 2 years and be accompanied by a fee ranging from $100 to $600. After a laboratory has been certified, it must notify HCFA within 6 months if it changes the types of tests it performs, which could alter the laboratory's classification.
   (5) Some examples of sanctions or penalties imposed by HCFA for noncompliance with the CLIA law are

Infraction	Penalty
Failure to enroll with HCFA	Denial or revocation of certificate
Nonparticipation in proficiency testing	A score of 0 (a score of 80% is required)
Failure to return the proficiency testing result	A score of 0

   In addition to the above, Medicare and Medicaid payments may be suspended or terminated and civil penalties of up to a $10,000 fine per violation or per day of noncompliance may be imposed. For CLIA condtions other than proficiency testing, newly regulated laboratories will not be subjected to penalties during the first inspection cycle unless it is determined that the laboratories' inadequacies pose immediate patient danger.
   (6) The law mandates quality assurance for nonwaived tests. Laboratories are required to establish policies and procedures through programs that assess test quality; identify problems and correct them; ensure precise, dependable, and punctual reporting of test results; and guarantee sufficient competent staff. In addition, laboratories must ensure that all quality control data are studied; and that if there is a complaint, an investigation must be

undertaken and appropriate action taken and recorded. It is a requirement that quality assurance records be maintained.

(7) The law mandates quality control for nonwaived tests. Laboratories are required to have an adequate supply of equipment to perform the number and types of tests they offer. A procedures manual must be available in the testing area and must include complete testing instructions. Documentation of maintenance programs for instruments, equipment, and test systems must be evident.

(8) The law establishes requirements for the correct collection, transportation, and storage of specimens and the reporting of results.

(9) The law mandates maintenance of records, equipment, and facilities of labs performing nonwaived tests.

(10) The law mandates personnel standards. There are requirements for personnel who perform nonwaived tests and they spell out the necessary qualifications and responsibilities required of them. Each person who does the tests must be licensed by the state, if required; have a high school diploma or equivalent; have adequate training; and be able to demonstrate an understanding of laboratory procedures, calibration of instruments, specimen collection, and quality control. Personnel must report test results accurately and with dependability. All high-complexity tests must be done by technologists and technicians except for cytology, which requires more stringent qualifications.

(11) The law mandates proficiency testing for nonwaived tests. The procedures and tests found in the waived category are exempt from proficiency testing, regardless of the type of laboratory in which the tests are performed. Moderate- and high-complexity test laboratories must enroll in proficiency testing programs that are approved by the Department of Health and Human Services. The proficiency testing samples are checked in the same manner as patient specimens. Unsatisfactory performance on a proficiency testing check can result in various penalties ranging from termination of the laboratory's license to operate to the termination of reimbursement from Medicare and Medicaid. January 1994 was the phase-in date for previously unregulated laboratories to enroll in proficiency testing, but proficiency testing will continue to be required for laboratories that were regulated by March 4, 1990.

(12) The law mandates unannounced on-site inspection. All laboratories in the moderate- and high-complexity category are subject to unannounced inspections by the Department of Health and Human Services or an agency assigned to the task by HHS. Laboratories that perform only waived tests must prove that tests are being done according to the manufacturer's directions. Inspections can involve employee interviews, observation of employees performing tests, and analysis of data and documentation of results. Violations of requirements by any laboratory can result in penalties. The cost of inspection is billed to the laboratory.

(13) The law mandates an annual listing of laboratories that have had action taken against them.

(14) The law mandates patient test management. All laboratories must have a strategy for properly receiving and processing specimens and for the precise reporting of the results. Written instructions regarding collection, safeguarding of specimens, and labeling of specimens must be available for patients. There must be a specific procedure for reporting life-threatening results and a follow-through to the person requesting the test. Test records must be kept for 2 years following the reporting of results.

(15) The law mandates documentation. The following documentation must be done and be available:

Specimen
  Patient preparation
  Specimen collection procedure
  Proper labeling technique
  Preservation of specimen if applicable
Proficiency Testing
  Corrective action taken
Quality Control and Quality Assurance
  Any corrective action taken
Problem and complaint log
Requisitions
  Patient name
  Name and address of laboratory
  Date and time of collection
  Name of test requested
  Diagnosis

Results
  Name and address of laboratory where test is
    done
  Test name
  Test results, including normal ranges listed on
    test results
  Disposition of unacceptable specimens must
    be released to authorized person
Log of Results
  Printouts from instruments report must be kept
  Identification of person performing test
  Patient identification number
  Specimen identification
  Date
  Time specimen is received in laboratory
  Specimen rejection log maintained

4. Quality control and quality assurance are regulations CLIA has established to ensure the highest standards for laboratory testing.

5. HCFA Form 116 is an application form that a laboratory must file to inform the U.S. Department of Health and Human Services about the laboratory's operation; it is a legal requirement.

6. A manual for a chemical hygiene plan for all employees should include the following information. The primary component of the OSHA standard is that a written chemical hygiene plan and program must be operational if chemicals are stored in a facility and handled by employees. Some examples of chemicals include, but are not limited to, stains, ethyl alcohol, sodium hypochlorite (household bleach), formaldehyde, fixatives, preservatives, injectables such as chemotherapeutic agents, and acetone. Many laboratory accidents result in chemical-related illnesses ranging from eye irritations to pulmonary edema.

There are three primary goals that an employer must accomplish to be in compliance with the OSHA standard for chemical exposure. The first is that there must be an inventory undertaken and a list compiled of all chemicals considered hazardous. The following information must be documented: the quantity of chemical stored per month or year; if the substance is gas, liquid, or solid; the manufacturer's name and address; and the chemical hazard classification. Second, a material safety data sheet (MSDS) manual must be assembled. (MSDSs oftentimes are supplied by the manufacturer when the chemicals are ordered and give information regarding whether or not a chemical is hazardous.) All other MSDSs must be requested from the manufacturer. The MSDSs must be alphabetized, indexed, and reviewed on a regular basis and modifications made. The manuals must be available to all employees. The various chemicals are labeled using the National Fire Protection Association's color and number method. Third, the employer is required to provide a hazard communication educational program to the employee within 30 days of employment and before the employee handles any hazardous chemicals. The training program should consist of location and identification of hazardous chemicals, how to read and understand the labels on the chemicals, where the MSDS manuals are kept, when to use personal protective equipment, and procedures to follow for chemical spills. The training sessions must be documented, signed by the employer, and permanently retained in the employee record.

January 1991 was the deadline for laboratories (including POLs) to have a chemical hygiene plan (CHP) in place. The requirements for a CHP include
- Employers must have an operational written plan (a manual) relevant to the safety and health of employees.
- Written instructions on the use of personal protection equipment must be available.
- Fume or biohazard hoods must be checked regularly.
- Training sessions must be held for employees regarding their right to know what hazardous chemicals exist in their work environment.
- It is the employer's legal responsibility to provide medical attention for an employee should an accidental chemical spill occur.
- The responsibility for executing training sessions, keeping manuals current, and documentation is designated to an employee.
- Instruction must be provided regarding disposal of hazardous waste produced in the workplace. (Usually this is a hazardous waste company contracted by the employer.)
- Each employee's record must have a written statement signed by the employer stating his or her responsibility to arrange for training for the employee as well as maintaining a safe work environment.
- Records and dates of all tests done.

ANSWERS TO WORKBOOK EXERCISES AND ACTIVITIES

Vocabulary Builder

A. 1. B.
  2. G.
  3. D.
  4. J.
  5. A.
  6. I.
  7. H.
  8. E.
  9. F.
 10. C.
B. 1. Acetone. A colorless, flammable liquid found in the blood and urine of diabetics caused by the breakdown of fatty acids.
  2. Chemotherapeutic agents. Agents used in the treatment of disease; the application of chemical reagents that are toxic to pathogenic microorganisms. Commonly used to describe agents (chemicals) used in the treatment of certain malignancies.
  3. Ethyl alcohol. Alcohol used to make a solution.

4. Aegis. Sponsorship, protection.
5. Formaldehyde. A colorless gas combined with methanol and used as a solution, such as a disinfectant, astringent, or a preservative for histologic specimen.
6. Forensic. Pertaining to the law.

Multiple Choice Questions

1. c. establish standards to ensure accurate test results
2. c. 1988
3. d. all of the above
4. d. training information for using the product/chemical
5. a. wash the area with water immediately

Investigation Activity

The instructor should record the list of chemical substances researched by the students for potential chemical hazards. Students must submit the MSDS or chemical hazard information they obtain from manufacturers to compile a proto-type of an MSDS manual. Class discussion can involve the types of hazards presented by various substances and the need for correct labeling and handling to reduce the risk of injury or accidents from improper usage or storage. In performing this activity, students achieve an awareness of the properties of chemical substances commonly used in the ambulatory care setting and the substances' potential hazards. Students gain a respect for chemical substances and recognize the need for care in handling and using them, and for performing duties in strict compliance with federal and state regulations and guidelines.

Learning Review

A. Waived tests: consult textbook Table 38-3 for the list of analytes currently on the CLIA '88 waived list.
B. Five specific duties of the medical assistant are
   1. Maintaining personnel records.
   2. Confirming employee hepatitis B status.
   3. Compiling a procedures manual for how tests are performed.
   4. Compiling an instrument log.
   5. Executing complete documentation.
C. 1. 4. Blue.
      3. White.
      2. Yellow.
      1. Fire.
   2. a. Chemical X is a combustible liquid that is corrosive or toxic and may be explosive if spark occurs or if heat-ed under confinement. Goggles, gloves, apron, and mask must be worn.
      b. Chemical Y is a noncombustible substance that may cause irritation and is nonreactive when mixed with water. Gloves must be worn.
      c. Chemical Z is combustible if heated and harmful if inhaled. It may react if heated or mixed with water. Goggles, gloves, and mask must be worn.

Chapter

39

Introduction to the Medical Laboratory

OVERVIEW

Medical assistants play an important role in laboratory testing, which provides important diagnostic information to physicians. Medical assistants may be responsible for patient preparation, obtaining specimens, and testing or sending specimens to an independent laboratory. Students learn about the departments inside a medical laboratory, the type of testing each department performs, and how to fill out a laboratory requisition form. They also learn about the importance of quality controls and safety standards and how to ensure that both are maintained. Standard precautions for infection control are mandatory in the laboratory setting.

PROFICIENCY EVALUATION OUTCOME ASSESSMENT

Students are evaluated on their knowledge of performance objectives. A working knowledge of the types of medical laboratories and the tests performed by each, as well as the proper procedures for collecting and processing patient specimens are covered. The importance of aseptic technique and standard precautions for infection control are emphasized. Students recognize the need to employ quality control and quality assurance programs to ensure accurate and reliable test results. Students demonstrate the ability to use and care for a compound microscope.

> Procedure 39-1   Using the Microscope

SUPPLEMENTARY RESOURCES

Medical Assisting Videos: Appropriate content is available on Delmar's Medical Assisting Videos, 2nd ed., for the following topics:

> Tape 13 Basic Information for Specimen Taking and Laboratory Work
> When the Physician Orders a Specimen
> Tape 14 Quality Control in Collecting and Processing Specimens
> Perform Microscopic Examination of Urine

ANSWERS TO TEXT REVIEW QUESTIONS

1. b. must be performed by certified laboratory professionals.
2. b. pathologist
3. b. studies blood and blood-forming tissues
4. d. all of the above
5. a. a written requisition
6. d. compound microscope

ANSWERS TO TEXT CRITICAL THINKING QUESTIONS

1. Physicians use accredited medical laboratories located within their business complex, which are in close proximity to their office, or with whom they have a contractual agreement. Specific laboratories have to be used because the patient's insurance often dictates what laboratory can do the patient's testing. It is best to check these factors before recommending a laboratory.

2. The kit test done at home could have been stored improperly or could be outdated. Also, the individual who does the home kit test is not as knowledgeable about quality control as are trained laboratory personnel. Pregnancy tests done in the medical office follow all the guidelines of quality control and are performed by trained personnel to give accurate results.

3. Clinical laboratory technologists have a bachelor's degree and one year of training in an accredited hospital. After education and training, they are qualified to take a national certification examination administered by an accredited agency. Clinical laboratory technicians have completed two years of formal education and training in an accredited hospital and have an associate's degree. After education and training, they are qualified to take a national certification examination administered by an accredited agency. Medical assistants have formal education and externship through community colleges, vocational-technical schools and private institutions. After education and training, they are qualified to take a national certification examination administered by an accredited agency.

4. Rather than order several separate tests, which often can be more costly, a physician has the option of ordering a group of tests called profiles. Profiles are packaged tests that give a complete analysis of the chemistry in various body systems or organs. Some common profiles are liver, kidney, and cardiac. By ordering a profile, the physician is getting a complete overview of a system and very often is saving the patient money.

5. When specimens are not processed and handled properly, or test kits and chemicals are mishandled, the test results can be inaccurate. The inaccuracy can lead to misdiagnosis and incorrect treatment of the patient. It is extremely important to store and handle kits properly and to follow all established guidelines for accurate results.

6. The medical assistant has been trained and educated to perform administrative duties, prepare patients, collect specimens, and perform certain tests. He or she is responsible for his or her own safety and the safety of the patient, and must ensure that the specimen is reliable and that the test performed is accurate. When all these aspects are considered, the test result will be accurate.

7. The date and time should always be on a specimen. The time of the specimen is important from several aspects, the promptness with which results are needed (STAT, routine, or the circumstances). Is it preoperative? Is it a timed blood sugar or fasting specimen? The time and date a specimen was drawn are important to the laboratory to ensure that the specimen was not mishandled and was delivered promptly and in the correct manner for the test required (such as icing or immediate removal of serum). All of these factors contribute to the accuracy and reliability of the results.

8. To obtain plasma, a blood sample tube with an anticoagulant must be used. The type of anticoagulant is designated by the color of the tube stopper. The anticoagulant needed in the tube for certain tests will be specified by the laboratory. If the medical assistant is unsure of which anticoagulant to use, it is best to call the laboratory.

9. To use and focus a microscope correctly, the medical assistant must be familiar with the components and functions of all parts of the microscope. Start by placing the slide on the stage of the microscope, and turn the light on to adjust the field under low power, using the coarse and fine adjustments. After the low power is in focus, the high and oil objectives can be used. If using the oil objective, remember to place a drop of cedar or mineral oil on the slide and only use the fine adjustment with high and oil objectives. After using the microscope, remember to clean it thoroughly.

10. A compound microscope magnifies an object using the lens of the objectives and eyepieces. The total magnification of the field is the product of the magnification in the eyepiece and the objective used. Most compound microscopes have a low objective with magnification of $10\times$, a high objective with magnification of $45\times$, and an oil objective with a magnification of $100\times$. The eyepiece, also called the ocular, magnifies the image formed by the lens of the objective. Eyepiece magnifications are usually $10\times$, but $20\times$ and $5\times$ are available. The magnification of the eyepiece and objective is marked on each piece. The eyepiece magnification and objective magnification are multiplied for total magnification of the object or field. If an ocular of $10\times$ is used with the high objective of $45\times$, the total magnification is $450\times$.

ANSWERS TO WORKBOOK EXERCISES AND ACTIVITIES

Vocabulary Builder

A.
1. objective
2. differential diagnosis
3. baseline
4. requisition

8. normal flora
9. quantitative tests
10. control test
11. glucose

15. serum
16. reagents
17. condenser
18. invasive

5.	diaphragm	12.	qualitative tests	19.	diagnosis
6.	assay	13.	biopsy	20.	clinical diagnosis
7.	profile	14.	asymptomatic	21.	electrolytes

B.
1. F.
2. H. See textbook Table 39–1 for diseases caused by parasites.
3. L.
4. D. Hgb: Hemoglobin; Diff: Differential White Blood Cell Count; ESR: Erythrocyte sedimentation rate; Hct: Hematocrit.
5. J.
6. A.
7. B. Some electrolytes include sodium, potassium, hydrogen, magnesium, calcium, bicarbonate, phosphate, and chloride.
8. I. See textbook Table 39–1 for a listing of infectious diseases.
9. K.
10. G.
11. E.
12. C. Two types of tests include chromosome studies and the Pap test.
13. M.

Learning Review

1. A. to confirm a clinical diagnosis.
   B. to prevent the exacerbation of diseases.
   C. prevention of diseases/disorders.
   D. to diagnose.
   E. to record an individual's state of health.
   F. to differentiate between two or more diseases.
   G. to detect asymptomatic conditions or diseases.
   H. to determine the effectiveness of treatments.
2. A. Five tests that can be performed in a physician's office laboratory (POL) are any five of the following: the hematocrit level test, hemoglobin level test, urinalysis, strep throat test, pregnancy test, blood sugar level test, and fecal occult blood test.
   B. 1. medical conditions.
      2. location of the patient.
      3. treatment methods.
3. A. L   F. T   K. L
   B. E   G. T   L. T
   C. T   H. E   M. L
   D. E   I. T   N. E
   E. L   J. L
4. A. The factors that can compromise the accuracy of test results include collection of specimen, methods of transporting and processing specimens, time limits of test, amount or age of specimen, time limits of test, using chemicals or reagents past their expiration dates, using test kits that have been exposed to extreme heat or cold, or using chemicals or reagents after their expiration dates.
   B. The purpose of a control sample is to ensure accurate test results by minimizing human errors, helping to make more accurate diagnoses, and providing a way to check for faulty testing methods or reagents. A control test sample is tested along with a patient's sample. The control sample has a known value or result that can be compared with the results of the patient's test. A health care worker can compare a sample of known value to a patient's sample and thereby more precisely determine the accurate result of the patient's test. The control sample can also be used to discover errors in testing methods. If a control sample does not test correctly, the health care worker knows to more closely examine the methods used and to check the reagents used, because these may be faulty or have expired.
5. A. 1. Do not consume food or drink in the laboratory.
      2. Wash hands frequently.
      3. Avoid touching eyes and mouth.
      4. Wear PPE.
   B. The contaminated surface should be immediately disinfected with 10 percent hypochlorite solution.
   C. Loose clothing and accessories should be avoided because they can easily catch fire or get caught on or in medical equipment.
   D. It is important to maintain laboratory equipment because faulty equipment can be dangerous; faulty equipment can cause fires or pieces could fly off during use and cause injury.

6. A. Examples of transmission include cuts and abrasions on the skin, chapped skin, open wounds, and hangnails. Standard precautions include handwashing, using lotions to protect against excoriated skin, wearing gloves, and appropriately dressing and bandaging open cuts and wounds.

   B. Examples of transmission include not washing the hands, especially after using the toilet or handling pathogenic substances; eating or drinking in contaminated areas; and eating or drinking food that has been contaminated or improperly cooked or prepared. Standard precautions include practicing aseptic handwashing technique; proper food preparation and cooking; and eating in designated areas.

   C. Examples of transmission include not washing hands and touching the face or inhaling infected droplets. Standard precautions include aseptic handwashing technique, keeping hands away from the face and eyes, and using PPE as required.

7. A. The purpose of a microscope is to allow health care professionals to see microorganisms that are much too small to be viewed without magnification.

   B. (1) light source; (2) eyepieces; (3) objectives; (4) condenser; (5) diaphragm.

   C. compound

   D. 1. The phase contrast microscope; this microscope is used for viewing specimens that are transparent and unstained.

      2. The fluorescent microscope; this microscope is used when viewing specimens that must be stained with a fluorescent dye.

      3. The electron microscope; this microscope is used to view extremely small organisms in great detail and in three dimensions.

   E. 1. The coarse adjustment, used to bring an object into view.

      2. The fine adjustment, used to sharpen the image.

   F. To properly care for a microscope, the medical assistant should

      1. Follow the manufacturer's and clinic's rules for the care and maintenance of the microscope.

      2. Carry the microscope with one hand securely supporting the base and the other hand holding the arm.

      3. Keep the microscope covered when it is not being used.

      4. Clean the lenses with special lens paper after each use.

      5. Always focus away from the lens to keep the lens from coming into contact with the slide.

      6. Use manufacturer's recommended oil only with the oil immersion lens.

Multiple Choice Questions

1. d. differential diagnosis
2. b. quantitative tests
3. c. microbiology department
4. d. bilirubin level
5. d. toxicological study

Investigation Activity

Use this investigation activity to encourage students to think about their own natural skills of observation and about their ability to pay attention to details. The activity helps students decide if they would enjoy working in a medical laboratory and whether their personalities match the working environment and level of precision required for accurate and reliable laboratory analysis.

ANSWERS TO WORKBOOK CASE STUDY QUESTIONS

NORTHBOROUGH REFERENCE LABORATORIES
128 Analysis Way
Northborough, OH 12468

☐ GROUP ACCOUNT ☐ PATIENT

Ordering Physician Signature

LAST NAME FIRST NAME MI	SEX	DATE OF BIRTH
Johnson, Abigail	F	3/1/20

PRIMARY CARE PHYSICIAN
Dr. Elizabeth King

ADDRESS 225 River Street   CITY Northborough   STATE OH   ZIP 12336

SPECIMEN INFORMATION

PHONE # Home 389-2631   SOC SEC # 011-11-1231

☒ STAT
Date of Collection 6/5/xxxx

Time of Collection 2:00 p.m.

COMPLETE SHADED BOX BELOW FOR PATIENT AND THIRD PARTY BILL ONLY

RESPONSIBLE PARTY   LAST NAME   FIRST NAME   MI

MEDICARE/MEDICAID ☐
021-45-6712-D

☒ Serum   ☐ Plasma
☐ Urine (Volume) _____
     Hours _____
☐ Other _____

ADDRESS   CITY   STATE   ZIP   PHONE #

INSURED NAME   INSURANCE CO. NAME/ADDRESS

CALL RESULTS TO:
Ellen Armstrong, CMA

Phone #:( ) 651-8000

INSURED'S EMPLOYER   RELATIONSHIP TO PATIENT   ☒ Self ☐ Spouse ☐ Dependent   CONTRACT #   GROUP #

Copy Results to:
Dr. Frank Jones
815 Heart Health Blvd.
Northborough, OH 12339

REASON FOR TEST (A DIAGNOSIS IS NECESSARY FOR ALL INSURANCE CLAIMS) SEE REVERSE FOR CODES

413.9 Angina; 250.00 Diabetes; 401.9 Hypertension

SPECIMEN CODES: G - GEL, L - LAVENDER, R - RED, B - BLUE, BK - BLACK, U - URINE

PROFILES (See Reverse for Contents)

☒ BIOCHEM BASIC	1G	☐ BIOCHEM PROFILE III	2G, 1L	☐ LIPID	1G
☐ BIOCHEM PROFILE I	1G, 1L	☐ ARTHRITIS	2G, 1BK	12-16 HOUR FAST REQUIRED	
☐ BIOCHEM PROFILE II	1G, 1L	☐ HEPATITIS	1G	☐ LIVER	1G
				☐ PRENATAL	1G, 1L, 1R

☐ THYROID	1G
☐ HYPERTHYROID	1G
☐ HYPOTHYROID	1G
☐ TORCH PROFILE	1G

INDIVIDUAL TESTS

☐ ALBUMIN	G	☐ FSH	G	☐ PROSTATE SPECIFIC ANTIGEN	G
☐ ALK. PHOSPHATASE	G	☐ GC CULTURE, SOURCE _____		☐ PT W/INR	B
☐ AMYLASE	G	☐ GLUCOSE	G	☐ PTT	B
☐ ANA SCREEN	G	☐ GLYCATED HEMOGLOBIN	L	☐ RHEUMATOID FACTOR	G
☐ BILIRUBIN, TOTAL	G	☐ hCG, BETA SUBUNIT QUANT.	G	☐ RPR	G
☐ BILIRUBIN, TOTAL + DIRECT	G	☐ HDL	G	☐ RUBELLA IgG ANTIBODY	G
☐ BILIRUBIN, NEONATAL	G	☐ HEPATITIS B SURF. ANTIBODY	G	☐ SEDIMENTATION RATE	BK
☐ BUN	G	☐ HEPATITIS B SURF. ANTIGEN	G	☐ SGOT	G
☐ CALCIUM, TOTAL	G	☐ HEPATITIS C ANTIBODY	G	☐ SGPT	G
☐ CBC W/AUTOMATED DIFF	L	☐ HIV ANTIBODY (SIGNED CONSENT REQUIRED)	G	☐ SPUTUM CULTURE	
☐ CBC W/MANUAL DIFF	L	☐ LACTIC DEHYDROGENASE	G	☐ STOOL CULTURE	
☐ CHLAMYDIA SCREEN, SOURCE _____		☐ LEAD, PEDIATRIC	L	☐ THROAT, GROUP A STREP CULTURE	
☐ CHOLESTEROL	G	☐ LH	G	☐ TOTAL PROTEIN	G
☐ CREATININE	G	☐ LIPASE	G	☐ TSH	G
☐ CULTURE, SOURCE _____		☐ LITHIUM	G	☐ URIC ACID	G
☐ ELECTROLYTES	G	☐ OVA & PARASITE PREP.		☐ URINALYSIS	U
☐ ESTRADIOL	G	☐ PHOSPHORUS	G	☐ URINE CULTURE	U
☐ FERRITIN	G	☐ PREGNANCY TEST, BLOOD	G	☐ VITAMIN B12	G
☐ FOLIC ACID	G	☐ PROGESTERONE	G		
☐ FREE T4	G	☐ PROLACTIN	G		

Chapter

40

Phlebotomy: Venipuncture and Capillary Puncture

OVERVIEW

Medical assisting students are presented with the techniques and procedures associated with venipuncture, the process of collecting blood. To obtain blood samples that will yield accurate and reliable test results, medical assistants will use proper clinical, administrative, and communication skills. The correct method of draw, order of draw, and the correct handling and processing of the sample after collection are essential components of the venipuncture procedure. When performing venipuncture, aseptic technique and standard precautions for infection control must be observed, particularly the correct handling and disposal of sharps.

PROFICIENCY EVALUATION OUTCOME ASSESSMENT

Students are evaluated for their understanding of performance objectives. Students should understand the principles of the circulatory system, as well as the principles of various equipment used for venipuncture procedures; demonstrate proficiency in drawing blood and an understanding of related interpersonal and communication skills; and recognize and be able to respond appropriately to adverse patient reactions to venipuncture, such as syncope, nausea, convulsions, cardiac arrest, and extreme pain. Students observe aseptic technique and standard precautions, including the proper handling and disposal of sharps.

SUPPLEMENTARY RESOURCES

Medical Assisting Videos: Appropriate content is available on Delmar's Medical Assisting Videos, 2nd ed., Tape 13, for the following topics:

Basic Information for Specimen Taking and Laboratory Work
When the Physician Orders a Specimen
Collect and Label a Blood Specimen
Butterfly Collection from Hand Vein
Collecting Tubes
Capillary Puncture

ANSWERS TO TEXT REVIEW QUESTIONS

1. d.   hemolysis
2. d.   prevent the blood from clotting
3. b.   avoid dripping blood out of the end of the needle
4. a.   hemoconcentration
5. b.   handwashing
6. b.   discarded intact in a sharps container
7. d.   red
8. b.   (light blue) sodium citrate
9. c.   ask another medical assistant to try
10. a.   collapse

ANSWERS TO TEXTBOOK CRITICAL THINKING QUESTIONS

1. It is best to try to calm patients by talking to them in a friendly and polite manner—explaining often what you are going to do, that the physician ordered the test, and that you are just trying to do your job in assisting with the physician's diagnosis. It is the health care professional's responsibility to provide excellent care to the patient by being skilled, polite, and friendly. Patients' responses regarding the quality of care at the physician's office will make a lasting impression spread by word of mouth to family and friends.

2. Plasma is the liquid portion of the blood that contains fibrinogen but not cells. It is composed of water and solutes, which contain nutrients. The cellular portion contains red blood cells, white blood cells, and platelets. To collect a plasma sample, the blood is drawn into one of the tubes containing an anticoagulant and is spun in the centrifuge. The blood separates into a cellular layer on the bottom of the tube and a straw-colored hazy liquid on top, which contains fibrinogen.

    Serum is essentially the same as plasma, except serum has converted fibrinogen to fibrin during the clotting process. The fibrin is like a web that traps the cellular elements into a mass known as a clot. The clot forms into a cellular mass and the liquid portion is serum. To collect a serum sample, blood is drawn into a tube that does not contain an anticoagulant.

3. The syringe and needle method is ideal for veins that are too fragile for blood collection with an evacuated system. With the syringe and needle, there is less risk of damaging thin, fragile veins. Vein collapse can be avoided by using the needle and syringe method and withdrawing a small amount of blood at a time. Often the vacuum in an evacuated tube can be too large and will collapse a thin, fragile vein.

4. Clots are formed when the fibrinogen in the liquid portion of the blood is converted into fibrin. The fibrin is like a web that traps the cellular elements into a mass. The liquid portion of this blood sample is serum. To stop the clotting process, the blood is drawn into a tube containing an anticoagulant.

5. The medical assistant should always try to leave the patient with a favorable impression of the physician's office and staff. If a patient has been treated properly, the office examination will be a good experience and will leave a favorable impression on the patient. The medical assistant, in handling this situation, has used professional skills to deal with the frightened patient, social skills in saying kind words and alleviating some of the fears, and technical skills in obtaining the blood sample.

6. If a patient is experiencing pain once the needle has entered the vein, it is best to try to slightly reposition the needle and loosen the tourniquet. If the blood sample cannot be obtained on the first attempt and the patient agrees to being stuck again, it is best to stick a vein in the opposite arm or below the site of the first one. The medical assistant should never attempt more than two venipunctures on a patient.

ANSWERS TO WORKBOOK EXERCISES AND ACTIVITIES

Vocabulary Builder

1. A. leukocytes
    B. aliquot
    C. edematous
    D. erythrocytes
    E. cannula
    F. luer
    G. hemolysis
2. A. plasma
    B. hypoglycemia
    C. venipuncture

H. tourniquet
I. viscosity
J. palpate
K. lipemia
L. phlebotomy
M. therapeutic
N. anticoagulant
F. hematoma
G. serum
H. thixotropic gel

D. additive
E. diurnal

I. thrombocytes
J. hemoconcentration

3. A. Integrity: normal structure without damage.
    B. Oxygenated: containing high levels of oxygen.
    C. Primary container: the container that directly contains the specimen.
    D. Dilate: to enlarge in diameter.
    E. Centrifuge: a device that spins tubes using centrifugal force to separate the fluid portion of blood from the formed elements.
    F. Buffy coat: the layer of white blood cells and platelets that forms at the interface between the plasma and red blood cells in an anticoagulated tube of blood.
    G. Constrict: to become smaller in diameter.

Learning Review

1. The first choice of location for venipuncture is the antecubital area, or the bend of the arm, which contains large veins near the surface of the skin. The median cubital vein is used most often, but the basilic, cephalic, and median veins can also be used. The second choice for venipuncture are the superficial veins in the hand. Drawing blood from these veins, however, is often painful for patients. The third choice for venipuncture are the veins in the wrist. Drawing blood from veins in this location is the most painful for the patient.

2. A. Tourniquets constrict blood flow, making veins more prominent.
    B. The tourniquet should be placed about 3" to 4" above the chosen puncture site.
    C. The tourniquet should remain on the patient's arm no more than one minute.
    D. Ideally, the tourniquet should be removed as soon as blood flow is established, but must be removed before withdrawing the needle or blood will be forced out of the needle hole and into surrounding tissue, causing heavy bleeding.

3. A. blue; B. lavender; C. gray; D. green.

4. The following are effects of these factors on blood test results.
    1. Exercise: Strenuous short-term exercise makes the heart work harder, which can increase the heart enzymes; long-term exercise can cause anemia. The increased production of heart enzymes and the presence of anemia can cause erroneous test results.
    2. Tourniquet: If a tourniquet is left on the arm for more than one minute, it can cause blood to pool at the venipuncture site (hemoconcentration). This reaction can cause inaccurate results.
    3. Volume of blood drawn: An insufficient amount of blood drawn causes a dilution factor, which can change the size of the blood cells and produce a variation in test results.
    4. Heparin: Incorrect use of heparin interferes with laboratory blood tests.
    5. Temperature of specimen: If testing requires that the specimen be chilled immediately, any delay in icing will alter results. The longer the delay, the greater the change in the results.

5. The following are techniques used to stimulate veins:
    1. Position arm lower than head.
    2. Reapply tourniquet.
    3. Massage arm using upward motion.
    4. Use blood pressure cuff instead of tourniquet.
    5. Warm the venipuncture site with warming device or warm washcloth.

6. Additives are used to improve the quality of the specimen or to accelerate specimen processing. Some serum tubes, for example, contain clot activators to speed the clotting process. Thrombin is an additive used to chemically increase the speed of clotting and the formation of the clot. Thixotrophic separator gel is an additive used to separate cells or clots from plasma or serum. Anticoagulants are used to prevent the clotting of blood. Anticoagulants contain chemical substances that remove calcium or inhibit the conversion of prothrombin to thrombin, actions that prevent coagulation. Oxalates, citrates, EDTA, and heparin are common anticoagulants. Color-coded tubes identify which anticoagulant is contained in the tube.

7. A. Medical assistants locate a suitable vein from which to obtain a blood sample by feeling and tracing the path of the vein several times. Use the tip of the index finger to palpate veins rather than the thumb, which contains a pulse and is less sensitive than fingers. Veins are soft and bouncy to the touch and do not produce any pulsing action. If a pulse is present, then the medical assistant has found an artery, not a vein. Medical assistants should not puncture arteries. Tendons have an appearance similar to veins, but do not have the same feel. Instead of feeling soft and bouncy, tendons are hard to the touch. If a tendon is mistaken for a vein and punctured, there will be no blood return. In addition, a tendon puncture will be very painful to the patient.
    B. 1. Artery; 2. Vein; 3. Vein; 4. Vein; 5. Artery; 6. Artery.

8. A. Syringe and needle method
    B. Butterfly collection set
    C. Punctur-Guard needle assembly
    D. Evacuated tube system

Multiple Choice Questions

1. b. centrifuge
2. a. fibrinogen
3. d. 15 degrees

4. b. put the patient at ease
5. c. fainting

Investigation Activity

Students' responses will vary according to their personal experiences with venipuncture. Engage students in a discussion of their "best" and "worst" blood tests. Ask them to identify specific factors they believe contributed to their positive or negative experience, for example, the personality or clinical skills of the technician, anxiety about the possible test results, fear or anxiety about the procedure, lack of knowledge about the procedure, the ambiance of the medical care setting, and pain or discomfort. Encourage students to examine ways in which their past experiences can help them develop social and clinical skills and techniques that will help their patients have positive experiences with venipuncture. Students explore their own feelings, fears, and concerns about performing this procedure on patients and form communication strategies for dealing with a variety of patient reactions. The goal of the activity is to help students feel confident about performing venipuncture, providing the best and most accurate clinical care to patients while respecting and empathizing with patients' responses through therapeutic communication.

ANSWERS TO WORKBOOK CASE STUDY QUESTIONS

1. Each specimen must have its own label attached to the specimen's primary container and must have the test that is to be performed written on each label. All labels must have the patient's complete name and identification number. Specimen labels should be verified against information entered on the laboratory requisition form to confirm accuracy.

2. All specimens must be in the appropriate anticoagulant. Anticoagulated blood collection tubes must be at least 75 percent full. All coagulation blood collection tubes must be at least 90 percent full. Anticoagulated blood specimens must be free of clots.

3. Wanda must dispose of all sharps in the designated sharps disposal container. She must then dispose of contaminated gauze and other items. After waste has been properly discarded, Wanda will remove and dispose of PPE, remove and discard gloves, and perform aseptic handwash.

Chapter

41

Hematology

OVERVIEW

Medical assisting students must have competent skill in performing hematology tests, the second most commonly performed tests in the physician's office laboratory (POL). Included in this competency is the study of hematology, including hematopoiesis and an understanding of the relationships of hematological tests to the pathology of the human body. Students learn the correct procedures for performing common hematological tests, observing all quality control guidelines, safety measures, and standard precautions to protect themselves and others and to ensure the accuracy of test results.

Proficiency Evaluation Outcome Assessment

Students are evaluated for their understanding of performance objectives. A thorough knowledge of the process of hematopoiesis and the study of hematology are demonstrated. Students possess the ability to perform hematological tests competently and are able to accurately document results. Specimens are collected and processed properly, with respect for the patient and attention to the patient's emotional needs. The principles of aseptic technique are observed, following all standard precautions. Quality control guidelines are followed in the testing process in compliance with CLIA '88. All equipment is safely operated and maintained. Students demonstrate a knowledge of both manual and automated instrumentation as required. Students recognize the importance of accurate, reliable hematological test results as a diagnostic tool for physicians.

> Procedure 41-1   Hemoglobin Determination (Manual Method Using a Spectrophotometer)
> Procedure 41-2   Hemoglobin Determination (Hemoglobin Analyzer)
> Procedure 41-3   Microhematocrit
> Procedure 41-4   White Blood Cell Count (Unopette® Method)★
> Procedure 41-5   Red Blood Cell Count (Unopette® Method)
> Procedure 41-6   Preparation of a Differential Blood Smear Slide★★
> Procedure 41-7   Staining a Differential Blood Smear Slide
> Procedure 41-8   Differential Leukocyte Count★★
> Procedure 41-9   Erythrocyte Sedimentation Rate

★*The student should master this procedure before continuing to subsequent procedures.*
★★*Reading skills depend on the student's competency of level or ability.*

Supplementary Resources

Medical Assisting Videos: Appropriate content is available on Delmar's Medical Assisting Videos, 2nd ed., Tape 13, for the following topics:

> Basic Information for Specimen Taking and Laboratory Work
> When the Physician Orders a Specimen
> Collect and Label a Blood Specimen
> Butterfly Collection from a Hand Vein
> Collecting Tubes
> Capillary Puncture
> Blood Smear
> Perform Hematological Tests and Record the Results

ANSWERS TO TEXT REVIEW QUESTIONS

1. d. erythropoietin
2. b. hematopoiesis
3. a. hemoglobin S
4. a. hematocrit
5. a. hemacytometer
6. c. neutrophil
7. b. anemias
8. d. ESR
9. a. iron deficiency anemia

ANSWERS TO TEXT CRITICAL THINKING QUESTIONS

1. White cells, red cells, and platelets will all show changes from normal as a result of disease and disorders. Infections such as appendicitis will cause an elevated white blood cell count with a high percentage of neutrophils. Viral infections, on the other hand, will cause a reduction in the white blood cells with an elevation in the percentage of lymphocytes. Anemias will affect the appearance of red cells. Red cells will reveal abnormalities related to size, shape, and hemoglobin content. Macrocytes (large cells) and microcytes (small cells) are evident, as well as anisocytosis and poikilocytosis. The amount of hemoglobin in the red cells can be checked by observing the width and color depth of the darker outer ring. Hypochromic cells are obvious from the thin, pale outer ring of color. Sickle cells may also be observed on a peripheral blood smear.

2. The erythrocyte indices measure the red blood cell size and hemoglobin content. These are measured by three indices and will increase or decrease in certain diseases. The mean corpuscular volume (MPV) measures the average volume of a red blood cell in the sample. The mean corpuscular hemoglobin (MCH) estimates the weight in hemoglobin in an average red cell in the sample. The mean corpuscular hemoglobin concentration (MCHC) is the average concentration of hemoglobin in the hematocrit (expressed in grams/deciliter). The MCH and MCV are increased in megaloblastic anemia, acute blood loss, and certain other disorders. A decrease will result from hypochromic and microcytic anemia. The MCHC will be increased in hereditary spherocytosis and decreased in iron deficiency anemia.

3. The physician will want to see the total white count, which will be elevated in appendicitis. Another hematological test that the physician may consider is the differential white blood cell count, which will show an increase in neutrophils in the case of bacterial infections such as appendicitis.

4. The test results of the sed rate can be altered by a number of factors; therefore, care must be taken to maintain an exactly vertical tube, exact timing of one-hour room temperature, a site free from vibration, drafts, or direct sunlight, and a quality specimen set-up within two hours of drawing.

5. Quality control in automated hematology is maintained with (1) careful workmanship, as in all other clinical procedures, and (2) by running daily, before testing a patient sample, two levels of controls. One must be a normal control and the other may be either an abnormal high or low control, and (3) prescribing to a proficiency testing program that is CLIA-approved.

ANSWERS TO WORKBOOK EXERCISES AND ACTIVITIES

Vocabulary Builder

1. O
2. N
3. M
4. L
5. E
6. F
7. K
8. J
9. I
10. H
11. F
12. D
13. C
14. B
15. A

Learning Review

1. Six general parameters included in a CBC are
   (1) Hemoglobin Determination.
   (2) Hematocrit Determination.
   (3) White Blood Cell Count.

(4) Red Blood Cell Count.
(5) Differential White Blood Cell Count.
(6) Erythrocyte Indices.
2. D. Iron Deficiency Anemia
3. Correct matching
   1. D.
   2. C.
   3. B.
   4. E.
   5. F.
   6. A.
   7. G.

4. A. Red Blood Cell Count: RBC mm³ = average number of cells × depth (mm) × dilution × area factor (mm)

   B. White Blood Cell Count: $\text{WBC/mm}^3 = \dfrac{\text{average number cells counted}}{\text{area counted (mm}^2)} \times \text{depth factor} \times \text{dilution factor}$

   C. Three features studied are general size of cell, nuclear characteristics, and cytoplasmic characteristics.
   D. Refer to textbook Figure 41-17.

5. List the formulas for the erythrocyte indices.

   MCH: Mean Corpuscular Hemoglobin (MCH) $= \dfrac{\text{Hemoglobin (in grams)}}{\text{RBC (in millions)}} \times 10$

   MCV: Mean Corpuscular Volume (MCV) $= \dfrac{\text{Hematocrit}}{\text{RBC (in millions)}} \times 10$

   MCHC: Mean Corpuscular Hemoglobin Concentration (MCHC) $= \dfrac{\text{Hemoglobin (in grams)}}{\text{Hematocrit}} \times 10$

6. A. The Westegren method differs from the Wintrobe method in that the blood sample is mixed with 3.8 percent sodium citrate solution before the tube is filled.
   B. The sedimentation rate varies with different states of health. Two factors that influence the sedimentation are the condition of the surface membrane of the red blood cells and changes in the level of fibrinogen in the plasma of the blood. The red blood cell is altered during certain disease conditions, affecting the rate at which the red blood cells fall in the tube. Red blood cells have an average life of 120 days, therefore this test can be used to determine the onset of illness.
7. A. The student is asked to identify at least five of the following advantages of automated hematology instruments: faster; less expensive; simple to operate; very accurate; can be calibrated; lend themselves to control testing; have printers to produce printed results; can store quality control results.
   B. The three regulations required by CLIA '88 for automated hematology instruments include calibration at regularly scheduled intervals with either a calibrator sample or normal control sample; two levels of control samples tested first each day on any parameter that must be performed before the patient's sample is tested; and enrolling in a proficiency testing program with a laboratory that is CLIA '88-approved.

Multiple Choice Questions

1. b. sternum
2. d. iron
3. c. platelets
4. b. hypochromic
5. a. hay fever or other allergic conditions

Investigation Activity

Use this investigation activity to increase students' awareness of the connection between hematological test values and the state of health or disease of patients. Students make the further empathetic connection to the patient who must undergo routine blood monitoring and become better able to support and encourage the patient through therapeutic communication. The medical assistant's knowledge of hematologic principles and the use of hematological testing as a vital diagnostic tool for physicians allows medical assistants to be better patient educators and to perform testing with a higher level of understanding, leading to a competency level that will consistently produce accurate, reliable test results.

ANSWERS TO WORKBOOK CASE STUDY QUESTIONS

Case 1

1. Dr. Reynolds will order a complete blood cell count.
2. The results to be expected in the case of influenza are as follows: Hematocrit test will show a normal red blood cell count. Hemoglobin test will show a normal hemoglobin count. White blood cell count will be below average. Lymphocytes will be above normal range. Differential count will show a normal differential count.

Case 2

1. Ellen will use a lavender-stoppered EDTA tube.
2. Dr. King will study the hemoglobin determination results closely. Any changes in the red blood cells could be indicative of a type of anemia.
3. Ellen should follow the same standard precautions that are observed routinely for these procedures. Standard precautions for infection control are instituted to protect health care professionals, patients, and visitors from the risk of transmission of pathogens, HIV included. Ellen should wear PPE, including gloves, gown, face mask, and goggles to protect against potential blood spills or splashes. All waste should be considered infectious and should be disposed of appropriately in biohazard waste containers. Sharps should be handled with care to avoid the potential for accidental needlesticks and should be immediately discarded after use in a sharps container, following the correct procedures. The work area should be properly cleaned and disinfected before the removal of PPE. Proper procedures for the removal and disposal of PPE should be observed. Perform aseptic handwashing techniques.
4. Students' responses will vary.

Chapter

42

Urinalysis

OVERVIEW

Urinalysis is an important tool in patient diagnosis or to follow the course of a disease. It is vital that medical assisting students understand both the importance of urinalysis and what it entails, including proper collection techniques for urine specimens, safety guidelines involved in collecting and handling specimens, and a knowledge of the measures that need to be taken to ensure a consistent quality control program. In addition, students must understand how to properly perform urinalysis and must be cognizant of factors that may intervene with urinalysis accuracy. Standard precautions must be observed when handling and analyzing urine specimens.

PROFICIENCY EVALUATION OUTCOME ASSESSMENT

Students are evaluated for their understanding of performance objectives. Students demonstrate an ability to communicate the significance of urinalysis as a diagnostic tool; a knowledge of how urine is formed and excreted in the human body; and an understanding of the critical role of safety guidelines, standard precautions, and quality control programs in urinalysis. Students will exhibit the ability to accurately perform a complete urinalysis, including physical, chemical, and microscopic examinations.

Procedure 42-1	Assessing Urine Volume
Procedure 42-2	Observing Urine Color
Procedure 42-3	Observing Urine Clarity
Procedure 42-4	Using the Refractometer to Measure Specific Gravity
Procedure 42-5	Performing a Urinalysis Chemical Examination
Procedure 42-6	Testing for Sugar in the Urine
Procedure 42-7	Microscopic Examination of Urine Sediment
Procedure 42-8	Performing a Urinalysis

SUPPLEMENTARY RESOURCES

Medical Assisting Videos: Appropriate content is available on Delmar's Medical Assisting Videos, 2nd ed., Tape 14, for the following topics:

Quality Control in Collecting and Processing Specimens
Collect and Label Random Urine Specimens
Perform a Routine Urinalysis and Record Results
Perform Microscopic Examination of Urine

ANSWERS TO TEXT REVIEW QUESTIONS

1. d. treat all specimens as if they were infectious
2. c. physical, chemical, and microscopic
3. a. random

4. b. glucose
5. a. reagent test strip
6. d. glucose, ketone, and protein
7. b. confirm positive results from initial testing
8. d. Acetest
9. c. blood

ANSWERS TO TEXT CRITICAL THINKING QUESTIONS

1. Proper collection is necessary to avoid contamination of the specimen and to ensure that urine components do not decompose before testing.
2. The urethral opening and surrounding tissues are cleansed and a midstream specimen is then collected into a sterile container.
3. A midstream specimen is a urine specimen collected during the middle of voiding.
4. Preservatives are necessary when a specimen cannot be refrigerated until tested or must be transported over a long distance before examination.
5. The first morning specimen is normally more concentrated than random specimens.
6. Urine is normally clear on voiding, but may become cloudy on cooling. This is the result of precipitation of crystals. Turbidity may also indicate the presence of cells or bacteria.
7. Normal specific gravity of urine ranges from 1.003 to 1.035.
8. For every 3° below 20° centigrade, you must subtract 0.001 from the measure specific gravity.

ANSWERS TO WORKBOOK EXERCISES AND ACTIVITIES

Vocabulary Builder

A. 1. D.   7. H.   13. Q.   19. T.
    2. I.   8. F.   14. G.   20. J.
    3. M.   9. C.   15. E.   21. R.
    4. U.   10. A. 16. K.   22. W.
    5. P.   11. S. 17. L.   23. V.
    6. B.   12. N. 18. O.

B. 1. Bilirubin.   6. Reagents.   10. Refractometer.
    2. Hematuria.   7. Ketoacidosis.   11. Urinometer.
    3. Glucose.   8. Circadian rhythm.   12. Supernatant.
    4. Leukocyte esterase.   9. Creatinine.   13. Tamm-Horsfall.
    5. Urobilinogen.

Learning Review

1. Terms are inserted into the paragraph as follows: urine, soluble, metabolism, homeostasis, filtration, waste products/salts/excess fluid, electrolytes/urea, glomerulus, tubule, nephron, milliliters.
2. Terms are inserted into the paragraph as follows: kidney, glucose/protein, blood, concentration, threshold, creatinine/amino acids.
3. Terms are inserted into the paragraph as follows: blood, kidney, urine, hydrogen/ammonium, secreted, sodium, drugs.
4. A. 96 percent water and 4 percent dissolved substances.
    B. (1) AB   (4) AB   (7) AB
       (2) N   (5) AB   (8) N
       (3) N   (6) AB   (9) N
    C. Six possible changes are (1) amount of urine excreted can rise or fall, (2) urine color can change, (3) urine appearance can vary, (4) urine odor can change, (5) cells may be present in urine, and (6) chemical constants in urine can change.
5. Five precautions are (1) treat all specimens as if they were infectious, handling them with gloved hands; (2) avoid splashes or creation of aerosols when handling or disposing of urine samples—wearing protective eye gear will prevent splashes from getting into the eyes; (3) process urine as soon as possible; (4) store urine specimens appropriately in a designated refrigerator that contains no food or drink items; and (5) dispose of urine appropriately, possibly in a special sink (run water to wash specimen into the drain) or toilet.
6. B.
7. C.

8. A.
9. B.
10. A.
11. CLIA regulations for medical assistants performing urine testing are (1) appropriate training in the methodology of test being performed; (2) understanding of urine testing quality control procedures; (3) proficiency in the use of instrumentation and being able to troubleshoot problems; (4) knowledge of the stability and proper storage of reagents; (5) awareness of factors that influence test results; and (6) knowledge of how to verify test results.
12. A. A proper label will include the patient's name, age, sex, identifying number, date, time of collection, and physician's name.
    B. Unlabeled or incorrectly labeled specimens are not tested. The medical assistant is required to determine whose urine is unlabeled. Then the patient is notified, and a new specimen is ordered.
    C. Four types of urine specimens are random (spot), fasting/timed, 24-hour, and catheterized.
    D. Four methods of urine collection are random, clean-catch, midstream, and catheterization.
13. A. The four steps of a physical examination of a urine specimen are (1) assess the volume of the urine specimen, (2) observe and record the color and transparency of the specimen, (3) note any unusual urine odor, and (4) measure the specific gravity of the specimen.
    B. The specific gravity of urine indicates the concentration of solids such as phosphates, chlorides, proteins, sugars, and urea that are dissolved in urine.
    C. Three methods of measuring the specific gravity of a urine specimen are (1) urinometer, (2) refractometer, and (3) reagent test strip (available in conjunction with chemical testing). Urine must be at room temperature to obtain an accurate urinometer reading. The refractometer is not as accurate as other methods but is balanced by the ease of use and reliability of the instrument; temperature does not have to be adjusted if it is between 60° and 100° F. Reagent test strips are convenient and measure results up to 1.030.
14. A. 1. F.   5. I.   8. A.
       2. H.   6. E.   9. D.
       3. B.   7. G.   10. J.
       4. C.
    B. Outdated strips or reagents should never be used. Strips should not be exposed to moisture, volatile substances, direct sunlight, or excess heat. Strips should not be removed from the container until the time of use. Test pads should not be touched or handled. Correct quality control procedures should be followed as required by CLIA and the facility where testing is performed. Follow manufacturer's instructions for proper storage.
15. 1. B. Clinitest.
    2. C. Sulfosalicylic acid test.
    3. D. Acetest.
    4. A. Ictotest.
16. A. 1. F.   4. E.   7. I.
       2. C.   5. G.   8. B.
       3. H.   6. A.   9. D.
    B. (1) See textbook Figure 42-15.
       (2) See textbook Figure 42-13.
       (3) See textbook Figure 42-9.
       (4) See textbook Figure 42-12.
17. Three crystals that may indicate disease states are (1) uric acid, (2) cystine, and (3) sulfa drug crystals.
18. A. Granular.   B. Cellular.   C. Hyaline.
    See textbook Figure 42-16 for illustrations.

Multiple Choice Questions

1. b. glomerulus
2. a. Pyridium®
3. d. sweet
4. c. meniscus
5. a. hyaline

Investigation Activity

Use this activity to encourage students to think actively about the importance of observing standard precautions and other safety precautions when performing procedures involving urine specimens.

Procedure: Clinitest for reducing sugars

Type of hazard: Health and Reactivity. Poison. May cause severe burns. Contains sodium hydroxide; not intended for internal use. Avoid contact with eyes, mucous membranes, skin, and clothing. Sensitive to air and water; excessive moisture from air or water may cause volatile chemical reaction resulting in bottle explosion.

PPE required: Gloves, eye shield

Proper techniques for safety: Consider all urine samples to be contaminated; handle all specimens with gloved hands. Take care not to spill or splash urine. Wipe up all spills with antiseptic cleaner. Wear eye shields, if necessary. Process urine specimens as quickly as possible; store urine specimens if necessary in a designated refrigerator not used for food or beverages. Do not touch the bottom of the test tube during the chemical reaction, as severe burns may occur. Do not refrigerate Clinitest tablets or place them in or near moist or wet environments.

What is done with used materials and soiled instruments? Disposable pipette, disposable urine collection container, and gloves are discarded in biohazard waste container. Urine is poured down a drain (possibly a special drain), which is rinsed with running water, or flushed in a toilet. The glass test tube is chemically sterilized. Clinitest tablets should be stored in the original container and kept in a dry place. The dessicant packet should not be removed from the container and the container lid should be kept tightly shut. Clinitest tablets should be stored and kept away from any possible contact with children. All manufacturer's instructions should be followed.

What chemical products are involved? Clinitest tablets. Distilled water.

What are the specific risks of the procedure? Burns can occur by handling the bottom of the test tube during the chemical reaction. Standard precautions must be followed when handling urine specimens, which may contain infectious materials.

Additional comments: Always check Clinitest tablets, whether from a bottle or foil packets, to observe that they are not discolored. Follow the 15-second time limit for testing carefully. Interference from other sugars or metabolized drugs may cause false-positive results. High levels of glucose yield a fast pass-through; the reaction must be watched very carefully.

ANSWERS TO WORKBOOK CASE STUDY QUESTIONS

Case 1

1. Wanda Slawson, CMA, should inform patient Wendy Janus to begin the 24-hour collection by emptying the bladder and not keeping the specimen. The provided container should be labeled at this time—directly after the bladder is emptied. Wanda should explain that each time Wendy urinates within the 24-hour period, she should urinate into the collection container. Wanda should instruct Wendy to keep the collection bottle refrigerated between voidings. Wanda should explain that at the end of the 24-hour period, the patient should urinate and write on the collection bottle label the exact "ended" time.

2. Wanda should be sure to ask Wendy if she has any questions and should make sure Wendy understands all steps of the 24-hour collection process by having her repeat them back to her correctly. If available, Wanda can also transmit the written instructions via fax or e-mail, following all proper procedures to protect patient confidentiality.

Case 2

1. Wanda should instruct the patient in the proper cleansing of the genital area; in this case, after thoroughly washing his hands, the patient should retract the foreskin of the penis (if not circumcised) using a sterile wipe. He should use a second Towelettes to wipe the urethral opening clean with a single stroke from the tip of the penis to the ring of the glans. This cleansing step should be repeated once more using a fresh pad. After cleansing the area, the patient should begin urinating, interrupting the stream to position the urine container for catching urine. Wanda should inform the patient that only the midstream needs to be collected. After collecting the urine, the patient should be instructed to secure the lid on the container.

2. Wanda should be sensitive to the boy's embarrassment and should relay the information in a professional and straightforward manner. Forcing the patient to maintain eye contact may heighten his discomfort. Wanda should look for clues in the patient's body language and tone to indicate his understanding of the verbal instructions.

Chapter

43

Basic Microbiology

OVERVIEW

Technology has changed vastly in health care in recent times. Laboratories have not been left behind. While many still plate organisms in the same manner as has been done for decades, new systems are emerging with more automation in the identification of cultures. The role of the medical assistant will vary according to the size and technology present. Some activities will remain very important and constant, such as the careful collection and processing of specimens; the need for knowledge of safety precautions, including standard precautions for infection control; and understanding the importance of always following the laboratory's established guidelines for procedures. Learning basic microbiology is an important step in advancing the quality of accurate diagnosis and treatment of patients.

PROFICIENCY EVALUATION OUTCOME ASSESSMENT

Students are evaluated for their understanding of performance objectives. Students obtain knowledge of microorganisms, how they grow, and the diseases they cause. Students discover how following laboratory procedures leads to better diagnostic abilities for the physician and more appropriate treatment for patients. Types of media are identified that encourage growth of specific microorganisms. Medical assisting students appreciate how enormous the microbiology field is and learn classifications and nomenclature relevant to the medical laboratory. Students discover the importance of caring for equipment. The practice of patient education in specimen collection is related to quality outcomes on tests. Students demonstrate an understanding of safety measures and recognize their responsibility to implement them. Students acknowledge the medical assistant's role in the laboratory and the support available for it to be safe, rewarding, and challenging.

SUPPLEMENTARY RESOURCES

Medical Assisting Videos: Appropriate content is available on Delmar's Medical Assisting Videos, 2nd ed., for the following topics:

Tape 5 Perform Medical Aseptic Technique of Handwashing
Infections in the Office
Tape 14 Quality Control in Collecting and Processing Specimens
Collect a Stool Specimen
Perform a Hemoccult Test
Collect a Sputum Specimen
Collect a Throat Culture
Perform a Strep Screen
Collect Vaginal Samples
Streak a Culture Plate
Make a Gram Stain

ANSWERS TO TEXT REVIEW QUESTIONS

1. c. spore
2. c. crystal violet, Gram's iodine, alcohol, safranin
3. b. will support the growth of all organisms and does not alter their appearance
4. b. *Neisseria meningitidis*
5. c. Gram-negative organisms that commonly reside as normal flora in the intestinal tract but can cause infection
6. c. *Staphylococcus aureus*
7. a. swab deep and place into an anaerobic container

ANSWERS TO TEXT CRITICAL THINKING QUESTIONS

1. Two ways to identify whether an organism is motile are the wet prep slide; special stain for flagella (Leifson); motility media.
2. If the iodine step in the Gram stain was omitted, the colonies would all be pink. Iodine is the mordant that holds crystal violet to the Gram-positive organisms. By not using iodine, all colonies would be decolorized by the acetone alcohol step.
3. An aerosol is a fine mist where particles are dispersed into the air. Aerosols could include airborne infectious particles. When working with aerosols or potential aerosols, work should be done in a biological safety cabinet or safety hood.
4. An acid-fast organism stains red against a blue or green background. The acid-fast organism is red due to the primary stain carbolfuchsin.
5. This question can have several answers, including:
Pathogenic: *Staphylococcus aureus*
Specimen source: boil or wound
Media, blood agar, Trypticase agar
Microscopic appearance: Gram-positive cocci in clusters
Disease: skin and wound infections
6. Stool for culture: Patient needs a clean container with a tight-fitting lid, the stool should not be contaminated with urine, often several specimens will be requested.
    Stool O & P: Patients sometimes need special containers. Often several specimens are requested for O & P examination. The specimen should be as fresh as possible and not contaminated with urine.
7. The female pinworm migrates toward the rectum at night and deposits several ova. The best time to collect the specimen is in the morning after awakening.

ANSWERS TO WORKBOOK EXERCISES AND ACTIVITIES

Vocabulary Builder

1. G.
2. L.
3. M.

10. D.
11. C.
12. B.

4.	H.	13.	P.
5.	J.	14.	Q.
6.	A.	15.	I.
7.	K.	16.	F.
8.	O.	17.	E.
9.	N.		

Learning Review

1. A. *Enterobius vermicularis; Trichomonas vaginalis*
    B. color, blood, consistency
    C. name, date, time/traveling
    D. adult worm, ova
    E. cellophane tape swab
    F. Personal protective equipment (PPE), infectious material
    G. handwashing, habit
2. Before opening the bags holding specimen containers, observe for leakage and contamination on the outside of the container. Before touching or handling the bags, wash hands and put on gloves.
3. Nine factors contributing to a laboratory's success:
    (1) Proper collection from infection site
    (2) Collection of specimen during infectious period
    (3) Sufficient amount of specimen
    (4) Appropriate sterile specimen container
    (5) Appropriate transport medium
    (6) Specimen labeled properly
    (7) Specimen brought to the laboratory in minimal amount of time
    (8) Specimen collected before antibiotics are administered
    (9) Specimen inoculated on proper media and placed into correct atmosphere
4. Students' answers will vary. They may state concerns regarding acquisition of infections. The resources to draw on include knowledge of disease transmission, infection control standards, safety regulations, and good communication skills with colleagues and supervisor.
5. Strep throat infection may be associated with kidney and heart infections and can lead to other conditions if not identified and treated rapidly. The enzyme immunoassay test or latex agglutination could be used. The five rules are (1) use the correct swab; (2) run positive and negative control with the test; (3) read and understand directions before the test; (4) observe expiration dates on kits; and (5) observe safety guidelines.
6. A. Capsule, some
    B. Cell wall, all
    C. Cytoplasmic membrane, all
    D. Nucleoid material, all
    E. Ribosomes, all
    F. Flagellum, some

Multiple Choice Questions

1. b. staphylococcus
2. d. spore
3. a. blood infection
4. a. rod shaped
5. b. pink

Investigation Activity

Instructors can use this activity to help students communicate their concerns about health, safety, and the workplace environment. Assertiveness rooted with the knowledge of disease and its transmission is a powerful tool for health care worker protection. Learning the chain of communication and developing problem-solving skills is a beneficial skill for the student. Medical assistants who make the connection between laboratory work, the public's health welfare, an understanding of the function of the CDC, OSHA, WHO, and local community health departments, in relationship to the medical laboratory, will be able to make a valuable contribution and perform their role effectively. This is a real opportunity to deal with confidentiality, ethics, and the individual's privacy versus public health needs. The opportunity is for recognizing a connection between accurate and reliable, high-quality diagnostic work in the laboratory and the world outside. Expand on the exercise by asking students to bring in newspaper or magazine clippings related to news events caused by outbreaks of infectious disease or topics of concern related to the transmission of infectious disease; for example, outbreaks of *Escherichia coli* (*E. coli*) at restaurants serving undercooked or spoiled meat products and/or articles about the "bacterial buffet" at the salad bar.

ANSWERS TO WORKBOOK CASE STUDY QUESTIONS

Case 1

1. Sputum specimen collection is correctly done by having the patient cough deeply and expectorate into a sterile container. The patient takes these containers home and obtains a specimen on awakening. Careful instruction is given so sterility is maintained and the patient does not obtain a poor specimen.
2. Depending on the offending organism, finding it on a single specimen could be difficult and the most concentrated sputum is present on awakening. The yield of the early morning specimen on three consecutive days increases the chances of identifying the problem and acquiring accurate treatment.
3. The physician has many possibilities in mind but the need to rule out tuberculosis is great. Acid-fast staining to look for possible *Mycobacterium tuberculosis* would be important. If an acid-fast staining test result indicates a strong possibility of *Mycobacterium tuberculosis*, a specimen should be sent to an outside reference laboratory for further analysis.

Case 2

1. To perform a Gram stain, the medical assistant will require gloves, laboratory coat, goggles and barrier or face shield, microscope, clean glass slide, distilled water, plastic squeeze bottle, loop or swab, paper towels, bibulous paper, patient specimen to be examined, heat, Gram stain kit, staining tray and rack.
2. Ellen must wash her hands before and after handling the patient specimen and only handle the specimen with gloved hands; wear PPE, including goggles, face shield, gloves, and lab coat; properly clean and disinfect the work area after preparing and Gram staining the smear; and properly dispose of all waste and PPE in the biohazard waste container.
3. *Staphylococcus* and *Streptococcus* are strains of Gram-positive bacteria and will appear purple after Gram staining is performed. *Staphylococcus* will appear in clusters while *Streptococcus* will appear in chains. See text.

Chapter

44

Specialty Laboratory Tests

OVERVIEW

Many laboratory tests are now performed in the ambulatory care setting by the medical assistant. Medical assisting students learn about laboratory safety procedures, medical terminology, and specimen collection and analysis. A basic understanding of the principles involved and proper sampling procedures are covered. Quality control programs, accurate documentation, and strict observance of standard precautions are stressed. Therapeutic communication with the patient, to gain cooperation in obtaining good specimens for analysis, is recognized as an important component of any laboratory testing.

PROFICIENCY EVALUATION OUTCOME ASSESSMENT

Students are evaluated for their understanding of performance objectives. The ability to perform laboratory tests that yield accurate, reliable results is demonstrated. Students understand the basic principles of the laboratory tests and possess the ability to read and interpret results and identify factors that may yield inaccurate results. The difference between normal and abnormal values is clearly recognized. Patient education and communication skills are explored as effective strategies for the medical assistant in obtaining good specimens for analysis and in providing information and support to patients during the testing process.

SUPPLEMENTARY RESOURCES

Medical Assisting Videos: Appropriate content is available on Delmar's Medical Assisting Videos, 2nd ed., Tape 13, for the following topics:

Basic Information for Specimen Taking and Laboratory Work
When the Physician Orders a Specimen
Collect and Label a Blood Specimen
Perform Blood Chemistry and Record the Results
Perform Immunologic Tests and Record the Results

ANSWERS TO TEXT REVIEW QUESTIONS

1. a. agglutination inhibition test
2. c. pelvic inflammatory disease
3. d. refrigerated at 4°C
4. b. infectious mononucleosis
5. d. hCG hormone
6. c. type O RBCs have A and B antigens on the cell
7. d. people without the Rh factor on their RBCs have naturally occurring antibodies called anti-D in their plasma
8. d. avoid the consumption of fats several days before the test
9. a. newborns
10. b. forearm three to four inches from bend of arm
11. a. 50–70 mg/dL

ANSWERS TO TEXT CRITICAL THINKING REVIEW QUESTIONS

1. The urine will contain the highest concentration of hCG.
2. African Burkitt's lymphoma, nasopharyngeal carcinoma, and chronic fatigue syndrome are other examples.
3. Individual males will have variable sperm counts, making a single analysis insufficient.
4. A positive skin test may be caused by an active case, an old inactive case, or vaccination with BCG.
5. The patient did not fast long enough or at all, or use of drugs such as contraceptives, salicylates, diuretics, and steroids.
6. Glucose levels return to, or below, fasting levels within two hours in nondiabetics. Diabetics will have glucose levels of 140 mg/dL or higher.
7. Saturated fats tend to raise blood cholesterol levels, increasing the risk of coronary heart disease.
8. Triglycerides serve as a source of energy. Excess triglycerides are deposited in the body as adipose tissue.
9. The patient should be instructed to remain on a stable diet for two weeks before collection of the blood sample. They should also fast for the last 12 to 16 hours and avoid consumption of alcohol for 48 hours before the test.
10. Urea in the blood is the nitrogenous end product of protein metabolism and is produced in the liver.

ANSWERS TO WORKBOOK EXERCISES AND ACTIVITIES

Vocabulary Builder

1. tine test, tuberculosis
2. Cushing's syndrome
3. immunoassay, human chorionic gonadotrophin, ectopic, hydatidiform, choriocarcinoma
4. antiserum, antibody, antigen, latex beads
5. hypoglycemia
6. agglutination
7. blood urea nitrogen
8. diabetes mellitus, insulin
9. low-density lipoprotein (LDL), high-density lipoprotein (HDL)
10. hemolytic anemia, bilirubin
11. triglyceride
12. semen
13. Mantoux test, wheal
14. infectious mononucleosis, Epstein-Barr virus, heterophile antibodies
15. phenylketonuria (PKU)
16. Guthrie screening test
17. hyperglycemia
18. purified protein derivative (PPD)
19. ABO blood group, Rh factor

Learning Review

1. A. Students list three of any of the following reasons for performing a semen analysis on a patient.
   1. To determine sperm cell counts before referring patients to fertility specialists.
   2. As part of a complete fertility workup.

3. To evaluate the effectiveness of a vasectomy.
4. To determine paternity.
5. To substantiate rape cases.

B. When a semen analysis is performed as part of a fertility workup, seminal fluid is analyzed to determine (1) total sperm count; (2) percent of motility; and (3) percent of normally formed sperm cells.

2. A. The four blood group categories are A, B, AB, and O.
   B. 1. A and B, none
      2. B, Anti-A
      3. Rh-, D
   C. The Rh type of most North Americans is positive. Most cases of hemolytic disease of the newborn can be prevented by administering RhoGAM, a concentrated solution of anti-D, to the Rh negative mother within 72 hours after delivery of an Rh positive baby.

3. B. smoking cigarettes
4. B. Refrigerated urine samples and test reagents should be allowed to come to room temperature before testing.
   D. First morning urine or urine with a specific gravity of at least 0.010 should be used.
5. C. 10 mm or more of induration.
6. A. blood
   B. reflectance photometry
   C. glycogen
   D. nondiabetic
   E. carbohydrates
   F. glycosylated hemoglobin determination
7. A. The cholesterol molecule consists of carbon, hydrogen, and oxygen. Most of the carbon atoms in the molecule are arranged into rings, rather than into long hydrocarbon chains as in most other lipids.
   B. Saturated refers to the number of hydrogen atoms attached to the molecule. Saturated fats are solid at room temperature; monounsaturated and polyunsaturated fats are liquid at room temperature. Examples of saturated fats are any fats of animal origin. Examples of monounsaturated fats are olive and peanut oils; some polyunsaturated fats are corn, safflower, sunflower, and many fish oils.
   C. Student answers will vary. See textbook Table 44-5.
   D. The adrenal cortex, the testes, and the ovaries use cholesterol to manufacture steroid hormones. Cholesterol is also an important component of bile and cellular membranes.

Multiple Choice Questions

1. a. carbohydrate
2. b. intravascular hemolysis
3. c. thyroid
4. d. less than 5 mm
5. a. after eating

Investigation Activity

Use this activity to help students relate laboratory analysis to specific patient diseases and conditions. Students are encouraged to explore the range of emotions experienced by patients who must have laboratory tests performed to confirm a suspected diagnosis. The patient's fears and concerns during the collection of the specimen(s) and the waiting period for results must be acknowledged and respected with empathy and compassion on the part of health care professionals, including medical assistants. Patient education and support throughout the testing process and when a diagnosis is confirmed are also important functions of the health care team. Medical assistants who are knowledgeable about the diseases and conditions for which they perform laboratory tests will be better prepared to assist physicians throughout the testing process and in the care and treatment of patients in the ambulatory care setting. The responsibility to perform laboratory analysis that yields accurate and reliable results is underscored for students when they realize the full impact of laboratory test results in determining the proper diagnosis and treatment of patients. Inaccurate test results necessitating a retest are stressful to patients. Inaccurate results also can lead to misdiagnosis and incorrect treatment of patients.

ANSWERS TO WORKBOOK CASE STUDY QUESTIONS

1. The glycosated hemoglobin determination is a blood test that measures how well the glucose level had been controlled over the past four to six weeks versus the conventional blood test, which shows only the current-day's status. Physicians can use this test to determine if diabetics are consistently adhering to their diet and health guidelines. An elevated finding of glycosated hemoglobin indicates poor glucose control in the assessment of glucose in the diabetic patient.

2. Glycosated hemoglobin (Hb A_1c) is a stable molecule formed when sugar and hemoglobin bind together on the RBC.

3. The medical assistant will draw blood and process the specimen properly for transport to an outside reference laboratory for analysis. The role of the medical assistant is to firmly, but empathetically, remind the patient that she must be truthful in her glucose level reporting. Bruce should not be overly critical of the patient, nor should he lecture or yell at her. Rather, Bruce should be persuasive and concerned in his tone and spoken language, conveying the importance of the patient's compliance with diet and health guidelines while letting her know that both she and health care team must work together to maintain an optimum state of health. If she feels a lapse of good dietary habits occurring, Mary should be encouraged to confide in her health care team and personal support system of friends and family to help her get through rough periods of temptation without damaging her health.

Chapter

45

The Medical Assistant as Office Manager

OVERVIEW

Medical assisting students are introduced to the responsibilities and duties of the office manager. This chapter introduces students to the staff member most likely to manage the daily operations of the medical practice. Duties from coordinating staff meetings, preparing meeting agendas and minutes, making travel arrangements, and compiling an Office Policy and Procedures Manual to processing payroll and establishing risk management protocols are discussed. Students recognize the potential of pursuing the long-term goal of becoming an office manager in an ambulatory setting.

PROFICIENCY EVALUATION OUTCOME ASSESSMENT

Students are evaluated for their understanding of performance objectives, demonstrating the ability to describe the duties of the office manager in the ambulatory care setting. These duties include supervising personnel; supervising student practicums; implementing time management techniques to boost office efficiency; organizing, updating, and reviewing the procedures manual; coordinating marketing functions; records and financial management; facility and equipment management; risk management; and liability coverage and bonding.

Procedure 45-1   Preparing a Meeting Agenda
Procedure 45-2   Making Travel Arrangements
Procedure 45-3   Making Travel Arrangements via Internet
Procedure 45-4   Supervising a Student Practicum
Procedure 45-5   Developing and Maintaining a Procedures Manual

SUPPLEMENTARY RESOURCES

Medical Assisting Videos: Appropriate content is available on Delmar's Medical Assisting Videos, 2nd ed., for the following topics:

Tape 1   Work as a Team Member
          Communication Skills
Tape 2   Apply Legal Concepts to Practice
          Practice Risk Management Measures to Prevent Professional Liability
Tape 3   Perform Administrative Duties
          Electronic Banking

ANSWERS TO TEXT REVIEW QUESTIONS

1. a. associate's degree
2. b. delegate the task to someone who is knowledgeable
3. c. understand and support the task

4. c. are more comfortable teaching, coaching, helping, leading, and inspiring others.
5. a. should address each agenda topic and include a brief summary of discussions, actions taken, name of person making motion, exact wording of motion, and motion approval or defeat
6. d. they have much to learn
7. c. provides detailed information relative to the performance of tasks within the health care facility
8. b. It assumes that the student is an employee who does not need to be introduced to patients.
9. a. marketing
10. d. equipment and supplies maintenance

ANSWERS TO TEXT CRITICAL THINKING QUESTIONS

1. The office manager should focus on the situation, issue, or behavior, not on the person(s). A discussion about solving the problem, not laying blame, is much more productive. Positive solutions may be more readily attained when discussing what was observed rather than what was told by someone else. Discussion should be with the individuals who have the authority and power to effect change.
2. Three benefits of a teamwork approach are: it improves efficiency of the office, builds morale, and results in getting more accomplished with the resources available.
3. The office manager promotes open and honest communication by example. Communication that is clear, diplomatic, tactful, and demonstrates respect for the feelings of others is vital to open and honest communication. Viewing challenges objectively and without bias or prejudice also promotes open and honest communication.
4. Answers to this question may vary, but the students should demonstrate a clear understanding of the various management styles and what teamwork means.
5. The office manager can help the extern feel more at ease the first day of "work" by scheduling an informational interview with the extern student before the practicum begins. A discussion of expectations, an establishment of a "work" schedule, a tour of the facility, and an introduction of key personnel helps the student relax and feel accepted the first day of "work."
6. Approaches a student might take to keep organized will vary. Examples include completing one task before beginning another; using an appointment book to schedule meetings and note deadlines; just doing it, without procrastinating; making an extra portion when preparing a meal and freezing it for a later date; and establishing short- and long-term goals to help maintain focus.
7. The single-physician office involves only a few staff and may be very specialized. With fewer employees, fewer copies of the manual would need to be produced and maintained. The multi-physician office involves many staff members and may serve a variety of specialties involving complex procedures. This will require a larger procedures manual, which must be maintained, updated, and distributed to various personnel and departments.
8. A procedure manual can quickly become outdated and require revisions. The addition of specialized equipment, new techniques and/or treatments, and added specialty services are examples of reasons for the revisions.
9. A press release may be used to announce the purchase of new equipment to perform specialty procedures, to introduce new staff members, to acknowledge expanded or remodeled office space, and to publicize seminars and patient teaching programs.
10. The risk management process includes the identification, analysis, and treatment of risks within the medical office. The risk management role of loss prevention includes, but is not limited to elimination of any procedure or hazard that could potentially be harmful to any patient, employee, employer, and visitors to the premises; a comprehensive safety program; employees working within the scope of training and qualifications for safety and insurability; and maintaining license and insurance coverage for physicians, employees, and the facility.

ANSWERS TO WORKBOOK EXERCISES AND ACTIVITIES

Vocabulary Builder

1. ancillary services
2. liability
3. "going bare"
4. benchmarking
5. professional liability insurance
6. minutes
7. work statement
8. bond
9. agenda
10. marketing
11. teamwork
12. negligence
13. practicum
14. benefit
15. extern
16. embezzle
17. risk management
18. procedures manual
19. malpractice

Learning Review

1. The student can choose five statements from the following list of office manager duties:
    1. Create and update the office procedures manual.
    2. Supervise office personnel.
    3. Assist in improving work flow and office efficiencies (time management).
    4. Supervise regular staff meetings.
    5. Supervise the purchase, repair, and maintenance of office equipment.
    6. Supervise the purchase and storage of office supplies.
    7. Supervise the purchase and storage of controlled substances.
    8. Approve financial transactions and account disposition; generate financial reports as needed.
    9. Prepare patient education materials and arrange patient/community education workshops as needed.
    10. Arrange and maintain practice insurance and develop risk management strategies.
2.
    1. D.
    2. B.
    3. E.
    4. A.
    5. C.
3. The student should select from the following list five out of the seven attributes needed to perform as a quality manager.
    1. People skills.
    2. Be truthful.
    3. Effective communication skills.
    4. Organizational skills.
    5. Objectivity.
    6. Problem-solving skills.
    7. Technical expertise.

Multiple Choice Questions

1. c. personality
2. b. management by exception
3. a. teaching and coaching
4. c. risk management
5. a. networking

Investigation Activity

Use this activity to get students thinking creatively about patient education techniques that can be related to public relations tools and activities. Students also use and expand their knowledge of basic nutritional principles in the exercise of preparing the patient newsletter. This activity can also be performed as a class or group project, with the newsletter "desktop published" on a computer. The class may divide into groups to prepare newsletters on different topics, in addition to nutrition. Some ideas include the importance of exercise in maintaining cardiovascular health; breastfeeding advice for expectant and new mothers; evaluating the home for health hazards and making suggestions for preventive measures, including first aid for emergencies; estrogen replacement therapy (ERT) and menopause; and strategies for making the home environment elder-friendly.

ANSWERS TO WORKBOOK CASE STUDY QUESTIONS

1. Information on the paycheck stub includes number of hours worked, including regular and overtime (if hourly); date of pay periods; date of check; gross salary; itemized deductions for federal income tax, Social Security (FICA) tax, and state, city, or local taxes; itemized deductions for health insurance and disability insurance; other deductions, such as uniforms, loan payments, and so on; and net salary.
2. The physician's office must have a federal tax reporting number, obtained from the Internal Revenue Service. In some states, a state employer number is also required.
3. The office manager must maintain employee payroll files and records in strict confidentiality. Payroll tasks are to be performed in a private environment and no payroll information is to be left open or out where another employee might have unauthorized access to it. The office manager will not discuss employee salaries and payroll information with any unauthorized staff member. Payroll records and files are to be kept in a locked cabinet.

Chapter

46

The Medical Assistant as Human Resources Manager

OVERVIEW

Medical assisting students are introduced to the duties of the human resources manager in the ambulatory care setting. The importance of good employee relations and the performance of employee-related duties, such as hiring, training and orientation, maintaining personnel records, implementing office policies, encouraging continuing education opportunities for employees, and mediating workplace conflicts, makes the human resources manager's position a challenging and rewarding one. Human resource managers are, above all, excellent communicators.

PROFICIENCY EVALUATION OUTCOME ASSESSMENT

Students are evaluated for their knowledge of performance objectives. Students demonstrate the ability to describe the duties and responsibilities of the human resources manager. Students realize the importance of developing strong communication skills and maintaining good relationships with employers and coworkers. Students understand that a good office manager and human resources manager facilitate the daily operation of the ambulatory care setting, providing a beneficial and efficient environment for all employees.

> Procedure 46–1   Develop and Maintain a Policy Manual
> Procedure 46–2   Preparing a Job Description
> Procedure 46–3   Interviewing
> Procedure 46–4   Orient and Train Personnel

SUPPLEMENTARY RESOURCES

Medical Assisting Videos: Appropriate content is available on Delmar's Medical Assisting Videos, 2nd ed., for the following topics:

> Tape 1   Work as a Team Member
> Career-seeking Skills
> Communication Skills
> Tape 3   Perform Administrative Duties
> Triage Skills

ANSWERS TO TEXT REVIEW QUESTIONS

1. d. both b and c
2. c. Can you supply a birth certificate or a Social Security card?
3. d. both b and c
4. a. resolving conflicts between personnel and dismissing an employee
5. d. all the above
6. d. protects employees from unsafe or unhealthy working conditions
7. c. usually is the result of poor communication or a misunderstanding
8. d. both b and c
9. d. all the above
10. d. all the above

ANSWERS TO TEXT CRITICAL THINKING QUESTIONS

1. No one understands or knows the job like the person performing that job. Job descriptions change and do not always indicate where the greatest amount of time is spent. That can be information supplied by employees.
2. References are checked either by phone or through a written document. Be prepared to ask specific questions and take notes on the response. Some former employers may respond to an open-ended question such as "Tell me about this applicant," but, increasingly, former employers are willing to supply only information related to the term of employment, reason for leaving, and so on.
3. Established policies and procedures for performance reviews leave no room for error. If the employee is clear about what is expected and the policy is well defined, there is no room for misunderstanding in discussing an employee's performance.
4. Physician-employers may be directly involved in personnel matters if the employee's performance is directly related to the physician's activities. Also, if illegal activity is involved, the physician-employer should be involved in the decision making. Physicians will be involved in personnel matters in most clinics, unless the clinics hire a very large number of employees.
5. An otherwise excellent employee who is a gossip and who has a negative attitude is worth trying to correct. Establish a review, identify the problem, determine a plan for correcting the problem, and set another review to determine if the correction has been achieved. Often employees are not aware there are problems until such a plan is put into place.
6. The first paragraph should simply state you have taken another position. Identify your leave date, being certain to allow time for your current employer to make the necessary adjustments. Explain what you have really appreciated about this position and what you will gain in the new position. Request an exit interview, and ask for a letter of reference for your file.
7. Employers are discovering that time off from work to care for an aging parent takes as much, if not more, time from work as caring for a small child. It would be good to identify a policy of how such leave could be taken. Some allow this time as sick days; others allow the employee to make up the work. Talk with hospital human resource managers and other physician-employers about their policies.
8. Both forms have merit. The sample form in the textbook requires that questions be asked and interpreted by an interviewer, who may interject personal feelings. The ABCs form can be done beforehand and brought to the exit interview.
9. Answers will vary. One is apt to find that specialized education and training is not necessarily rewarded in the health care field. Most likely the plumber and the automobile mechanic will receive the highest hourly wage.
10. Employees can be rewarded in many ways. If their salary is competitive, involve them in decision making, provide any necessary training, encourage their participation in professional organizations, pay their registration to a national AAMA meeting, or provide their uniforms. To make them feel special, remember their birthdays and hire-date anniversaries, take them to lunch on occasion, or tell them how much you personally appreciate their dedication and hard work.

ANSWERS TO WORKBOOK EXERCISES AND ACTIVIES

Vocabulary Builder

1. evaluation
2. overtime
3. salary review
4. exit interview
5. conflict resolution
6. letter of reference
7. work history
8. résumés
9. educational history
10. involuntary dismissal
11. mentor
12. networking
13. letter of resignation
14. probation
15. job description

Learning Review

1. The student should list four topics from among the six that follow.
    1. The mission statement of the practice
    2. Biographical data on each physician
    3. Employment policies
    4. Wage and salaries policies
    5. Benefits to be awarded
    6. Employee conduct expectations
2. A. Incorrect. Accompany employee to his or her desk to pack belongings.
    B. Correct.
    C. Incorrect. Take no longer than 10 minutes for the dismissal.
    D. Correct.
    E. Correct.
    F. Incorrect. Listen to employee's opinion and emotions; it is not necessary to agree.
    G. Incorrect. Escort employee out of the facility; do not allow employee to finish the work of the day.
    H. Correct.

3. 1. Necessary work experience
    2. Necessary skills
    3. Necessary education
    4. Any special certification or licensure needed
4. The student will choose items from the following: applicant's name, telephone number, education and training, work experience, special skills, professional demeanor and general impressions, voice and mannerisms, responses to questions regarding work habits, ability to problem-solve when given a scenario, any health-related or work-related problems the applicant discloses, and interviewer's personal impressions and recommendations.

Multiple Choice Questions

1. b. networking
2. b. inappropriate
3. d. sexual harassment
4. a. a confirmation letter
5. d. ADA

Investigation Activity

Use this activity to encourage students to relate their school performance to the kind of performance evaluation that will be held by employers. Students become aware that their skills and behaviors are being observed by supervisors and that a good performance in the workplace will be required for advancement and pay increases. Discuss student reactions to filling out the Self-Performance Rating Form. Evaluate the importance of each skill listed on the form to success on the job or in the classroom.

Discuss methods for improving weak areas and building upon personal strengths.

ANSWERS TO WORKBOOK CASE STUDY QUESTIONS

1. Other conflict resolution techniques include, but are not limited to, temporarily assisting employees having a difficult time, encouraging employees to admit mistakes, acknowledging job stressors, giving positive verbal feedback, exhibiting honesty at all times, showing zero tolerance for negative comments or actions, celebrating successes and the completion of major projects, keeping employees informed of changes that impact them, encouraging an open-door policy, respecting employee confidences, and encouraging continuing education. Physician-employers can contribute by hosting occasional employee lunches. Office managers and human resource managers can set a good example by working hard and being role models for other employees.
2. Effective communication keeps the staff satisfied and working well together, ensuring that potential problems and challenges will be aired and addressed in a timely fashion.

Chapter

47 Preparing for Medical Assisting Credentials

OVERVIEW

Although certification examinations are not legally required for medical assistants, all students should recognize the benefits and advantages of certification and recertification. Membership in the AAMA or in the AMT is also suggested. Students are encouraged to understand the certification process and to prepare fully and promptly for the certification examination.

PROFICIENCY EVALUATION OUTCOME ASSESSMENT

Students are evaluated for their understanding of performance objectives. A thorough knowledge of the requirements for certification and the logistics of applying for and taking the certification examination should be demonstrated. Students recognize that the process does not end with passing the certification examination, but remains an ongoing process of growth in the medical assisting profession through recertification and continuing education activities.

SUPPLEMENTARY RESOURCES

Medical Assisting Videos: Appropriate content is available on Delmar's Medical Assisting Videos, 2nd ed., Tape 1, for the following topics:

Examinations and Certification through AAMA
RMA/AMT

ANSWERS TO TEXT REVIEW QUESTIONS

1. d. earn the CMA credential and maintain it
2. a. a comprehensive test based on tasks medical assistants perform daily
3. a. discounted rates on legal representation
4. b. reexamination or CEU method
5. a. October 1 for January exam and March 1 for June exam
6. c. AMT
7. d. Categories 1 or 2
8. a. are offered at Cogent testing center locations

ANSWERS TO TEXTBOOK CRITICAL THINKING QUESTIONS

1. The purpose of the certification examination is to establish and evaluate a consistent standard of competency on which hiring physicians can depend and to encourage continuing education by practicing medical assistants. Certified medical assistants typically earn increased respect and recognition from their professional peers. Certification also demonstrates a commitment and ability to assume added

responsibility. Employers may recognize the value of the credential by paying higher salaries and offering more benefits to CMAs.

2. Recertify by taking the certification exam and passing or submit CEUs and earn the recertification seal every five years.

3. Graduate of schools accredited by the ABHES and may be eligible to sit for the examination by a combination of work and training programs or by verification of five years of work experience without formal training.

4. Recertification may be achieved by either reexamination or by the continuing education method.

5. Continuing education courses are offered by local, state, and national AAMA groups. Guided study programs are also available through the AAMA's "Quest for Excellence" program. *The Professional Medical Assistant*, the official bimonthly publication of the AAMA, provides articles designated for continuing education credits.

6. The advantages of membership in the AAMA include: (1) CEU opportunities are available to members, (2) quarterly newsletter received, (3) credit card privileges, (4) group insurance plans, (5) legal advice, (6) a loan program, and (7) discounted airline and car rental programs.

ANSWERS TO WORKBOOK EXERCISES AND ACTIVITIES

Vocabulary Builder

1. C.	3. B.	5. D.	7. A.
2. E.	4. H.	6. G.	8. F.

Learning Review

1. The three major areas tested are
   1. General medical knowledge, including terminology, anatomy, physiology, behavioral science, medical law, and ethics.
   2. Administrative knowledge, including medical records, management, collections, and insurance processing.
   3. Clinical knowledge, including examination room techniques, medications, injections, pharmacology, laboratory procedures, and specimen collection.
2. A. continuing education
   B. credentials, five years
   C. 60 points
   D. local, state, and national AAMA groups
3. A. AAMA Certification Department, 20 North Wacker Drive, Suite 1575, Chicago, IL 60606-2963, telephone, 312-424-3100.
   B. A Candidate's Guide to the AAMA Certification Examination
   C. Program: AAMA's "Quest for Excellence"
   Publication: *The Professional Medical Assistant*

Multiple Choice Questions

1. b. medical ethics
2. a. NBME
3. d. 12 months

4. b. 60
5. d. all of the above

Investigation Activity

Use this activity to encourage students to prepare properly for the CMA certification examination and to identify areas of strength and weakness for study concentration. As a class, discuss students' reactions to taking the sample examination and strategies for overcoming any anxiety or fears students may associate with the examination process for certification. Use the sample examination to focus students on the seriousness of proper study habits and preparation techniques. Students who prepare properly will approach the certification examination with confidence and are likely to perform more successfully.

ANSWERS TO WORKBOOK CASE STUDY QUESTIONS

1. Michele can approach Karen and Jane to ask for more externship tasks that deal with collections and insurance processing, explaining that she needs more experience and knowledge in this area to prepare for her certification examination. She may also ask the professionals to drill her on the job with critical thinking questions related to these types of administrative duties. Michele will take care, however, not to disrupt the office routine or allow her study needs to impose on the time and productivity of the office staff.
2. Students' responses will vary. Students are encouraged to identify their study weaknesses and to devise a program for strengthening their knowledge in weak areas.

Chapter

48

Employment Strategies

OVERVIEW

Medical assisting students are introduced to techniques that will help them prepare for a job search. Skills include researching prospective employers and employment opportunities, performing self-assessment evaluations, composing effective résumés, and developing techniques for successful interviews.

PROFICIENCY EVALUATION OUTCOME ASSESSMENT

Students are evaluated for their knowledge of performance objectives. The ability to distinguish between résumé styles and choose the appropriate style should be demonstrated, as well as the ability to draft and compose an effective résumé using accomplishment statements. Students learn interview techniques and are reminded of the importance of cover letters and follow-up letters to a successful interview process. The method of choosing employment references is discussed. At all times, display professionalism.

SUPPLEMENTARY RESOURCES

Medical Assisting Videos: Appropriate content is available on Delmar's Medical Assisting Videos, 2nd ed., Tape 1, for the following topics:

> Your Career as a Medical Assistant
> Display Professionalism
> Career-seeking Skills
> Communication Skills

ANSWERS TO TEXT REVIEW QUESTIONS

1. a. is a summary data sheet or brief account of your qualifications and progress in your career
2. d. should be someone who knows you or has worked with you long enough to make an honest assessment of your capabilities and integrity
3. d. when you have extensive specialized experience
4. b. introduces you to a prospective employer and captures their interest in you as a candidate for the position
5. b. requires you to think before answering questions, listen carefully, and ask for clarification if uncertain of the question
6. d. a, b, and c
7. d. all of the above
8. d. all of the above
9. d. all of the above
10. b. having poise and good appearance

ANSWERS TO TEXT CRITICAL THINKING QUESTIONS

1. Students' responses will vary according to their individual experience, situation, and job search needs. Students demonstrate the ability to distinguish between chronological, functional, and targeted résumés in evaluating the style best suited to their individual needs.

2. Methods of researching prospective employers include collecting patient brochures from medical practices listing hours, staff, and a mission statement or philosophy of the practice; looking through the yellow pages for practices in your geographic area; using the Internet; visiting a local employment agency; checking bulletin boards in community centers such as laundromats, churches, and health clubs; contacting the local chamber of commerce; contacting the local AAMA chapter; networking with professionals; utilizing the job placement center at your college campus or contacts your instructors may have; telling your personal physicians about your job search; and consulting the newspaper want ads.

3. 1. A poor appearance (not dressed properly, poorly groomed) displays a negative image on the facility employing you and does not reflect professionalism. No one enjoys being around others who have body odor and who look unkempt.
   2. Acting like a know-it-all does not display professionalism and drives away clients.
   3. When medical assistants cannot express themselves clearly because of poor voice, diction, or grammar, clients may not understand or may misinterpret physician instructions.
   4. When there is a lack of planning for work—no purpose or goals—the office does not run efficiently. Time wasted is dollars out of the practice's income and will not be tolerated. Short-term and long-term goals assist in achievements.
   5. A lack of confidence or poise may lead to loss of clients.
   6. When there is no interest or enthusiasm for the job, others are turned off.
   7. Not being active in school extracurricular programs may be interpreted as a lack of interest in general and no established goals. It may also cause others to think that you are not a team player.
   8. If you are interested only in the best dollar offer, you may send a message that you will only work until a better-paying job comes along.
   9. A poor school record (academic, attendance) may send a message that you are incompetent or that you have underlying problems.
   10. If you are unwilling to start at the bottom and work your way up, the employer may think you have a know-it-all attitude. There is value in understanding all of the workings of an office.
   11. Making excuses or hedging on an unfavorable record may indicate you are not willing to own up to mistakes. Employers want employees they can trust.
   12. A great deal of tact is required when working with patients who are ill and may have a short fuse. It is best to remember not to take things personally and to be as diplomatic and tactful as possible to create a positive image.
   13. Medical offices need employees who are mature in their thinking and problem-solving strategies.
   14. If you are not curious about the job, it may be interpreted as a lack of initiative.
   15. The medical community is very traditional; it is best not to burn any bridges. You never know when a client will be referred to another office that you have spoken of negatively.

4. Preparing a budget will vary from student to student. It is important that all of the key expenses have been itemized.
5. Numerous application forms are collected and brought to class for review and discussion.

ANSWERS TO WORKBOOK EXERCISES AND ACTIVITIES

Vocabulary Builder

1. F.
2. C.
3. J.
4. G.
5. A.
6. K.
7. M.
8. B.
9. L.
10. I.
11. D.
12. H.
13. E.

Learning Review

1. A. clear speakers and writers
   B. 1. Former instructor 2. Physician 3. Externship supervisor
      Students' listings of professional reference choices will vary.
2. Target Résumé: Entries 1, 4, and 5 are advantageous.
   Chronological Résumé: Entries 2, 3, and 5 are advantageous.
   Functional Résumé: Entries 1, 3, and 5 are advantageous.

3. Students should choose four of the following seven guidelines:
   1. Address your letter to a specific individual whenever possible. You may need to make a telephone call to obtain the name and correct spelling.
   2. Keep the letter short, use correct grammar and spelling, and follow standard business letter format.
   3. The first paragraph should state your reason for writing and focus the reader's attention.
   4. The second paragraph should identify how your education, experience, and qualifications relate to the job and refer to the enclosed résumé.
   5. The last paragraph should close with a request for an interview.
   6. Do not reproduce cover letters. An original letter should be sent to each individual.
   7. The cover letter and résumé should be mailed in a business-size envelope that matches its contents or in an 8½″ × 11″ manila envelope containing your return address.
4. The student should choose four of the following six items:
   1. Answer every item completely.
   2. Read all the directions carefully.
   3. Use black ink to complete the form.
   4. Print clearly and make no errors.
   5. Be sure to list any volunteer or externship experience that relates to the position you are seeking.
   6. Carry a completed copy of your résumé, reference list, and cover letter with you to complete the application on the spot, if necessary.
5. A. 1. Think, positive and professional
      2. Listen
      3. Ask, clarification
   B. 1. Salary 2. Vacation 3. Sick leave 4. Retirement benefits

Multiple Choice Questions

1. a. networking
2. c. ten years
3. b. chronological résumé
4. b. confidence and appearance
5. c. follow-up letter

Investigation Activity

Students' responses will vary. Consult textbook Figure 48-4 for a complete listing of suggested power words useful in drafting effective accomplishment statements. Use this exercise to build students' confidence and to encourage them to evaluate their skills, knowledge, experience, and achievements in the context of drafting a professional résumé.

ANSWERS TO WORKBOOK CASE STUDY QUESTIONS

Students' responses will vary. Use the case study to promote students' self-awareness and encourage them to seek employment in settings that are challenging and desirable to them as individuals.